Methods in Immunology and Immunochemistry

VOLUME III

Reactions of Antibodies with Soluble Antigens

Methods in
IMMUNOLOGY
and IMMUNOCHEMISTRY

Edited by

CURTIS A. WILLIAMS
THE ROCKEFELLER UNIVERSITY
NEW YORK, NEW YORK

MERRILL W. CHASE
THE ROCKEFELLER UNIVERSITY
NEW YORK, NEW YORK

Volume III
Reactions of Antibodies with Soluble Antigens

1971

ACADEMIC PRESS   New York and London

ACADEMIC PRESS, INC.
111 Fifth Avenue, New York, New York 10003

United Kingdom Edition published by
ACADEMIC PRESS, INC. (LONDON) LTD.
Berkeley Square House, London W1X 6BA

LIBRARY OF CONGRESS CATALOG CARD NUMBER: 67-22779

PRINTED IN THE UNITED STATES OF AMERICA

Topical Listing of Contents

Chapter 13. Precipitation Reactions

Chapter 15. Hapten Reactions and Kinetics of Interaction with Antibodies

Contributors to Volume III

Numbers in parentheses indicate the pages on which the authors' contributions begin.

FREDERICK ALADJEM (108), Department of Microbiology, University of Southern California, School of Medicine, Los Angeles, California

A. C. ALLISON (188),* Clinical Research Centre Laboratories, National Institute for Medical Research, Mill Hill, London, England

ELMER L. BECKER (174, 229), Walter Reed Army Institute of Research, Walter Reed Army Medical Center, Washington, D.C.

JOHN J. CEBRA (58, 427), Department of Biology, Johns Hopkins University, Baltimore, Maryland

MERRILL W. CHASE (321), The Rockefeller University, New York, New York

H. G. MICHIN CLARKE (287),† Medical Research Council, National Institute for Medical Research, Mill Hill, London, England

ALFRED J. CROWLE (357), Division of Immunology, Webb-Waring Institute for Medical Research, Denver, Colorado

RICHARD A. DAMMKOEHLER (407), Washington University Computing Facilities, St. Louis, Missouri

WALTER B. DANDLIKER (435), Department of Biochemistry, Scripps Clinic and Research Foundation, La Jolla, California

D. A. DARCY (200),‡ The Chester Beatty Research Institute, Institute of Cancer Research, Royal Cancer Hospital, London, England

---

* Present address: Clinical Research Centre, Harrow, Middlesex.
† Present address: Serum Protein Section, Clinical Research Centre, Harrow, Middlesex.
‡ Present address: The Chester Beatty Research Institute, Belmont, Sutton, Surrey.

G. C. EASTY (339), The Chester Beatty Research Institute, Institute of Cancer Research, London, England

HERMAN N. EISEN (395), Department of Microbiology, Washington University, School of Medicine, St. Louis, Missouri

RICHARD S. FARR (66), Department of Clinical Biology, Scripps Clinic and Research Foundation, La Jolla, California and National Jewish Hospital and Research Center, Denver, Colorado

I. FINGER (138), Department of Biology, Haverford College, Haverford, Pennsylvania

A. FROESE (412), Department of Chemistry, McGill University, Montreal, Canada

TOM L. GALLAGHER (407), Washington University Computing Facilities, St. Louis, Missouri

JOSEPH F. HEREMANS (213), Hôpital Saint-Pierre, Louvain (Leuven), Belgium

STELLAN HJERTÉN (364), Institute of Biochemistry, University of Uppsala, Uppsala, Sweden

G. M. HOCHWALD (343), Department of Neurology, New York University School of Medicine, New York, New York

FRED KARUSH (383), Department of Microbiology, School of Medicine, University of Pennsylvania, Philadelphia, Pennsylvania

SALLY S. KARUSH (383), Department of Microbiology, School of Medicine, University of Pennsylvania, Philadelphia, Pennsylvania

J. KOHN (168, 273), Queen Mary's Hospital, Roehampton, London, England

CHARLES A. LEONE (86), The Graduate School, Bowling Green State University, Bowling Green, Ohio

I. W. LI (94), The Rockefeller University, New York, New York

JAMES E. McGUIGAN (395), Department of Microbiology, Washington University, School of Medicine, St. Louis, Missouri

PAUL H. MAURER (1), Department of Biochemistry, Jefferson Medical College, Philadelphia, Pennsylvania

FELIX MILGROM (370), Department of Microbiology, State University of New York at Buffalo, School of Medicine, Buffalo, New York

JOHN J. MUNOZ (146), National Institute of Allergy and Infectious Diseases, Rocky Mountain Laboratory, Hamilton, Montana

ABRAHAM G. OSLER (73), Department of Medical Immunology, Public Health Research Institute of the City of New York, New York, New York

JACQUES OUDIN (103, 118, 160), Department of Analytical Immunochemistry, Institut Pasteur, Paris, France

ALFRED POLSON (180, 186), Council of Scientific and Industrial Research and University of Cape Town Virus Research Unit, University of Cape Town, Cape Town, South Africa

M.D. POULIK (279), Department of Pediatrics, Wayne State University, College of Medicine, Detroit, Michigan

JOHN R. PREER, JR. (225), Department of Zoology, Indiana University, Bloomington, Indiana

B. RUSSELL (186), Council of Scientific and Industrial Research and University of Cape Town Virus Research Unit, University of Cape Town, Cape Town, South Africa

A. H. SEHON (375, 412), Faculty of Medicine, Department of Immunology, Winnipeg, Manitoba, Canada

HARRY SMITH (367), Department of Microbiology, The University of Birmingham, Birmingham, England

G. J. THORBECKE (343), Department of Pathology, New York University School of Medicine, New York, New York

JOSE URIEL (294), Laboratoire de Chimie des Proteines, Institut de Recherches Scientifiques sur le Cancer, Villejuif, France

CURTIS A. WILLIAMS (94, 103, 209, 234, 237, 321, 343), The Rockefeller University, New York, New York

YASUO YAGI (463), Department of Biochemistry Research, Roswell Park Memorial Institute, Buffalo, New York

Preface

The rapid growth of research in immunochemistry and immunology warrants the initiation of an open-end treatise dealing with methodology. The increasing number of applications of immunological methodology to problems in other areas of biology dictates an organization, content, and style which will be helpful to the nonspecialist and specialist alike. Our aim, therefore, has been to open our colleagues' notebooks to bring together detailed procedures that are hard to retrieve from original literature. But the presentation and discussion of reliable methods are intended to provide confidence and guidance, not rigidity. The solution of research problems often demands inventive modifications and sometimes the development of new and specialized approaches. Accordingly, contributors were asked to include not only the details of procedures they had found most satisfactory in their own laboratory, but also critical remarks about common pitfalls and interpretation of results, references to alternative methods, and mention of applications to other problems. While not all topics are easily suited to this format, we feel that insofar as our general objectives are achieved, these volumes represent high potential energy.

Other publications have appeared with similar titles. Some are intended primarily for teaching purposes, others have appeared as reports of symposia. Many are excellent aids to workers in laboratories. None we have seen to date, however, encompasses the scope of the present volumes. Volume I is concerned with typical preparative methods employed in handling antigens, antibodies, and laboratory animals. Volume II presents general chemical and physicochemical methods of great usefulness for immunological reasearch. Volume III deals with antigen–antibody and hapten–antibody reactions *in vitro*, in free solution, and in gels. Volume IV covers agglutination reactions, complement-fixation and complement components, and neutralization reactions (toxins, enzymes, bacteria, animal viruses, bacteriophage). Volume V includes methods and interpretation of approaches to study the immune response. Unavoidably, some important general topics as well as many specific methods had to be postponed for subsequent volumes, which will treat hypersensitivity, transplantation, immunogenetics, immunity to parasites, and histochemistry, in addition to updating material already presented and introducing new fields of interest.

It would clearly be impossible to compile high quality material of this scope without the enthusiastic support and creative advice of the advisory editors. Their contributed sections, their help in suggesting topics and authors, and in some cases their assistance with the editing are not only greatly appreciated by us but, we are certain, also will be appreciated by the users of these volumes.

CURTIS A. WILLIAMS
MERRILL W. CHASE

New York, New York
September, 1970

Contents of Other Volumes

CHAPTER 13

Precipitation Reactions

A. The Quantitative Precipitin Reaction* †

1. THEORETICAL CONSIDERATIONS

a. PRECIPITIN REACTION

Of the many *in vitro* methods available for estimating the concentration of antibody in serum or other fluids, only the quantitative precipitin reaction gives an accurate measure in absolute weight units. When a proper assessment of the factors influencing the reaction is made and rigorous criteria of quantitative analysis are employed in analysis of the washed specific precipitate consisting of antigen and antibody, antibody values in absolute weight units can be obtained.‡

The quantitative estimation of antibody, as developed by Heidelberger and Kendall[1-4] is based on the observations that upon the addition of increasing amounts of soluble antigen to a series of tubes containing a constant volume of antisera, the amount of precipitate formed increases to a maximum and then decreases (Table I). The composition of the

* Section 13.A was contributed by Paul H. Maurer.

† Research Career Awardee (K6, AI-15, 210) of the National Institute of Allergy and Infectious Diseases, National Institutes of Health.

‡ Applications of the quantitative precipitin reactions are listed in the following symposia: Serological Approaches to Studies of Protein Structure and Metabolism, W. H. Cole, ed., Rutgers Univ. Press, New Brunswick, New Jersey, 1954; Serological and Biochemical Comparisons of Proteins, W. H. Cole, ed., Rutgers Univ. Press, New Brunswick, New Jersey, 1958; Immunochemical Approaches to Problems in Microbiology, M. H. Heidelberger and O. J. Plescia, eds., Rutgers Univ. Press, New Brunswick, New Jersey, 1961; Molecular and Cellular Basis of Antibody Formation, J. Šterzl, ed., Czechoslovak Acad. Sci., Prague, 1965; Symposium: Regulation of the Antibody Response, B. Cinader, ed., Charles C Thomas, Springfield, Illinois, 1968.

[1] M. Heidelberger and F. E. Kendall, *J. Exptl. Med.* **50**, 809 (1929).
[2] M. Heidelberger and F. E. Kendall, *J. Exptl. Med.* **62**, 697 (1935).
[3] M. Heidelberger and F. E. Kendall, *J. Exptl. Med.* **62**, 467 (1935).
[3a] M. Heidelberger and F. E. Kendall, *J. Exptl. Med.* **61**, 563 (1935).
[4] M. Heidelberger and F. E. Kendall, *J. Exptl. Med.* **65**, 647 (1937).

TABLE I

ADDITION OF INCREASING AMOUNTS OF EGG ALBUMIN TO 1.0 ML
OF AN UNDILUTED RABBIT SERUM AT 0° (COURSE I)[a]

Ea N added (mg)	Ea N pptd. (mg)	Total N pptd. (mg)	Antibody N by difference (mg)	Ratio antibody N : Ea N in ppt.	Antibody N pptd. calcd. from Eq. (3)[b] (mg)	Tests on supernatant
0.009	Total	0.156	0.147	16.2	0.137	Excess A
0.015	Total	0.236	0.220	14.2	0.225	Excess A
0.025	Total	0.374	0.349	14.0	0.343	Excess A
0.040	Total	0.526	0.486	12.2	0.499	Excess A
0.050	Total	0.632	0.582	11.6	0.582	Excess A
0.065	Total	0.740	0.675	10.4	0.677	Excess A, trace Ea
0.074	Total	0.794	0.720	9.7	0.714	No A or Ea
0.082	Total	0.830	0.748	9.1	0.738	No A, <0.001 Ea N
0.090	0.087	0.826	0.739	8.5	0.746	Excess Ea
0.098	0.089	0.820	0.731	8.2	—	Excess Ea
0.124	0.087	0.730	0.643	7.4	—	Excess Ea
0.135	(0.072)	0.610	(0.538)	(7.5)	—	Excess Ea
0.195	(0.048)	0.414	(0.366)	(7.6)	—	Excess Ea
0.307	(0.004)	0.106	—	—	—	Excess Ea
0.490	—	0.042	—	—	—	—

[a] Values in parentheses are considered uncertain. From Heidelberger and Kendall.[2]
[b] Equation (3) [Eq. (4) of Section 1.a] is derived in Heidelberger and Kendall.[3-4]

various precipitates is plotted in Fig. 1, *precipitated* AgN being plotted against total N of the precipitate (curve *IV*), against total Ab-N of the precipitate (curve *III*), and against the Ab-N/Ag-N ratio (curve *I*). An analysis of the supernatant fluids of the precipitates indicates the presence of three zones as shown in Table I with the ovalbumin (Ea)-rabbit and anti-Ea system. The nomenclature of the zones describes the results noted upon adding more antigen or antibody to the supernatants. The region where the addition of antigen, but not antibody, leads to more precipitate formation is termed the region of *antibody excess* (the precipitate contains all the added antigen plus some antibody). This is followed by an *equivalence zone* where neither antigen nor antibody can be detected (i.e., all is found in the precipitate), and finally a region of reduced precipitation, *antigen excess*, where soluble complexes of Ag and Ab* are formed. At the

* Abbreviations used in text: Ab, antibody; Ag, antigen; BGG, bovine γ-globulin; BSA, bovine serum albumin; DNP, dinitrophenyl; Ea, ovalbumin; HGG, human

beginning of the antigen excess region, all the antibody and most of the antigen is in the precipitate.

Quantitative analysis of precipitates is generally expressed in terms of nitrogen (N); thus, by subtracting the antigen N added from the total N precipitated in the equivalence zone, a measure of antibody N in the serum is determined. The curve obtained above is referred to as a "calibration curve" and the serum as a "calibrated serum."

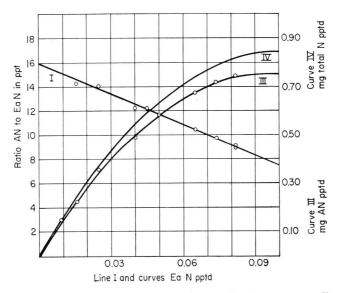

Fig. 1. Quantitative course of the precipitin reaction between egg albumin and rabbit anti egg albumin. AN = antibody nitrogen. From Heidelberger and Kendall.[2]

When the ratio of AbN:EaN in the antibody excess zone is plotted against the antigen N added, a straight line is obtained which can be expressed by Eq. (1).

$$\frac{\text{AbN precipitated}}{x} = a - bx \tag{1}$$

or

$$\text{AbN precipitated} = ax - bx^2 \tag{2}$$

γ-globulin; HSA, human serum albumin; ^{131}I-BSA, iodine-131-labeled bovine serum albumin; N, nitrogen; Pn III, pneumococcus type III; RGG, rabbit γ-globulin; RSA, rabbit serum albumin; S III, pneumococcal capsular polysaccharide type III; Tg, thyroglobulin; TMV, tobacco mosaic virus.

where x = antigen N added, a = the intercept on the y axis, and b = the slope.[2] The equation of the above reaction, therefore, becomes

$$AbN\ pptd = 15.8x - 0.083x^2 \tag{3}$$

The application of mass law considerations of bimolecular reactions between antigen and antibody led Heidelberger and Kendall[3] to derive Eq. (4).

$$AbN\ pptd = 2Rx - \frac{R^2}{A}x^2 \tag{4}$$

where A = the amount of antibody N precipitated at the midpoint of the equivalence zone, R is the ratio of A to the amount of antigen N precipitated at that point, and x = amount of antigen N added at any point. By comparing these two equations, it is evident that $a = 2R$ and $b = R^2/A$. $2R$ or a has been referred to as the initial combining ratio (i.c.r.) of antibody with antigen. In Eq. (1), the constant a depends on certain characteristics of the antibody, and b on the characteristics as well as on the amount of antibody present. Therefore, in order to compare different antisera by the use of such equations, the antibody content factor is eliminated by dividing the values for *antibody precipitated* and *antigen added* by the amount of maximum precipitable antibody. The limitations and exceptions to the foregoing ideal situations are many. Therefore, every system has to be studied by itself.

Antibody in any serum is very heterogeneous, and different molecules of antibody may have different affinities for antigen. Also, the distribution of antibody activities among the several immunoglobulin classes can affect in unknown ways the reaction with antigen that leads to precipitation. The question of whether γA, γG, or γM immunoglobulins show different precipitin characteristics, or whether one class may inhibit the precipitation of another, is also not known. Different types of precipitin curves are obtained with different antigens. The narrow equivalence zone found in many native protein–antiprotein systems when the antigen is of molecular weight 40,000 to 160,000 is not obtained with polysaccharide antigens (Fig. 2),[3a, 5] or with aggregated denatured proteins, such as denatured ovalbumin[6] or gelatin,[7] or with macromolecules, such as tobacco mosaic virus.[8] Among the recently studied synthetic polyamino

[5] E. A. Kabat and D. Berg, *J. Immunol.* **70**, 514 (1953).
[6] C. F. C. MacPherson and M. Heidelberger, *J. Am. Chem. Soc.* **67**, 585 (1945).
[7] P. H. Maurer, *J. Exptl. Med.* **100**, 497 (1954).
[8] I. Rappaport, *J. Immunol.* **78**, 246 (1957).

acid antigens, some have exhibited very sharp equivalence zones whereas others have indicated a rather broad zone in reaction with the specific antibody.[9, 9a] All the reasons underlying the shapes of the curves are not known, but an important factor is the solubility of the antigen–antibody complex, which is determined by the nature of the antigen. The solubility of the antigen has been demonstrated to play a role in the horse-anti-HGG system.[10] A recent study of Lindqvist and Bauer[10a] compared the precipitation behavior of 7 S with 19 S rabbit antibody against diazobenzidine BSA. In contrast to the reaction of 7 S γG anti-BSA, the macroglobulin

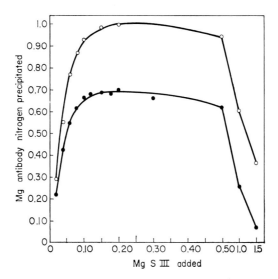

FIG. 2. Quantitative course of the precipitin reaction between pneumococcal capsular polysaccharide S III and a rabbit anti-S III serum. ● First-course serum (dilution 1:6). ○ Third-course serum (dilution 1:1.5). From Heidelberger and Kendall.[4]

γM antibody–antigen complexes showed no evidence of solubility in extreme antigen excess. One hundred times the concentration of antigen at equivalence did not diminish precipitation of γM whereas three times the antigen concentration at equivalence resulted in more than 85% decrease in precipitation of 7 S anti-BSA.

Simple equations which have been obtained in other systems, such as

[9] P. H. Maurer, B. F. Gerulat, and P. Pinchuck, *J. Biol. Chem.* **239**, 922 (1964).
[9a] P. H. Maurer, B. F. Gerulat, and P. Pinchuck, *J. Exptl. Med.* **119**, 1005 (1964).
[10] C. A. Williams, *Bull. Soc. Chim. Biol.* **36**, 1407 (1954).
[10a] K. Lindqvist and D. C. Bauer, *Immunochem.* **3**, 373 (1966).

HSA,[1],[11] thyroglobulin,[12] and the S III system,[5] have not held with the dextran–antidextran system in man[4] and rabbit anti-TMV sera[13, 14] for reasons presented below. Modified equations have been developed for these precipitin systems.[15] The type of precipitin curve obtained even with the same animal varies with different courses of immunization.[2] A broadening of the equivalence zone, and a change in the a and b values (Table II) have, among other things, indicated that antibody is formed against more determinant groups which increases the $2R$ value or that there is a change in the characteristics of the antibody (e.g., increase in heterogeneity). The equation or precipitin curve describes only the average behavior of the heterogeneous antibody population against the same antigen.

TABLE II

EQUATION OF PRECIPITIN REACTION OF RABBIT SERUM[a]

	Equation calculated for 1 mg of antibody N	
Course	Anti-Ea sera	Anti-S III sera
1	mg Ab N pptd. $= 15.8$ Ea N $- 62.4$ (Ea N)^2	mg Ab N pptd. $= 14.9$ S $- 46.2$ S^2
2	mg Ab N pptd. $= 20.4$ Ea N $- 104$ (Ea N)^2	mg Ab N pptd. $= 15.6$ S $- 60.8$ S^2
3	mg Ab N pptd. $= 24.8$ Ea N $- 154$ (Ea N)^2	mg Ab N pptd. $= 16.8$ S $- 70.6$ S^2

[a] From Heidelberger and Kendall.[2]

Of crucial importance to the calculation of the antibody content of a serum is the requirement that, at the point of maximum precipitation, most of the antigen added should be in the precipitate. Stated differently, if a system consists of a single antigenic substance and its homologous antibody, the supernatants obtained in the equivalence zone should give negative tests for excess of both antigen and antibody; also, up through the region of slight antigen excess, supernatant tests should not be positive for both antigen and antibody.[16] Positive tests for both antigen and

[11] E. A. Kabat and M. Heidelberger, *J. Exptl. Med.* **66**, 229 (1937).

[12] H. E. Stokinger and M. Heidelberger, *J. Exptl. Med.* **66**, 251 (1937).

[13] S. Malkiel and W. M. Stanley, *J. Immunol.* **57**, 31 (1947).

[14] I. Rappaport, *J. Immunol.* **82**, 526 (1959).

[15] E. A. Kabat *in* "Experimental Immunochemistry" 2nd ed. (E. A. Kabat and M. M. Mayer, eds.). Thomas, Springfield, Illinois, 1961.

[16] F. E. Kendall, *J. Clin. Invest.* **16**, 921 (1937).

antibody indicate that the antiserum contains a mixture of antibodies and that more than one antigenic component is present. This principle has been used to tremendous advantage in immunochemistry to detect impurities in antigens, and the presence of antibodies against such constituent impurities in the antigenic material. However, many examples have been reported in recent years to indicate that the above behavior in supernatants does not always obtain even with purified antigens. Feinberg reported the formation of a rabbit anti-BSA serum produced by immunization with complete Freund's adjuvant that precipitated only 46% of the ^{131}I-BSA at equivalence.[17] In *antibody* excess, the ^{131}I-BSA formed soluble complexes with antibody. With a horse anti-HSA system, it was noted that 17 to 28% of ^{131}I-HSA did not precipitate in the equivalence region.[18] A guinea pig antiserum against insulin precipitated only 47% of the ^{131}I-labeled insulin.[19] With a canine antiserum against BSA, incomplete precipitation of ^{131}I-BSA in antibody excess was noted and ascribed to inhibition by admixed nonprecipitating antibody.[20] For different sera, the maximum amount of antibody precipitated 30 to 80% of the antigen, but, after ammonium sulfate fractionation of the antiserum, the fraction precipitated at one-third saturation precipitated the antibody completely in antibody excess. The "nonprecipitating" antibody was a β_2-globulin. In rat antibody systems against Ea, HGG, and a hapten-BGG conjugate the maximum antibody was precipitated in 20% antigen excess.[21] In several chicken antibody systems, even though all the antigen was precipitated in antibody excess, at maximum precipitation of antibody only 50 to 65% of the ^{131}I-labeled antigens were in the precipitates.[22] Similar findings with antisera against the gelatins,[7] polypeptidyl gelatins,[23] or synthetic polymers of amino acids[9, 9a, 24] may be explained as being related to the heterogeneous nature of the degraded or synthetic antigens. However, this explanation cannot apply to the antisera against highly purified antigens. It is reasonable to assume that there may be considerable antibody heterogeneity against a single antigenic molecule leading to different types of antigen–antibody complexes with different solubility products. Not all of them may be included in the complex lattice network formed by antigen–antibody interactions.

[17] R. Feinberg, *J. Immunol.* **81**, 14 (1958).
[18] P. Burtin, *Bull. Soc. Chim. Biol.* **37**, 977 (1956).
[19] V. E. Jones and A. C. Cunliffe, *Nature* **192**, 136 (1961).
[20] R. Patterson, W. W. Y. Chang, and J. J. Pruzansky, *Immunology* **7**, 150 (1964).
[21] R. A. Binaghi and B. Benacerraf, *J. Immunol.* **92**, 920 (1964).
[22] I. D. Aitken and W. Mulligan, *Immunology* **5**, 295 (1962).
[23] R. Arnon and M. Sela, *Biochem. J.* **75**, 103 (1960).
[24] M. Sela, H. Ungar-Waron, and Y. Schechter, *Proc. Natl. Acad. Sci. U.S.* **52**, 285 (1964).

TABLE III

ADDITION OF INCREASING AMOUNTS OF DIPHTHERIC TOXIN TO
300 UNITS OF HORSE ANTITOXIN[a,b]

I	II	III Supernatants[g]		IV	V[h]	VI[h]
Lf units toxin added	Toxin[c] nitrogen added (mg)	Toxin total Lf	Antitoxin total units	Nitrogen in precipitate (mg)	Antitoxin nitrogen in precipitate (IV-II)	Ratio A-nitrogen: T-nitrogen (V-II)
50[d]	0.023	—	190[f]	0	0	—
100[d]	0.046	—	95[f]	0	0	—
150[e]	0.069	—	—	0.386	(0.474)	(6.9)
175	0.081	—	Trace[g]	0.554	0.473	5.8
200	0.092	—	—	0.564	0.472	5.1
225	0.103	—	—	0.579	0.476	4.6
300	0.138	—	—	0.612	0.474	3.4
400	0.184	Trace[g]	—	0.661	0.477	2.6
425	—	—	—	—	—	(2.4)
450	0.207	Trace[g]	—	0.652	—	—
500[e]	0.230	100[f]	—	0.359	—	—
600[d]	0.276	240[f]	—	0	0	—

[a] From Pappenheimer and Robinson.[25]

[b] Antitoxin having (A) had 300 antitoxic units and 8.11 mg nitrogen per milliliter. Toxin (T) had 0.00055 mg nitrogen per Lf unit.

[c] The nitrogen (column IV) precipitated by 200 Lf of toxin subtracted from that precipitated by 400 Lf and divided by 200 gives 0.00048 mg of nitrogen per Lf of toxin. The figure used in column II, however, is 0.00046 mg of nitrogen per Lf, the average obtained from six titrations including the above.

[d] No flocculation.

[e] Incomplete flocculation.

[f] Determined by flocculation.

[g] By intracutaneous rabbit test.

[h] Figures in parentheses were calculated for the ends of the neutral zone assuming 150 Lf and 425 Lf and complete flocculation.

b. FLOCCULATION REACTION

This special type of precipitin reaction (Table III, Fig. 3) is characterized by flocculation over a narrow range of antigen concentration and the formation of soluble antigen–antibody complexes in both antibody and antigen excess.[25, 26] It was originally believed to be a property of horse antitoxin sera. However, this type of curve has been found with horse

[25] A. W. Pappenheimer, Jr. and E. S. Robinson, *J. Immunol.* **32**, 291 (1937).
[26] G. Ramon, *Compt. Rend. Soc. Biol.* **86**, 661, 711, and 813 (1922).

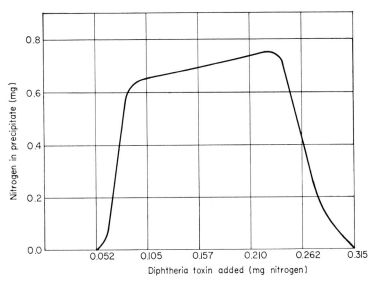

Fig. 3. Quantitative toxin–horse antitoxin reaction. From Pappenheimer and Robinson.[25]

antisera against other antigens such as ovalbumin,[27] HSA,[28] HGG,[10] hemocyanin,[29] and a human antiserum against thyroglobulin[30] and sheep antiserum against synthetic polypeptides.[30a] Throughout the range of flocculation (straight-line portion of the curve from antibody excess to antigen excess), all the antigen and antibody were precipitated; i.e., negative tests for both were found in the supernatants. The nature of this "toxin–antitoxin" type of curve has been debated and, in some instances, ascribed to the presence of trace impurities in the antigen leading to multiple antigen–antibody systems. In the studies of Pope et al.[31, 32] as purification of the toxin was continued and antisera were absorbed with nontoxin proteins, the straight-line portion of the curve (broad equivalence zone) was no longer evident and was replaced by a symmetrical flocculation curve (Fig. 4). However, with highly purified antigens, such as RSA[33] and HSA, the heterogeneity of the antibody population in these

[27] M. Heidelberger, H. P. Treffers, and M. Mayer, J. Exptl. Med. **71**, 271 (1940).
[28] D. Gitlin, C. S. Davidson, and L. H. Wetterlow, J. Immunol. **63**, 415 (1949).
[29] S. B. Hooker and W. C. Boyd, Ann. N.Y. Acad. Sci. **43**, 107 (1942).
[30] I. M. Roitt, P. N. Campbell, and D. Doniach, Biochem. J. **69**, 248 (1958).
[30a] P. H. Maurer, unpublished experiments (1968, 1969).
[31] C. G. Pope, M. F. Stevens, E. A. Caspary, and E. L. Fenton, Brit. J. Exptl. Pathol. **32**, 246 (1951).
[32] C. G. Pope and M. F. Stevens, Brit. J. Exptl. Pathol. **34**, 56 (1953).
[33] M. Heidelberger, H. P. Treffers, and J. Freund, J. Exptl. Med. **86**, 83 (1947).

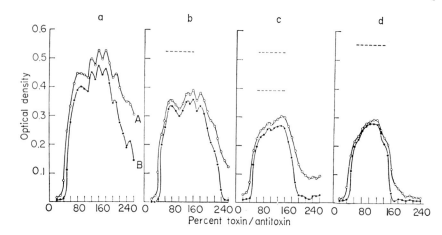

Fig. 4. Alteration in the precipitin reaction by purification of reagents. Curves a: Reaction between crude toxin and the original preparation of antitoxin ("peptic-antitoxin" after treatment with pepsin). The first flocculating mixture is at 100% toxin. O, Total density; ●, floccule density. Curves b: The reaction of the peptic-antitoxin with crude toxin after absorption with antigens present in culture filtrate containing iron in excess. Dotted line = maximum density from panel a. Curves c: The reaction between the original peptic antitoxin and a toxin with a purity of 2560 Lf per milligram of protein N. Dotted lines are maxima from curves a and b, respectively. Curves d: The reaction between absorbed antitoxin and purified toxin (2560 Lf per milligram of protein N). From Pope and Stevens.[32]

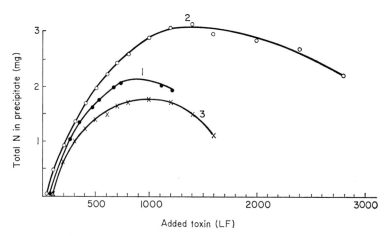

Fig. 5. Quantitative precipitin curves with diphtheria toxin and antitoxic sera. Curve 1: Serum unfractionated. Curve 2: 0–33% saturation $(NH_4)_2SO_4$ precipitate. Curve 3: 33–50% saturation $(NH_4)_2SO_4$ precipitate. From Relyveld and Raynaud.[34]

sera may also explain this behavior. Relyveld and Raynaud[34] showed that certain horse antitoxin sera could be fractionated so that both precipitin and flocculation curves were observed with the same serum (Fig. 5). The antibody precipitated at 33% saturation with ammonium sulfate gave the precipitin curve, and the antibody precipitated between 33 and 50% saturation gave the flocculation curve. The antibody in the former instance was a γ-globulin and in the latter a β_2-globulin (T component). In the studies of Treffers et al.[35] the flocculating antibody against RSA was present in the water-soluble portion of the globulin fraction, whereas the precipitin type of antibody was in the water-insoluble fraction of this fraction.

2. FACTORS INFLUENCING THE AG–AB REACTION AND VALUES FOR ANTIBODY N

Consideration should be given to the following factors as they can affect the proper estimation of antibody. However, as will be shown with the examples below, there may be no uniformity in the effect of these variables on different sera.

a. PRECIPITIN REACTION

i. Area of Curve and Amounts of Antibody

Owing to the several zones in the precipitin reaction, one must be sure that the estimation for antibody is being made in or near the equivalence zone. Too little or too much antigen may fail to precipitate all antibody (cf. Table I). Also, since the mass action laws apply, it is necessary that sufficient antibody be present to exceed the solubility product of Ag–Ab precipitates (1 to 2 μg N per ml). This factor becomes of major importance when micro methods are employed for analysis of precipitates.

ii. Effect of pH

In general, the precipitin reaction is insensitive to pH in the range pH 6.6 to 8.5.[36] The effect of pH on the maximum antibody precipitated with the Ea–rabbit anti-Ea system is shown in Fig. 6. At pH 4.9 and 9.6, one-half of the maximum antibody was precipitated and at pH 4.2 and 9.5, all of the precipitate was soluble. Similarly, maximal values were obtained in the dextran–antidextran system at pH's of 6 to 9.[37] The systems most sensitive to pH are the reactions of antibody with synthetic polymers of

[34] E. H. Relyveld and M. Raynaud, *Ann. Inst. Pasteur* **93**, 246 (1957).
[35] H. P. Treffers, M. Heidelberger, and J. Freund, *J. Exptl. Med.* **86**, 83 (1947).
[36] W. J. Kleinschmidt and P. D. Boyer, *J. Immunol.* **69**, 247 (1952).
[37] H. J. Gould, T. J. Gill, and H. W. Kunz, *J. Biol. Chem.* **239**, 3071 (1964).

amino acids. Gould *et al.*[37] and Gill and Doty[38] indicated that in some instances pH 7.6 was better than 6.5, but usually reactions conducted at pH 6.8 to 8.9 did not lead to reduced antibody values (Fig. 7). The greater the number of charged groups involved in the antigenic determinants, the greater may be the effect of pH. Therefore, studies with charged haptenic determinants may be most sensitive and control of pH of paramount importance. However, with a neutral hapten such as 2,4-DNP,

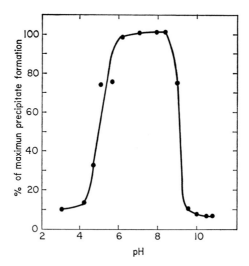

FIG. 6. Effect of pH on precipitation of rabbit anti egg albumin by egg albumin. From Kleinschmidt and Boyer.[36]

maximum precipitation occurred at pH 7.3 with little change over the region pH 6 to 9.[39]

iii. Effect of Salt Concentration (Ionic Strength)

Studies on the effect of varying the concentration and type of electrolytes on the precipitin reaction of *horse* and *rabbit* antiserum indicate that each system must be studied individually. Electrostatic interactions are not always necessary for Ag–Ab reaction, but electrolytes do contribute to the stabilization of the reaction and electrostatic interactions are affected both by pH and salt concentrations.

In precipitin reactions with *horse* and *rabbit* antipneumococcal sera, increasing the salt concentration from 0.15 M to 0.95 M led to a decrease of about 70% in the antibody precipitated with *rabbit* sera, but only about

[38] T. J. Gill and P. Doty, *J. Biol. Chem.* **236**, 2677 (1961).
[39] G. W. Siskind, *J. Immunol.* **92**, 702 (1964).

30% decrease with the *horse* sera, as shown in Table IV.[40] With the Ea–anti-Ea system in rabbits, the effect of increasing NaCl concentration was minimal,[41] yet in this system potassium halide salts showed tremendous effects (Fig. 8). Inhibition of precipitation by the anions decreased in the following order: $CNS^- > I^- > Br^- > Cl^- > F^-$.[36] This effect seemed to be inversely related to the energy of hydration of the ions. In

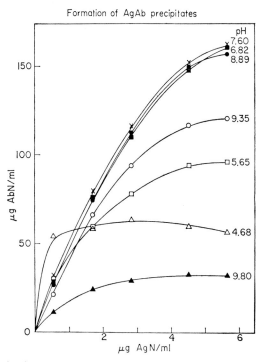

Fig. 7. Precipitation curves for the reactions of polyglutamyl[56]-lysyl[38]-tyrosine[6], poly(glu[56]lys[38]tyr[6])$_n$, with rabbit antibody at various pH values. From Gould *et al.*[37]

the antipneumococcus system, divalent cations $MgCl_2$ and Na_2SO_4 showed but little effect.

In the absence of salt (i.e., H_2O at pH 7.0) HSA-rabbit antibody precipitate dissolved whereas at pH 6.0 the complex precipitated even in the absence of salt.[42] Nonspecific precipitation of nonantibody globulin was, however, associated with the reaction at pH 6.0. A similar need for the proper ionic medium was shown with the TMV system. Although

[40] M. H. Heidelberger, F. E. Kendall, and T. Teorell, *J. Exptl. Med.* **63**, 819 (1936).
[41] J. Oudin and P. Grabar, *Ann. Inst. Pasteur* **70**, 7 (1944).
[42] A. Kleczkowski, *Immunology* **8**, 170 (1965).

TABLE IV

EFFECT OF THE CONCENTRATION OF SODIUM CHLORIDE
UPON THE REACTION BETWEEN S III AND ANTIBODY
OF HORSE AND RABBIT ORIGIN AT 37° AND 0°[a]

Pneumococcal S III used (mg)	Horse antibody[b]					Rabbit antibody[b]	
	0.1 M NaCl	0.15 M NaCl	0.51 M NaCl	0.93 M NaCl	1.79 M NaCl	0.15 M NaCl	0.93–0.98 M NaCl
0.02	0.54	0.50	0.42	0.39	0.36	—	—
0.05	1.13	1.03	0.90	0.84	0.75	0.43	0.24
0.075	1.41	1.41	1.29	1.15	1.03	0.60	
0.10	1.75	1.66	1.54	1.28	1.22	0.77	0.34
0.15	1.78	1.86	1.62	1.50	1.45	1.04	0.39
0.20[c]	1.82	1.85	1.70	1.58	1.51	1.18	0.41

[a] From Heidelberger et al.[40]
[b] Values are expressed as milligrams of antibody nitrogen precipitated.
[c] Excess S III.

TMV *combines* with rabbit antibody in the absence of salt, salt is needed for *precipitation* to occur. Here, too, precipitation could occur at pH 6.0 in a salt-free medium, but much of the precipitate was nonspecific globulin. At pH 6.5, with a pseudoglobulin fraction of rabbit anti-Ea there was *increased* precipitation in the region of antigen excess in 0.09% NaCl

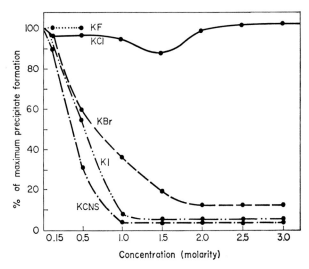

FIG. 8. Effect of various ions on the Ea–anti-Ea system. From Kleinschmidt and Boyer.[36]

or in diluent lacking NaCl.[43] Decreasing the ionic strength in an anti-2,4-DNP system from 0.1 to 0.01 had no effect on the maximum precipitation of *antibody* but did decrease the amount precipitated in antigen excess.[39] In a study with *rat antibody*, there was only a slight decrease in precipitation at high salt concentration (1.5 M) and no effect of reducing the ionic strength to 0.001.[21] With *mouse antibody* to Ea, precipitation occurred best at 0.85% NaCl and decreased slightly at 12% NaCl.[44] A still greater effect of ionic strength was shown with the *charged* synthetic polymer systems. At pH 7.6, as the ionic strength increased from 0.15 to 2.1, the

TABLE V

EFFECT OF pH AND IONIC STRENGTH ON PRECIPITATION
OF RABBIT ANTIBODY BY 18 μg OF N
poly(L-Glu^{56}-L-Lys^{38}-L-Tyr^6)$_n$ AT 4° FOR 5 DAYS[a]

pH	Final [NaCl]	Antibody N pptd. (μg/ml)
6.5	0.15	156
7.6	0.15	185
10.0	0.15	130
7.6	0.12	186
	0.15	185
	0.31	164
	0.51	149
	1.1	111
	2.1	18

[a] From Gill and Doty.[38]

precipitation decreased as indicated in Table V.[38] However, a similar effect was not evident with an *uncharged* synthetic polymer.[44a]

iv. Effect of Temperature

With most rabbit antisera, the amount of antibody precipitated is slightly greater at 0° than at 37°.[2, 5] In general, it can be stated that most precipitin reactions can be set up at 37° for about 0.5 hour, but subsequent incubation should be at 0°. If the serum contains enzymes that can inactivate the antigen at 37°, then the latter temperature should not be employed.

The greatest effect of temperature of incubation was noted with rabbit

[43] F. Aladjem and M. Lieberman, *J. Immunol.* **69**, 117 (1952).
[44] R. L. Anacker and J. Muñoz, *J. Immunol.* **87**, 426 (1961).
[44a] M. Sela and S. Fuchs, *Proc. Symp. Mol. Cellular Basis Antibody Formation, Prague, 1964* p. 43. Academic Press, New York, 1965.

antisera against synthetic polypeptides.[37, 38] There was little difference between incubation at 37° for 1 hour followed by 4° for 5 days, and holding at 0° for 5 days. However, with the charged polymers, the amount of AbN precipitated decreased from 185 μg of N at 4° to 147 at 25° and 71 μg of N at 37°, respectively, when the holding period was 15 hours. In other words, a decrease of 40% occurred upon storage at 37°. With horse antipneumo-coccal[2, 3] and anti-RGG sera[35] there was a great temperature effect which was not noted in a horse anti-Ea system. Conducting the former reaction at 0° can lead to precipitation of 13% more Ab than at 37°. With horse

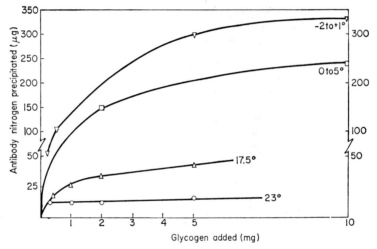

FIG. 9. Precipitation of antipneumococcus serum type XII horse serum by glycogen at various temperatures. From Heidelberger et al.[45]

sera where 0° is the temperature of choice, cross-reactions can be multiplied as well[45] (Fig. 9). In a mouse anti-Ea system, there was little difference between the values obtained at 4° or 37°.[44] With antitoxin of low affinity for diphtheria toxin, toxin was neutralized much better by incubation at 37° than at 0°, and mixtures shown to be neutral at 37° would become toxic if transferred to the cold room.[46]

v. Rate of Mixing and Addition of Antigen and Antibody

If small amounts of antigen are added with rapid mixing to a very large excess of antibody (molar excess of about 200:1), considerably reduced or no precipitation occurs (prozone phenomenon) from formation of soluble

[45] M. Heidelberger, A. C. Aisenberg, and W. Z. Hassid, J. Exptl. Med. **99**, 343 (1954).
[46] N. K. Jerne, Acta Pathol. Microbiol. Scand. Suppl. **87**, 1 (1951).

complexes in antibody excess. This has been documented by Nisonoff and Winkler[47] with the Ea system and by Forster and Weigle[48] with the anti-BSA but not with anti-BGG system. The greatest reduction in precipitation was brought about by adding antigen slowly and stirring the mixture rapidly. The report of Neff and Becker[49] that addition of antigen to antibody leads to greater precipitation than in the reverse order is still to be confirmed, especially since removal of complement abolished this effect.

vi. Complement in Sera

Small amounts of complement may persist in rabbit, guinea pig, and human sera for many months at $0°$[50] and add to specific precipitates and

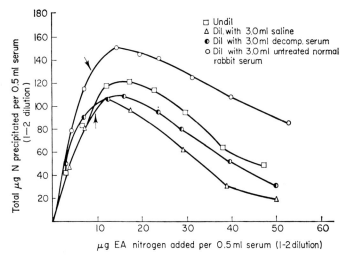

FIG. 10. Effect of decomplementation on precipitin curves of an anti-Ea serum. From Maurer and Talmage.[51]

increase its weight and contribute to apparent values for antibody N.[51-53] The amount of complement N present in fresh sera may vary from 5 to 50 μg of N per milliliter serum. In addition to augmenting specific precipitates (Fig. 10), complement has the ability to shift the solubility

[47] A. Nisonoff and M. Winkler, J. Immunol. **81**, 65 (1958).
[48] O. Forster and W. O. Weigle, J. Immunol. **90**, 935 (1963).
[49] J. C. Neff and E. L. Becker, J. Immunol. **73**, 286 (1954).
[50] P. H. Maurer and W. O. Weigle, J. Immunol. **71**, 284 (1953).
[51] P. H. Maurer and D. W. Talmage, J. Immunol. **70**, 135 (1953).
[52] P. H. Maurer and D. W. Talmage, J. Immunol. **70**, 435 (1953).
[53] H. F. Deutsch and J. E. Morton, Arch. Biochem. Biophys. **64**, 19 and 26 (1956).

equilibrium and precipitate the soluble antigen–antibody complexes formed in antigen excess. Also, the $2R$ (initial combining ratio) values are increased[51] (Table VI). The extent of error by not decomplementing sera is greatest when sera containing low levels of antibody are employed and several milliliters of sera have to be used to obtain single values. The errors introduced in not removing complement are greater with rabbit and guinea pig sera than with human sera.

The method of removal or inactivation of the complement present in sera also affects the antibody N values. The method least deleterious to the antibody is to absorb complement on an unrelated specific precipitate

TABLE VI

EFFECT OF VARIOUS DILUENTS ON INITIAL COMBINING
RATIOS ($2R$) TWO SPECIMENS OF RABBIT ANTISERA[a]

Diluent	Initial combining ratios	
	Anti-Ea	Anti-BSA
Undiluted[b]	16.6	12.6
Normal rabbit serum[c]	21.0	17.8
Decomplemented rabbit serum[c]	17.6	12.3
0.15 M NaCl[c]	17.3	11.9

[a] From Maurer and Talmage.[51]

[b] 0.5 ml of 1:1 dilution of serum.

[c] 3.0 ml of diluent was used with the anti-Ea system, and 4.0 ml with the anti-BSA system.

formed at equivalence (usually rabbit antibody) in the amounts of 100 μg of N per milliliter of serum.[54] This can be accomplished either with a preformed specific precipitate or by a precipitate formed by reacting the antibody and antigen in the serum, which subsequently will be analyzed for another antibody. It is important to use a precipitate which does not react (or cross react) with the major serum constituents (i.e., do not use an anti-HSA serum to decomplement human serum). EDTA (ethylenediaminetetraacetic acid) 0.02 M, which prevents guinea pig and human complement from adding to antigen–antibody precipitates, has but little effect on rabbit complement even in aged sera.[50] The method of "decomplementing" sera by inactivation for 30–60 minutes at 56° may affect the antibody adversely (Table VII). Antibody in human[54] and guinea pig

[54] M. Heidelberger, C. M. Mac Leod, S. J. Kaiser, and B. Robinson, *J. Exptl. Med.* **83,** 303 (1946).

TABLE VII

EFFECT OF METHOD OF REMOVAL OF HUMAN COMPLEMENT ON PRECIPITABLE
ANTIBODY TO PNEUMOCOCCAL POLYSACCHARIDES[a]

	Micrograms of antibody N per 4 ml		
	Complement removed by		
Antibody estimated	Ea–anti-Ea	Heat, 56°C, 30 min	Heat, 56°C, 50 min
Anti-C[b]	36	2	0
Anti-I	8	3	0
Anti-II	10	2	0

[a] From Heidelberger et al.[54]

[b] In another pool anti-C was reduced from 14 to 6 and 0, respectively; in a third, from 57 to 30 and 22.

sera[55] are affected more by heating than are rabbit and horse sera,[56] losing their ability to *precipitate*, although they may coprecipitate with unheated antibody. It is believed that heating causes the formation of albumin-globulin complexes which do not precipitate with antigen alone.[57] If the serum is fractionated and the albumin is removed before heating, there is little effect on the precipitating activity of the antibody.[58, 59]

vii. Velocity of the Reaction

Although the combination between antigen and antibody is very rapid (it need not lead to precipitation), the amount of time needed for precipitation to occur depends on the amount of aggregated complexes present. With strong antisera (about 100 to 300 μg of antibody N per milliliter of serum), 2 days at 0 to 5° is usually sufficient for complete precipitation. With less than 100 μg of antibody N, it is usual to incubate the reaction mixture at 0° for 6 to 8 days with daily mixing. With some systems such as gelatin–antigelatin, about 10 days at 0° may be required. The *rate of precipitation* is greatest near equivalence proportions and least in the region of antigen excess[60] (Fig. 11). The effect of time on completion of precipitation of the same antibody with different amounts of antigen is shown in Fig. 12. The curve with 1 μg enzyme required a week for maxi-

[55] J. J. Pruzansky and S. M. Feinberg, *J. Immunol.* **88**, 256 (1962).

[56] M. Cohn and A. W. Pappenheimer, *J. Immunol.* **63**, 291 (1949).

[57] A. Kleczkowski, *Brit. J. Exptl. Pathol.* **22**, 188 and 192 (1941).

[58] F. C. Bowden and A. Kleczkowski, *Brit. J. Exptl. Pathol.* **23**, 178 (1942).

[59] F. S. Farah, A. K. Kurban, and H. T. Chaglassian, *J. Immunol.* **93**, 300 (1964).

[60] M. Schlamowitz, *J. Immunol.* **80**, 176 (1958).

mum precipitation. Although more N is precipitated, in the presence of complement, the rate of precipitation is decreased. Often when one is analyzing weak sera and therefore needs several milliliters of serum for each analysis, it may not be possible to see the precipitate until after centrifugation since the precipitate may not settle readily through the dense serum medium. Because of the occasional need to incubate for long periods of time, it is essential to have appropriate preservative added to

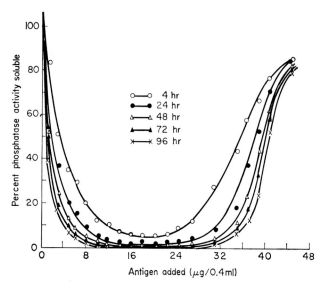

Fig. 11. Influence of time on the precipitin curve of dog intestinal phosphatase (DIP) with its antiserum (0.10 ml). From Schlamowitz.[60]

the serum to prevent bacterial growth. (See Vol. I, Chap. 2 for discussion of preservatives.)

viii. Nonspecific Factors Affecting Precipitation

(a) *Lipids.* When lipids are removed from serum with ether in the cold, there is no change in the level of antibody precipitable, although the velocity of precipitation may be reduced.[61] If the lipids are removed by large volumes of alcohol–ether mixture, precipitation is inhibited.[62] It has been observed that, with properly delipidated sera, it is possible to obtain greater precipitates after centrifugation which yield higher AbN/AgN ratios. It has been postulated that serum lipids prevent complete precipi-

[61] F. Tayeau, F. Faure, E. Neuzil, and R. Pautrizel, *Trans. Faraday Soc.* **6,** 106 (1949).
[62] M. Heidelberger and R. C. Krueger, "Plasma Proteins," p. 334. Thomas, Springfield, Illinois, 1950.

tation of a portion of the antibody. However, removal of lipids also prevents coalescence into floccules; this therefore necessitates high speed centrifugation to bring down the antigen–antibody aggregates.[63] Whether the increased precipitation might be related to "denaturation" of the serum proteins has not been completely investigated.

(b) *Macromolecules.* Because interactions of highly charged macromolecules with serum proteins may lead to precipitation, it is sometimes necessary to establish the specificity of the reaction and to be able to ascribe some biological activity to the serum protein being precipitated. Many polymers containing high concentrations of excess lysine precipitate serum

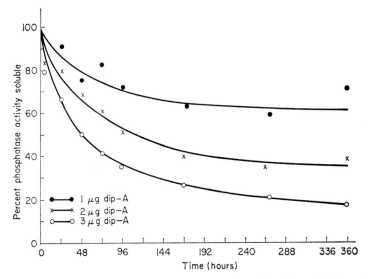

Fɪɢ. 12. Effect of time on completeness of precipitation of dog intestinal phosphatase with antibody (0.20 ml). From Schlamowitz.[60]

proteins nonspecifically, i.e., poly(L-Lys^{70}L-Ala^{30})$_n$.[9a]* The same obtains with other positively charged macromolecules, such as ricin, the chemically modified methylated albumin,[64] and polyhaptenic dyes.[65] Nucleic acids, high molecular weight proteins, and bacterial extracts may also interact with serum proteins. High concentrations of amino acids may inhibit the precipitation of antigen and antibody.[36]

[63] M. Heidelberger, *Bacteriol. Rev.* **3**, 49 (1939).

* For nomenclature employed for synthetic polymers of amino acids and procedures for preparation, see Vol. I, Chap. 1.E.7.

[64] J. Sri Ram and P. H. Maurer, *Arch. Biochem. Biophys.* **83**, 223 (1959).

[65] J. L. Morrison, *Can. J. Chem.* **31**, 216 (1953).

ix. Storage of Serum

Methods of storage and preservation are discussed in detail in Vol. I, Chap. 2.C.4. It is recommended to store serum refrigerated at 0 to 5° or in the frozen state. Lyophilization of human sera was observed to have a deleterious effect on measurements of antibody[66]; with rabbit sera, irregular effects of lyophilization have been noted on solubility and freeing of lipids.

x. Dilution Effects on the Quantitative Precipitin Reaction

The maximal amount of precipitable antibody is determined by mixing undiluted decomplemented antiserum with small volumes of antigen, added preferably from standardized micropipets. The total recovery of precipitated antibody is lessened not only by solubility of Ag–Ab precipitates and by dissociation of antibody from the precipitate during washing procedures carried out with limited amounts of cold saline [Section (a) below], but much more markedly by increasing the reaction volume with diluent [Section (b) below].

(a) *Effects of Washing Ag–Ab Precipitates.* Because nonspecific serum proteins are trapped within centrifuged specific precipitates, it is necessary to wash the precipitates adequately several times with cold (1 to 3 ml) 0.15 M NaCl or saline phosphate or saline borate solution before analyzing the precipitates (see footnote to Section 13.A.3.b.i). It is customary to wash precipitates two to three times with 2 to 3 ml of saline—sufficient even when 3 to 5 ml of undiluted serum are used for analysis—and to neglect any losses incurred by solubility of Ag–Ab precipitates. The loss is, of course, proportionately greater when small amounts of precipitate are being analyzed, and appropriate corrections should be made on the basis of experience with the particular system. As an example, Kabat et al.[67] found that a precipitate of human blood group A substance and anti-A antibody containing only 25 μg of N, when washed 6 times with 3.0 ml of ice-cold saline, lost 3.0 μg AbN per 2 washings. A larger bulk precipitate of specific catalase–anticatalase washed at 0° and 37° showed a solubility of 0.22 μg of N per milliliter of saline.[68] In a rabbit antipolymer system, essentially no difference in the antibody N value was reported after 2 or 5 washings at 0°,[38] yet here the solubility of the precipitates may have been decreased by the presence of complement in the undiluted serum.

The use of large volumes for washing, approximating "equilibrium"

[66] M. Heidelberger and M. M. Di Lapi, *J. Immunol.* **61**, 153 (1949).
[67] E. A. Kabat, C. H. Bendich and A. E. Bezer, *J. Exptl. Med.* **83**, 477 (1946).
[68] H. F. Deutsch and A. Seabra, *J. Biol. Chem.* **214**, 455 (1955).

conditions, incurs much greater losses and should be avoided. Haurowitz *et al.*[69] washed repeatedly with 10-ml portions of saline at 3° and 27° and measured the antibody content of successive washes. The greatest loss occurred in the first two washings and was referable to dissociation of antibody from the precipitate, since the Ab/Ag ratios in the precipitates after extraction at 3° measured, respectively, 5.0, 4.5, 4.3, 4.1, 3.9, and 3.8. The actual losses with repeated washings with 10 ml saline of a precipitate formed by mixing 1.0 mg of radioactive arsanilazo beef serum pseudoglobulin and 7.35 mg of purified Ab were 495, 364, 243, 185 μg at 3.5°, whereas at 28° the losses were 585, 400, 285, 206, 222 μg. Boyd,[70] also, had found that the solubility of the precipitate declined with

TABLE VIII

SOLUBILITY IN SALINE[a] OF THRICE-WASHED
PRECIPITATES (HEMOCYANIN–HORSE ANTIHEMOCYANIN)[b]

Extraction	Volume of extractant, milliliters saline per gram precipitate nitrogen		
	333	878	1660
1	0.0379	0.0210	0.0211
2	0.0169	0.0032	0.0036
3	0.0082	0.0038	0.0024
4	0.0056	0.0021	0.0026
5	0.0036	—	0.0011
6	0.0004	—	0.0001

[a] Values expressed as milligrams of nitrogen per milliliter.
[b] From Boyd.[70]

repeated washings, was largest with the first washing, and varied with the sample of antiserum (Table VIII).

These observations may be related to different degrees of heterogeneity in the binding constants of the various antibody molecules. Accordingly, if antigen–antibody complexes dissociate in saline, it may be possible to precipitate all the antibody in the equivalence zone only if it is highly "avid" antibody.

(b) *Effect of Volume of the Reaction Mixture.* The maximal amount of precipitated antibody found with undiluted, decomplemented antiserum

[69] F. Haurowitz, R. Sowinski, and H. F. Cheng, *J. Am. Chem. Soc.* **79**, 1882 (1957).
[70] W. C. Boyd, "Fundamentals of Immunology," 3rd ed. Wiley (Interscience), New York, 1956.

is lessened when antiserum (rabbit[51, 71, 72] or sheep[73]) is diluted before or during analysis or when the volume is increased deliberately[2]; the major effect occurs during the initial dilution (Table IX). The finding reflects the presence of weakly bound antibody molecules (heterogeneity of Ab) as was seen in Section (a) above on saline extraction of Ag–Ab precipitates, or increased possibility for intraparticulate interactions on dilution, as well as solubility of the Ag–Ab aggregates. (Appropriate concentration of the supernatants will lead to recovery of the nonprecipitated portion of antibody.)

TABLE IX

DECREASE IN PRECIPITABLE ANTIBODY ATTRIBUTABLE TO DILUTION EFFECTS

Immune sera	Antibody recovered in precipitates (μg AbN/ml antiserum)								Reference
	Dilution of antiserum								
	1:1[a]	1:4	1:6	1:10	1:12	1:16	1:20	1:40	
Rabbit anti-BSA	300	240	—	—	—	228	—	—	Maurer and Talmage[51]
Rabbit anti-Ea	400	—	—	273	—	—	—	167	Kabat and Schorr,[71] cf. Talmage and Maurer[72]
Sheep antitestosterone-BSA	3830	2660	—	—	2000	—	665	—	Zimmering et. al.[73]

[a] 1:1 signifies "neat," i.e., undiluted, serum.

The reduction in precipitability of antibody (either in serum or as the γ-globulin fraction) obeyed the following formula:

$$A_{\mathrm{app}} = A_1 e^{-b(f-1)}$$

where A_{app} is the apparent Ab at the dilution tested, A_1 is the Ab concentration of the undiluted test solution at which the dilution factor, f, equals 1. The term b is a measure of the degree of variation of the precipitation of Ab with dilution, and represents the slope of the straight line obtained by plotting log A_{app} vs. f.

When the volume of the reaction mixture was increased by adding saline, the decrease in the amount of precipitated antibody was of the

[71] E. A. Kabat and J. M. Schorr, Unpublished data quoted in Kabat.[15]

[72] D. W. Talmage and P. H. Maurer, *J. Infect. Diseases* **92**, 288 (1953).

[73] P. E. Zimmering, S. M. Beiser, and B. F. Erlanger, *J. Immunol.* **95**, 262 (1965).

order of 1 to 2 μg of AbN per milliliter for horse[74] and human[67] antisera, and much greater, about 3 to 10 μg N per milliliter, for rabbit antibody (Table X).

(c) *Effect of Diluent on the Reaction.* Generally, there is little difference in the results when one uses as diluent 0.15 M NaCl adjusted to pH 7.5, a 0.15 M saline—0.01 M phosphate buffer at pH 7.5, 0.15 M saline–borate buffer at pH 8, 5% serum albumin, or decomplemented normal serum. Fresh serum should be avoided as it will contribute complement to the precipitates. An unexplained finding of Schlossman and Kabat[75] is that the addition of normal human serum to purified human antibody reduced the amount of antibody precipitated from 4.0 to only 2.8 μg of Ab–N. Human γ-globulin or HSA also caused a significant decrease in antibody N precipitated as compared to saline solution.

xi. Effect of Serum Enzymes

As serum may contain active enzymes, one has to ensure that the antigen is not digested by serum enzymes. For example, in the reaction of glycogen with rabbit antipneumococcal sera types IX and XII, as in Fig. 9, serum amylase digested the glycogen-antibody precipitates even at 0°.[76] Long periods of incubation, therefore, had to be avoided. This same problem did not arise with a horse antiserum that was low in amylase content.[77] In studies with anti-RNA antibodies, it has been found necessary to remove the RNase from the serum with bentonite[78] or an anti-RNase serum.[24] A reverse situation may also exist in studies with anti-enzymes. In studies with antibodies against such proteolytic enzymes as trypsin and papain,[79] it is important to have inhibitors present or use the inactive form of the enzyme so that the antigen does not digest the antigen–antibody complex or compete with other protein substrates.

With this latter system (papain–antipapain) the precipitin curve shows two peaks—one due to papain–antipapain and the other to papain–anti-digested antibody complexes. When cysteine and EDTA are added to the reaction mixture, the damaged antibody is further reduced. A single peak is obtained, however, if inactive mercuripapain is used in the reaction.

The recent findings of the degradation of IgG to F_{ab} and F_c fragments upon storage at 37° or even 0° has been attributed to the action of plasmin.

[74] J. W. Goodman and E. A. Kabat, *J. Immunol.* **84**, 333 and 347 (1960).

[75] S. F. Schlossman and E. A. Kabat, *J. Exptl. Med.* **116**, 535 (1962).

[76] M. Heidelberger, H. Jahrmarker, and F. Cordoba, *J. Immunol.* **78**, 427 (1957).

[77] M. Heidelberger, H. Jahrmarker, B. Bjorklund, and J. Adams, *J. Immunol.* **78** 419 (1957).

[78] E. Barbu and J. P. Dandeu, *Compt. Rend.* **256**, 1166 (1963).

[79] R. Arnon, *Immunochemistry* **2**, 107 (1965).

TABLE X

EFFECT OF VOLUME ON TOTAL N PRECIPITATED IN HOMOLOGOUS ANTIGEN–ANTIBODY SYSTEMS: VOLUME ADJUSTED WITH SALINE[a]

Species of antiserum	Antiserum to	Volume serum used (ml)	Antigen added (μg)	Total volume (ml)												Solubility (μg N/ml)
				Total N precipitated (μg)												
				1.0	1.5	2.0	2.5	3	4	4.5	5	6	8	9	10	
Horse	Pn XII	0.03	15	58	—	—	—	—	54	—	—	—	—	—	53	0.6
	Pn XIV	0.5	25	—	189	190	—	192	186	—	186	—	—	—	—	1.0
Human	Hog A	1.5	100	—	—	—	26.1	—	24.1	—	—	19.5	—	—	—	1.9
	Dextran	0.5	4	—	30.4	—	—	28.5	—	27.5	—	24.6	—	—	—	1.3
Rabbit	Pn III	1.0	100	—	—	550	—	—	—	—	—	—	—	—	494	7
	Pn III	1.0	60	—	—	496	—	—	—	—	—	—	—	474	—	3
	Hen Ea	1.0	98 (μg N)	—	—	1180	—	—	—	—	—	—	—	1150	—	4
	Horse Sa	1.0	250 (μg N)	—	—	642	—	—	—	—	—	—	584	—	—	10
	Hog Tg	1.0	158 (μg N)	252	—	—	—	—	—	—	238	—	—	—	—	3[b]

[a] From Kabat.[15]

[b] A value of 1 μg N/ml was obtained if dilutions were made in normal rabbit serum.

This proteolytic activity which can be prevented by the addition of inhibitors such as ε-aminocaproic acid may lead to changes in the precipitin behavior of fractionated antibody upon storage.

xii. State of Aggregation (Molecular Weight) of Antigen

An investigation of the reaction of human serum albumin and its mercury dimer with anti-HSA serum showed that the monomer and dimer gave identical curves up to the equivalence zone. However, in antigen excess the dimer gave more precipitation, i.e., was less effective in inhibiting precipitation.[80] The same effect was noted in the dextran–antidextran,[4] gelatin–antigelatin,[7] and denatured Ea-anti-Dn-Ea systems[6] wherein the low molecular weight fractions caused inhibition more rapidly than the "native" high molecular weight fractions. The low molecular weight fractions, however, are more effective per unit weight in precipitating the antibody.

xiii. Effect of Solvents on the Precipitin Reaction

Ordinarily, one does not analyze for antibody in the presence of non-aqueous solvents. Solvents are employed to learn the nature of the attractive forces in the Ag-Ab reaction and their action on the antibody followed by removal before reaction with antigen. This section gives data obtained in the presence of the solvents, a limited number of which have been studied for effects on the *precipitin* reaction.

A recent study by Bata et al.[81] shows the effect of varying concentrations of urea on the precipitin reaction of rabbit anti-BSA serum. Inhibition of the precipitin reaction was progressively enhanced in media containing increasing concentrations of urea. The effect was largest in the equivalence zone (Fig. 13).

Grant[82, 83] noted that 20% dioxane reversed some antigen–antibody reactions, even completely, but other workers reported no effect of 25% dioxane.[84]

Ethanol in about 10% concentration increased the amount precipitated presumably by precipitating soluble complexes.[85, 86]

The action of a variety of solvents on a charged synthetic polymer system showed that all of the solvents, at the concentration employed,

[80] L. Levine and R. K. Brown, *Biochim. Biophys. Acta* **25**, 329 (1957).
[81] J. E. Bata, L. Gyenes, and A. Sehon, *Immunology* **1**, 289 (1964).
[82] R. A. Grant, *Brit. J. Exptl. Pathol.* **40**, 6 (1960).
[83] R. A. Grant, *Brit. J. Exptl. Pathol.* **41**, 45 (1961).
[84] J. J. Cebra, D. Givol, and E. Katchalski, *J. Biol. Chem.* **237**, 751 (1962).
[85] R. A. Grant, *Brit. J. Exptl. Pathol.* **34**, 50 (1953).
[86] P. Grabar and J. Oudin, *Ann. Inst. Pasteur* **69**, 195 (1943).

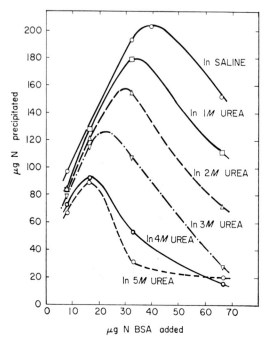

Fig. 13. The effect of different concentrations of urea on the precipitin reaction. From Bata et al.[81]

had some effect on the precipitin reaction with the exception of 20% dimethyl sulfoxide.[37] * The major effects in reduction of precipitation were 15% by 15% dimethyl formamide, and 40% by 15% dioxane (Table XI). The values were calculated by the areas under each precipitin curve, and the effect, when present, occurred both at equivalence and in antibody excess.† From these studies, it was inferred that the *major forces* involved

---

* These findings with DMSO cannot be assumed to obtain with all antigen–antibody systems. Williams and Hafleigh[86a] found significant reduction of precipitation by 10% DMSO in the antigen-excess zone with an HSA rabbit-anti-HSA. The magnitude of the effect varied with the time of incubation and the antiserum employed. One pooled antiserum gave reduced precipitate in 10% DMSO over the entire range at 24 hours, but normal precipitate values after 4 days of incubation.

[86a] C. A. Williams and A. S. Hafleigh, Unpublished data (1965).

† This method of calculation has not been adequately evaluated. It has resulted in some false impressions concerning the amounts of Ab in any serum not precipitable by homologous antigen. Percent of cross reactions observed between heterologous polymers and an antiserum against a copolymer of poly(L-Glu^{96}-L-Tyr^{4})$_n$ have been reported as follows: poly(L-Glu^{59}-L-Lys^{41})$_n$—360%, poly(L-Glu^{56}-L-Lys^{43}-L-Tyr^{1})$_n$—475%, poly(L-Glu^{56}-L-Lys^{38}-L-Tyr^{6})$_n$—350%, poly(L-Glu^{62}-L-Lys^{33}-L-Phe^{5})$_n$ —250%.

in the interaction were electrostatic. However, in a study of the influence of nonaqueous solvents, homologous and heterologous reactions of an uncharged synthetic polypeptide antigen and of a charged one showed no significant differences with respect to pH and ionic strength with antisera

TABLE XI

EFFECT OF SOLVENTS ON ANTIBODY-SYNTHETIC POLYPEPTIDE INTERACTION[a,b]

Solvent	Final concentration (gm/100 ml[c])	Extent of precipitin reaction (%)
NaCl-phosphate (control)	0.15 M	100
Urea	12	45
Formamide	50	10
Dimethyl formamide	15	85
Acetamide	5	65
N-Methyl acetamide	40% saturated	75
N,N-Dimethyl acetamide	15	70
N-Butyl acetamide	15	40
Acetone	15	75
Acetonitrile	15	30
Methanol	7.5	125
Ethanol	7.5	130
Isopropyl alcohol	7.5	105
n-Propyl alcohol	7.5	75
Ethylene glycol	50	35
1,4-Butanediol	25	40
Glycerol	25	25
Dioxane	15	60
Tetrahydrofuran	15	55
Chloroethanol	10	25
Dimethyl sulfoxide	20	95
Sodium dodecyl sulfate[d]	2.2	60

[a] From Gould et al.[37]

[b] Antigen, poly(L-Glu^{56}-L-Lys^{38}-L-Tyr^6)$_n$.

[c] Except as noted.

[d] Temperature, 20°.

to the two antigens.[87] However, 15% dioxane and 15% dimethyl formamide which *did not* decrease the amount of precipitate in the charged system reduced it to only 10% of its value in the uncharged system. Similarly, 4 M urea reduced the amount of precipitate in the *charged* system to 60% and of the uncharged to 8%. This would indicate that electrostatic interactions are not always necessary for the Ag–Ab inter-

[87] E. Hurwitz, S. Fuchs, and M. Sela, Unpublished data (1965).

actions, but when charged groups are present they may contribute to the stabilization of the Ag–Ab bond.

More recently, Hawkins[88] showed that polyhydroxy compounds such as glucose, fructose, mannitol, and glycerol reduce the *velocity* of the precipitin reaction at concentrations of 0.3 M and above, and only slightly affect the amount of complex finally precipitated. However, other nonionic solutes such as formamide, N-methyl formamide, and N,N–dimethyl formamide even at concentrations of 0.02 M are powerful inhibitors of the rabbit anti-BSA system. The extents of inhibition noted were 47%, 54%, and 50%, respectively. It is not known how these substances block the combination of antigen and antibody or otherwise inhibit the flocculation of antigen–antibody complexes.

xiv. Action of Reducing Agents

Reducing agents such as mercaptoethanol (MEA) have been used to differentiate between the 19 S and 7 S classes of immunoglobulins. Initially, it was believed that 0.1 M MEA abolished the activity only of 19 S antibody. The recent findings of Adler[88a] indicate that 0.1 M MEA reduces the *precipitating* activity and rate of precipitation of 7 S antibody in mouse sera. This effect is greater on 7 S antibody in early (2–4 week) sera than in later bleedings, i.e., a reduction of 38 to 55% vs. 26%. A more drastic loss of precipitating activity of MEA-treated 7 S chicken antibody has been reported by Rosenquist and Gilden.[89]

b. Flocculation Reaction

As indicated in Section 13.A.1, the flocculation reaction—a special case of the precipitin reaction usually obtained in horse antiprotein reactions—may be affected by the same experimental conditions as the precipitin reaction. Precipitation of horse anti-HSA serum held for varying periods at 1°, 37°, and 45° is shown in Fig. 14. Greater precipitation occurred after 4 days at 1°, or 37° for 1 hour plus 3 days at 1° than after 1 hour at 37° or 45°.[90] Burtin[91] has indicated that 2 days at 37° gave more precipitation than at 0°. Treffers *et al.*[35] found no differences within the region of maximum flocculation, but in the antibody and antigen excess regions noted that more precipitation was obtained at 0° when the mixtures were held for 7 and 14 days rather than for 3 days. As for the effect of volume, increasing a 3-ml reaction, giving 527 μg AbN precipitated in the zone of maximal flocculation, to 10 ml led to a decrease of 6 to 10 μg of N in the

[88] J. D. Hawkins, *Immunology* **9**, 107 (1965).
[88a] F. L. Adler, *J. Immunol.* **95**, 39 (1965).
[89] G. L. Rosenquist and R. V. Gilden, *Biochim. Biophys. Acta* **78**, 543 (1963).
[90] D. Gitlin, *J. Immunol.* **62**, 437 (1949).
[91] P. Burtin, *Bull. Soc. Chim. Biol.* **36**, 335 (1954).

precipitate. In the antibody-excess and antigen-excess regions, however, differences were as great as 92 and 110 μg of N, respectively. In this study, an unusual temperature effect was noted. In mixtures held at 0° for 7 days or at 37° for 3 hours, the points of maximum precipitation coincided. In this regard, the system resembled the horse diphtheria toxin–antitoxin and egg albumin–antialbumin reaction rather than the carbohydrate–anticarbohydrate system in the horse. More N was precipitated in antibody excess at 0° than at 37°, and the reverse was true in the region of

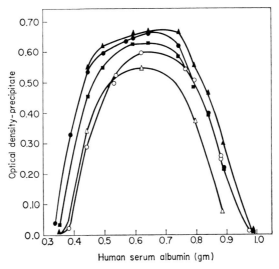

FIG. 14. The effect of varying conditions of incubation on the precipitation of HSA by horse antibodies to crystallized HSA. △, 37° for 1 hour; ○, 45° for 1 hour; ■, 37° for 1 hour followed by 1 day at 1°; ● 37° for 1 hour followed by 3 days at 1°; ▲ 4 days at 1°. From Gitlin.[90]

antigen excess. These effects may be due to basic differences in the rate at which the two types of antibodies attain equilibrium or difference in solubilities of the complexes at the two temperatures. It has also been shown that equilibrium is reached more rapidly in antigen excess than in antibody excess. The solubility of antigen–antibody complexes in antigen excess has also been shown to be governed by the solubility of the antigen.

c. CHICKEN ANTIBODY REACTION

Characteristics of the antibody response in chickens, purification of the immunoglobulins, and physiochemical studies have been cited by Benedict in Vol. I, Chap. 2.D.2. Particular differences from mammalian antiserum include a high lipid content in serum, often greatly increased precipitation with antibody in the presence of high (8%) concentrations of NaCl, the association or aggregation of nonantibody protein with Ag–Ab precipitates, especially when formed in high salt, and a tendency of γG to precipitate during dialysis against buffers of ionic strengths commonly used in chromatographic separations.

Owing to these circumstances, quantitative precipitin studies must deal with precipitates of fairly complex nature. In early bleedings, γM macroglobulin is present, and it precipitates best in low salt concentration. Early γG antibody precipitates best in high salt concentration, but γG produced by booster injections is not very sensitive to salt concentration. Benedict *et al.* concluded, for example, that "the varying amounts of high and low salt precipitins between different sera and the inclusion or exclusion of the macroglobulin components in precipitates seem to depend on the varying ratios of these three types of antibodies and probably on the coprecipitation of normal proteins."[92]

In each of two systems, anti-RGG and anti-BSA, the precipitate was found to contain two antibodies of the same electrophoretic mobility, one of 600,000 molecular weight, the other of 180,000. Both antibodies precipitated with antigen in either 0.9% or 8% NaCl, but the precipitate found in 8% NaCl was larger and contained more of the 180,000 type, together with another, non antibody component.[93]

i. Effect of Salt Concentration

The increased precipitation seen with fowl antiserum in concentrations greater than 0.15 M (0.9%) NaCl, termed "low salt," was studied in the edestin–antiedestin system. Precipitation increased up through a concentration of 10% NaCl and decreased at 12% NaCl.[94] At this high concentration of salt, serum blanks tend to give high readings. A straight line was not found when the quotient (AbN/AgN) was plotted against added AgN. The type of curves obtained with an avian antibovine serum albumin system is shown in Fig. 15.[95] Little difference was found whether reactions were run at 0° or at room temperature. In the presence of 0.15 M NaI, the precipitation was greater than with 0.15 M NaCl; and at 1.5 M concentration of NaCl, the reverse situation obtained.[96]

ii. Precipitation Curves

An intensive investigation of fowl antisera, using ^{131}I-labeled anti-BSA and anti-BGG and 1, 4, and 8% NaCl was undertaken by Aitken and

[92] A. A. Benedict, R. T. Hersh, and C. Larson, *J. Immunol.* **91**, 795 (1963).
[93] E. Orlans, M. E. Rose, and J. R. Marrack, *Immunology* **4**, 262 (1961).
[94] J. Muñoz and E. L. Becker, *J. Immunol.* **68**, 405 (1952).
[95] M. Goodman and H. R. Wolfe, *J. Immunol.* **69**, 423 (1952).
[96] M. Goodman, H. R. Wolfe, and R. Goldberg, *J. Immunol.* **72**, 440 (1954).

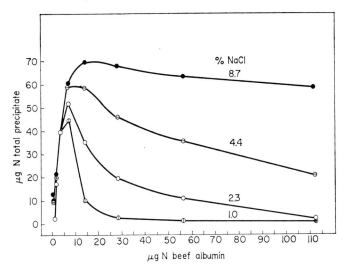

Fig. 15. Effect of salt concentration on total nitrogen precipitated (minus control), by BSA from pooled pheasant anti-BSA serum. From Goodman and Wolfe.[95]

Mulligan.[22] Increasing the salt concentration is found to lead to increased precipitation of both the antigen and antibody (see Vol. I, Chap. 2.B.3). Of interest was the finding that complete precipitation of antigen occurred only in extreme antibody excess.[22] In the region of maximum precipitation of antibody, only 50% and 65% of antigens BSA and BGG were precipitated. Therefore, there was no equivalence point as is found with many rabbit antisera.

iii. Effect of Time of Incubation

A study of the effect of temperature and length of incubation on the amount of precipitate formed in the avian BSA–anti-BSA system showed precipitation to be maximal after *3 hours at 37°* followed by centrifugation at 22°.[97] Centrifugation at 4° yielded less precipitable antibody N. Lengthening the incubation period (at either high or low temperatures) led to reduction in amount of original precipitate. It has not been determined as yet whether these effects may be related to the release of coprecipitated material.

iv. Effect of Aging of Sera

Allowing sera to age for 1 week at 4° or −20° led to a decrease in the Ab N as determined in 8% NaCl and an increase when the test was performed in 1% NaCl.[98]

[97] H. R. Wolfe, A. P. Mueller, and J. C. Neess, *Immunology* **2**, 195 (1959).
[98] N. Gengozian and H. R. Wolfe, *J. Immunol.* **78**, 401 (1957).

v. Nature of Coprecipitating Material in Immune Precipitates

The coprecipitating protein is not solely complement even though fixation of fowl complement by fowl antibody coincides with a considerable increase in the weight of the precipitates[99] and with increased precipitation in the equivalence and antigen-excess regions.[98]

Nonantibody macroglobulin (s_{20} = 21) analogous to complement constitutes part of the precipitate found in the presence of fresh normal serum[100] and is incorporated more in 1% NaCl than in 8% NaCl.[99] This component can be removed from the antiserum by absorption with a heterologous antigen–antibody system and then restored by normal fowl serum.[99] Versene (0.0025 M) was found to reduce the total protein precipitated, both in 0.9% and 8% NaCl,[92] but apparently not always.[99] Whichever the effect of Versene, it seems to be the same with a given antiserum whether fresh or aged.[98]

Although coprecipitating α-globulin has been reported in precipitates,[101] none was found by other workers when specific precipitates formed in 8% NaCl were redissolved.[102]

vi. Effect of Dilution

The effect of dilution is similar to that noted with rabbit sera: i.e., the initial dilution decreases the extent of precipitation.

In the antibovine serum albumin system, increasing the volume of the reaction mixture from 1 to 10 ml reduced the amount of antibody precipitated in 1% NaCl (30 μg of N vs. 2 μg of N), but a lesser effect was noted in 8% NaCl (43 μg of N vs. 36 μg of N).[96] In another study also, increasing the volume of the reaction mixture from 1 to 4 ml led to a loss of 20 μg of N out of 100 to 450 μg of Ab N.[103]

3. QUANTITATIVE DETERMINATION OF ANTIBODY

Although there are many tests both *in vitro* and *in vivo* for the detection and estimation of antibody activities, the quantitative precipitin reaction for measurement of antibody has become the conventional assay procedure. Its major advantage is that it is the only method which allows an absolute measurement in weight units of the number of precipitating antibody molecules present in a serum.

The need for the quantitative precipitin reaction was foreshadowed by

[99] E. Orlans, M. E. Rose, and K. H. Clapp, *Immunology* **5**, 656 (1962).
[100] T. Makinodan, N. Gengozian, and R. E. Canning, *J. Immunol.* **85**, 439 (1960).
[101] H. F. Deutsch, J. C. Nichol, and M. Cohn, *J. Immunol.* **63**, 195 (1949).
[102] J. Banovitz and H. R. Wolfe, *J. Immunol.* **82**, 489 (1959).
[103] N. Gengozian and H. R. Wolfe, *J. Immunol.* **77**, 172 (1956).

many studies that suggested heterogeneity in the antibody population within certain sera, notably antitoxic and antihapten sera. Yet the complexity of immunoglobulin classes and the intraclass heterogeneity, not suspected at the time when the quantitative precipitin reaction was being developed, would not have been revealed solely by measurement of total antibody, or by partial absorption of antibody, or by detection of nonprecipitating antibody that was able only to coprecipitate. The further developments of antigen–antibody reactions in gel media and of immunoelectrophoresis were requisite to our present understanding.

Because of molecular heterogeneity and the distribution of antibody activity among immunoglobulins having different characteristics with regard to antigen precipitation, it must be realized that the quantitative precipitin reaction may not be measuring all the antibody in any serum. Nevertheless, disciplined immunochemistry provides a quantitative approach to many aspects of *in vitro* and *in vivo* immune reactions.

Before analyzing a serum quantitatively for precipitating antibody or preparing a "calibrated" antiserum, it is important to establish the presence and approximate concentration of precipitating antibody, and the amount of antigen needed to yield a precipitate, the antibody leaving no excess or minimal antigen or antibody in the supernatant. It is essential also to ascertain the "purity" of the system, as by agar diffusion (see Section 13.A.3.a.iii) to determine that no contaminating precipitating systems are present as a result of impurity of antigen and production of antibodies to the impurities.

Tests for ascertaining the presence of Ab are given in Sections 13.A.3.a.i and ii below. Various techniques are described below (Sections iv, v, vi) for locating optimal precipitation ratios. When these are known, one can proceed to design the mixtures that will be used in Section 13.A.3.b below. Sometimes the preliminary combining ratio will give a direct indication of the amount of antibody. Thus if one is dealing with a known system, such as the BSA–anti-BSA system in which one can assume a 5.5:1 ratio of AbN/AgN at equivalence, and if, for example, 10 μg of BSA N gave the optimal precipitate with 0.5 ml of a 1:4 dilution of serum, then 1 ml of the serum is estimated to contain about 440 μg of AbN. Antisera do vary in combining ratio, however, 5.5:1 being a reasonable average.

a. PRELIMINARY QUALITATIVE AND SEMIQUANTITATIVE TESTS

i. *Interfacial Ring Test*

The interfacial ring test is used primarily to detect antibody. The technique is to carefully overlay a clear, undiluted specimen of immune serum with antigen without mixing the two solutions. The reaction of antigen with antiserum at the liquid–liquid interface gives rise to a visible ring of precipitate when the concentration of antigen is appropriate, and it may detect as little as 1 μg of antibody protein. Although the test is not overly dependent upon a critical ratio of antibody and antigen, it is best, if the antibody concentration is low, to test initially with a low antigen concentration, i.e., 1 μg/ml. Clear tubes are used, 6 $\times$ 50 mm or narrower. Excellent tubes can be made of 40-mm lengths of 3 mm o.d. (1.6 mm i.d.) soft-glass tubing, one end sealed by heating with a microburner. Antiserum (0.1 to 0.3 ml for a 6-mm diameter tube, 0.02 to 0.05 ml for a 3 mm diameter tube) is introduced with a Pasteur pipet or needle and syringe. No air pocket or surface bubble should be present (these can be removed by brief centrifugation). An equal volume of antigen is overlaid carefully without mixing. Normal rabbit serum and preimmunization serum should be included as controls, as well as the immune serum overlaid with saline. The tubes are incubated upright, either at room temperature or in the cold, and the interface is observed for the development of turbidity or a sharp ring in the antibody layer. This should appear shortly, and always within 24 hours. The bottom of the tubes should be observed, as Ag–Ab precipitate may form and settle overnight. The technique is rapid and indicates the presence of at least 3 to 5 μg of antibody N per milliliter of serum, but gives little information about the combining proportions of antigen and antibody. Dilutions of antiserum can also be set up by this procedure provided normal serum is used as the diluent; the antiserum layer must be of greater density than the antigen.

ii. The Swift–Wilson–Lancefield Capillary Tube Test[103a]

A modification of the interfacial ring test employs disposable capillary tubes (75 mm $\times$ 1.3 to 1.5 mm diameter) in which, by capillarity, antiserum is taken up to a height of about 22 mm followed directly and contiguously by an approximately equal amount of antigen solution. This is conveniently carried out by placing separate drops of antiserum and antigen dilution on a glass slide; the capillary tube, polished to remove fingermarks, is inclined to a horizontal position, touched first to the drop of antiserum and then to the drop of antigen, both rising by capillarity. A final column of air (about 6 mm) is taken into the tube by tilting it downward. The top of the tube is closed with a forefinger, and the base is plunged downward into modeling clay. In this system, the antiserum (of heavier specific gravity) is at the top and the initial interface between antigen and antibody is cone-shaped, affording many ratios of Ag to Ab.

[103a] H. F. Swift, A. T. Wilson, and R. C. Lancefield, *J. Exptl. Med.* **78**, 127 (1943).

The system was devised originally for carbohydrate reactions and for tests of streptococcal M-substance. Further mixing occurs owing to the specific gravity of serum, and precipitate usually appears within 10 minutes. Later, the precipitate sinks and rests on the lower air–liquid interface. The method gives much more information about antibody content than the simple interfacial test. The order of adding the reagents can be reversed if only slight mixing is preferred. It is useful to use a trench cut in a wooden block (e.g., $\frac{5}{16}$ inch wide by $\frac{1}{4}$ inch deep) to hold the plasticene. Positions along the plasticene are marked by attaching a strip of quad-ruled paper along the block and scoring the plasticene correspondingly. Rapid scoring is possible with a comb having alternate teeth snapped off to match paper ruled at 5-mm intervals.

iii. Agar Diffusion Methods (see also Chapter 14)

The Oudin (single diffusion) or Preer (double diffusion) procedures may give an estimate of (a) the number of antigen–antibody systems present and (b) the quantity of antibody present. The *sensitivity* of the Oudin procedure in detecting antibody (Chap. 14, Sections B.1 and C.8) is of the order of 5 to 10 μg AbN/ml. The Preer technique (Chap. 14, Sections B.2 and C.7) uses less serum (0.02 ml) and is slightly more sensitive in detecting antibody; compared with Ouchterlony tests in agar plates, the Preer test is considerably more sensitive since there is no loss of effective antibody by radial diffusion. The major purpose in screening sera by agar diffusion methods is to test for the presence of two or more bands of precipitate, which would indicate the presence of more than one antigen–antibody system and suggest that quantitative analysis may not be in order until a more purified antigen is obtained. Antibody against one component may be analyzed even in highly complex antisera; i.e., it is possible to analyze an antiserum against whole human serum quantitatively for anti-HSA or anti-HGG if highly purified albumin or γ-globulin is employed. Methods for antigen purification are discussed in Vol. I.

iv. Dilution for Ascertaining Optimal Proportions

A method based upon mixing small amounts of antiserum with selected *antigen dilutions* and observing precipitation, described in Vol. I, Chap. 2.C.1, gives further information about the response of the animals. Readings can be made within 60 minutes. By centrifuging these tubes and testing the supernatant for residual antigen and residual antibody by the Swift–Wilson–Lancefield capillary tube technique (Section 13.A.3.a.ii above), much of the preliminary information described below can be ascertained, so that subsequent steps in determining the quantitative precipitin curve can be taken readily.

It has been pointed out, for a carbohydrate–anticarbohydrate system, that antigen and antibody will precipitate in constant ratios when concentrations of antibody and antigen are varied widely and if neither reactant is highly concentrated. To determine this ratio in a practical sense, the smallest concentration of Ag capable of showing a precipitate in antibody excess is first determined. Various dilutions of antiserum are then tested against this amount of antigen, the supernatants being examined to locate the tube devoid of both antibody and antigen.[104]

A technique which estimates the equivalence by determining the ratio of antigen to antibody which *flocculates* most rapidly is described under neutralization reactions (see Chap. 18.A).

The preliminary assessment of the combining ratio should be determined on a minimal amount of antiserum. The use of several small tubes is suggested above. Another technique is to add several concentrations of antigen serially to 0.1 to 0.5 ml of serum and centrifuge the precipitate off after each addition of antigen, and continue until no further precipitation occurs. The total amount of antigen added gives only a rough estimate of the amount of antigen needed in the equivalence region because usually more total antigen is needed to precipitate total antibody when added at once than when added serially in several smaller portions (the so-called Danysz phenomenon). Additional tubes may then be set up to determine more accurately the area of slight antigen excess. In both instances, the washed precipitate may also be analyzed for protein so as to give some further indication of the method to follow for the quantitative analysis.

Weak antisera (2 to 10 μg of AbN per milliliter of serum), for example, most human antisera, require use of more serum, such as 3.0-ml aliquots in 8-ml conical centrifuge tubes. It is necessary to use very small additions of antigen at first and so avoid antigen excess; further increments are then added, the tube being centrifuged when the amount of precipitate warrants clarification. The specific antigen is added serially, precipitates are allowed to form, and the centrifuged supernatant is transferred to another tube for further testing.

v. P-80 Analysis

When a labeled antigen is available, such as a radioactive antigen or an antigen with enzymatic activity,[60] the region of slight antigen excess may be determined easily, either by counts of the radioactivity or determination of the biological activity in the supernatant, and without need for decomplementation. And, if one is dealing with antiserum against a well

---

[104] D. S. Martin, *J. Lab. Clin. Med.* **28,** 1477 (1943).

characterized antigen, such as BSA, BGG, or Ea, whose combining ratio at equivalence is known, it is possible to calculate the approximate antibody content of the serum. This has been the basis of the P-80 (80% precipitation of added antigen) analysis for antibody of Talmage and Maurer[72] based upon Eisen and Keston's[105] initial use of ^{131}I-labeled antigens for determining antibody content.

A preliminary test is made to determine the amount of labeled Ag needed to give a definite antigen excess. Depending on the amount of antibody, 0.5 ml of serum will require between 1 and 100 μg of AgN. A starting point can be determined readily on small amounts of serum by the procedure described in Vol. I, Chap. 2.C.1. Several portions of 0.5 ml of serum are then put up with appropriate amounts of AgN. The tubes are tapped to mix well, incubated at 37° for 30 minutes, refrigerated overnight, and then centrifuged in the cold at 2000 rpm for 30 minutes. The supernatants are decanted, and the tubes are drained carefully. The two fractions of each serum (supernatant and precipitate) are counted separately to determine approximately what percentage of antigen has been precipitated.

Final determinations are then run on 4 to 6 accurately measured 0.5-ml portions of serum with several amounts of antigen extending over the region of antigen excess as indicated by the results of the preliminary tests. Final determinations are kept at least 2 days in the refrigerator, and the precipitates are washed once with 1 ml of cold 0.85% saline. The washing is added to the tube containing the corresponding supernatant. After counting is completed, the log of the antigen added per milliliter is plotted against the precipitated fraction of antigen. The concentration of antigen where 80% of the antigen is precipitated is P-80. This point, although arbitrary, allows one to measure also non-avid antibody with which a value for "P-100" (complete precipitation) is difficult to attain.

vi. Turbidimetric Analysis (see Vol. II, Chap. 10.B and Vol. III, Chap. 13.D and E)

A rapid semiquantitative method for analysis of antibody is based upon rapid measurement of the early increase in turbidity of an antiserum when mixed with antigen.[106] Each system has to be calibrated accurately, especially as to time of reading, since many nonspecific factors affect the rate of aggregation of the particles. When one arrives with these techniques at the optimal proportion of antigen and antibody (antiserum), and if one knows this ratio for the specific system under

[105] H. N. Eisen and A. S. Keston, *J. Immunol.* **63**, 71 (1949).
[106] R. L. Libby, *J. Immunol.* **34**, 71 (1938).

study, it is possible to estimate roughly the antibody content of the serum.

b. QUANTITATIVE ANALYSIS FOR ANTIBODY

i. Setup, Incubation, and Washing of Precipitate

All the factors that influence the antigen–antibody interaction should be borne in mind—pH, salt concentration, complement, dilution effects on antiserum, volume of reaction mixture, temperature and time of reaction, etc. (see Section 13.A.2.a).

Antigen and antibody solutions should in general have preservative added (see Vol. I, Chap. 2.C.4.a), and the serum and antigen solutions should be freshly clarified by centrifugation. If the antiserum has been diluted quantitatively for the analysis, it should be kept for several days in the cold and recentrifuged before use. Sera should be centrifuged at 3000 to 10,000 rpm in a high-speed angle rotor head or in an ultracentrifuge for several hours in the cold to remove particulate matter and allow lipid to rise to the surface of the tube where it can be aspirated off. Filtration of serum through a Millipore filter (Vol. I, Chap. 2.C.5.b, for filtration and use of wetted filters) has been found to cut down appreciably on high blanks in microanalyses. With sera, such as human, in which relatively large volumes are needed for sufficient precipitation to analyze by micro procedures, it is advisable to centrifuge the sera overnight in the cold. All sera and solutions should be kept cold during all operations.

After the approximate antibody content of the serum is known (Section 13.A.3.a above) one can plan the amount of serum to be used per reaction tube in the determination of a quantitative curve. If the antiserum volume required is between 0.5 ml and 5.0 ml of serum, calibrated Ostwald-Folin pipets should be used in measuring volumes. For smaller amounts of serum, calibrated micropipets should be employed. If the analysis is intended to determine total precipitable antibody, undiluted serum should be used in a minimal total volume. If, however, one wishes to calibrate a serum for determination of antigen by a uniform routine test, then diluted antiserum may be used. It is more important that the amounts of added protein or N containing antigens be known accurately than it is for polysaccharide added. The amounts of antibody that may be determined accurately by the precipitin reaction range from a few hundred to about 2 to 5 μg of N, depending on the volumes employed and the method used to assay the precipitates.

The appropriate volume of antiserum (0.5 to 5.0 ml) is transferred into 8-ml conical centrifuge tubes. Depending on the method of analysis, this tube may have calibration marks at various volumes such as 2.5 or or 1.0 ml for the Folin-Ciocalteau method (see Vol. II, Chap. 12.A.7). For ultramicro procedures (10 μl up to 1 ml of serum), 3-ml conical centrifuge tubes with calibrated markings at 0.4 ml or 1.0 ml can be employed. Antigen solutions are added in duplicate to the serum tubes and rapidly mixed by a rotary motion produced by drawing fingers down the side and under the tube, or by twirling in a test tube rack. Mechanical agitators may be used if care is employed to avoid frothing and splattering. The total volume of reactants in all tubes should be equalized by addition of 0.15 M NaCl. The tubes are closed with rubber caps.

As a practical example, after the ratio of Ag and Ab for complete or nearly complete precipitation has been determined by small-scale tests, eight ratios of Ag:Ab are set up, say on 0.5-ml portions of serum. The amount of serum is selected to give a quantity of precipitate that is conveniently assayed by the method of choice. To one tube, antigen is added in the previously determined equivalence ratio; the antibody excess zone is examined in four tubes by additions of 20, 40, 60, and 80%, respectively, of the equivalence amount of antigen, and the antigen excess part of the curve is explored in three tubes receiving, respectively, 1.5, 2.0, and 2.5 times as much antigen. In all tubes, the volume containing the various concentrations of antigen is held constant. A convenient reaction volume for 8-ml conical centrifuge tubes is 2.5 ml. Duplicate tubes are strongly advised.

Each precipitin analysis should have appropriate controls. These include antiserum plus saline, normal serum plus antigen, and pre-immunization serum plus antigen. It is also advisable periodically to set up known amounts of antigen and antibody to check on the method of analysis and to have known standards to be used in further calculations.

The tubes are incubated at 25° or 37° for 30 minutes to 1 hour, and then stored at 0 to 5° for 2 to 10 days depending on the level of antibody being analyzed and the volume of the reactants involved. With high levels of antibody (150 μg of AbN), 2 days of incubation should be sufficient, 4 days for amounts of 20 to 100 μg of AbN, and 7 to 10 days for antibody levels below 20 μg of N. Maximum precipitation in the antigen excess region usually takes longer than in the other regions. During this period the tubes are carefully mixed twice daily to resuspend the precipitates. Different antigen–antibody systems form different types of precipitates. Polysaccharides and gelatins form gelatinous, and, at times, transparent precipitates which are difficult to break up, whereas with most protein systems the aggregates resuspend easily.

After the incubation period the tubes are centrifuged in the cold for

1 hour at 2000 to 2500 rpm. This should be done even if no precipitates are visually present, as some very fine particles may not settle easily in the presence of serum. The tubes are removed from the centrifuge and placed in a cold bath. Supernatants are poured off by decanting into other centrifuge tubes with a continuous motion without touching the bottom of the precipitin tube. The decanted supernatants are examined for the presence of any precipitate that may have come over and recentrifuged if necessary. Supernatants are saved for testing as described in Section 13.A.3.b.3. The tubes containing the precipitates are drained for 2 minutes while inverted on a towel in a test tube rack. If strict temperature control of the precipitates is necessary during this draining procedure, one may work in a cold room or a cold box similar to the one used by Heidelberger and Rebers.[107]

Before being washed, precipitates are broken up by a rotary motion similar to that used for mixing the antigen and antibody. The tubes are placed in a rack in a cold bath and 0.2 to 0.5 ml of cold saline (saline–phosphate or saline–borate)* is added to the precipitates. The precipitates are suspended in the saline. An additional volume of cold saline, 1 to 2.5 ml, is added from the pipet with swirling to wash down serum proteins and any precipitates adhering to the wall of the tube. The volume of saline used in this and subsequent washes depends on the amount of antibody being analyzed and the volume of undiluted serum employed in each analysis. The tubes are mixed to resuspend the precipitate and capped with fresh rubber caps. After 20 to 30 minutes in the cold bath (new equilibrium conditions should not become established), the tubes are recentrifuged and the above procedure of decanting and washing the precipitates is repeated 2 or 3 times. (A more extensive procedure of recentrifuging the original supernatants and the supernatant of the first washing is sometimes employed.[15]) The washed precipitates are then analyzed by one of the procedures described below. These assay procedures are described in detail in Vol. II, Chap. 12.A.

ii. Methods for Analysis of Precipitates

(a) *Protein N Determination.* The method for estimation of protein which serves as the standard is the Markham[108] procedure for analysis

---

[107] M. Heidelberger and P. A. Rebers, *J. Am. Chem. Soc.* **80,** 116 (1958).

* Solutions used in washing precipitates include: (1) physiological saline: 0.15 M NaCl, pH adjusted to 7 to 7.5 with 0.01 M NaOH or 0.01 M HCl; (2) phosphate–saline: 0.01 M phosphate, pH 7.5, and 0.15 M NaCl, prepared by adding 1 ml of 1 M phosphate solution (16 ml of 1 M $NaH_2PO_4 \cdot H_2O$ + 84 ml of 1 M $Na_2HPO_4 \cdot 7H_2O$) to 100 ml of 0.15 M NaCl solution; (3) saline–borate buffer, pH 8, prepared by adding 165 ml of 0.16 M NaOH to 1 liter containing 10.27 gm of boric acid (0.2 M) and 7.8 gm of NaCl.

[108] R. Markham, *Biochem. J.* **36,** 790 (1942).

of N (see Vol. II, Chap. 12, Section A.3). In this procedure the precipitate is dissolved in a small amount of 0.5 M NaOH and transferred to microKjeldahl flasks; it is digested with H_2SO_4 in the presence of Cu^{++} and the formed $(NH_4)_2SO_4$ is analyzed as volatile NH_3. The technique is suitable for analyzing 10 to 100 μg of N with an accuracy of ± 2 μg of N. When the antigen contains N, its contribution to the weight of the precipitate must be subtracted. For example, if 120 μg of total N were precipitated by 20 μg of antigen N at the point of slight antigen excess, then the antibody content of the aliquot analyzed is 100 μg of N. The antibody N antigen N ratio at this point is 5. When the antigen contains no N, as is the case with many polysaccharides, then the total precipitate N is assumed to be antibody N.

(b) *Biuret Method.* The biuret reagent leads to the formation, in alkali, of a blue complex of copper with peptide nitrogen. A modification of the Weichselbaum[109] procedure, introduced by Dittenbrandt,[110] allows a spectrophotometric analysis of 20 to 400 μg of N (see Vol. II, Chap. 12.A.6). This is the least sensitive of the spectrophotometric methods. To the washed precipitate, 1.5 ml of the biuret reagent is added, and after solution the volume is brought up to the 2.5-ml mark. After incubation, the color is read in a spectrophotometer at 555 mμ. In this colorimetric method, as well as in any other one, it is essential to have calibration curves with known standards of the specific γ-globulin species as well as the antigen being studied. It is necessary to subtract the contribution to the optical density of the antigen (as well as the blanks) from the total absorbancy before calculating the antibody equivalence. Typical extinctions for different antibodies and some antigens are given in Table XII.[111] *

(c) *Absorption (Ultraviolet and Visible) Spectrophotometry.* The specific precipitates can be dissolved either in 0.25 N acetic acid as outlined by Gitlin[90] or in 0.1 N NaOH as described by Eisen.[112] The final volume of the dissolved precipitates may be 1.0 or 2.5 ml. The acid solution is read at 277 mμ and the alkaline solution at 287 mμ. With the use of 1.0-ml volumes, special cuvettes are used to provide a 10-mm depth, and standard calibration curves must be determined for standard proteins when measured in the special cuvettes. Both methods can measure 5 to 100 μg of N, the measurement at 277 mμ is slightly more accurate but about 4% less sensitive than measurement in alkali.

[109] T. E. Weichselbaum, *Am. J. Clin. Pathol., Tech. Sect.* **10**, 40 (1946).

[110] M. Dittenbrandt, *Am. J. Clin. Pathol.* **18**, 439 (1948).

[111] F. C. McDuffie and E. A. Kabat, *J. Immunol.* **77**, 193 (1956).

* These values are presented as a guide. It is important that each investigator establish his own absolute extinction values, based on his own nitrogen determinations or protein dry weights corrected for moisture and ash (see Vol. II, Chap. 12.A.1).

[112] H. N. Eisen, *J. Immunol.* **60**, 77 (1948).

TABLE XII

Color Values and Ultraviolet Absorption of Proteins and Antibodies Determined by Various Methods[a]

Protein	E, Biuret OD μg N/2.5 ml	Ultraviolet light absorption E (277 mμ) in 0.25 N HAc OD μg N/ml	Ultraviolet light absorption E (287 mμ) in 0.1 N NaOH OD μg N/ml	E, Folin-Ciocalteu OD μg N/10 ml	E, Ninhydrin OD μg N/2.6 ml
Hen ovalbumin	0.00078	0.0045	0.0048	0.0110	0.0187
Human serum albumin	0.00072	0.0043	0.0060	0.0083	0.0317
Human γ-globulin (II$_{1,2}$)	0.00079	0.0090	0.0105	0.0125	0.0216
Rabbit antibody to:					
Pneumococcal polysaccharide, type XIV	0.00092	0.0098	0.0103	0.0157	0.0188
Hen ovalbumin	0.00091	0.0102	0.0102	0.0146	0.0163
Human γ-globulin (II$_3$)	0.00091	0.0097	0.0103	0.0176	0.0176
All rabbit antibodies	0.00091	0.0099	0.0103		0.0176
Horse antibody to:					
Pneumococcal polysaccharide, type XIV	0.00084	0.0085	0.0104	0.0159	
Standard deviation of E for rabbit antibodies	0.00002	0.0005	0.0008	0.0012	0.0020
Range of sensitivity (μg N)	20–400	5–100	5–100	2–30	1–20

[a] From McDuffie and Kabat.[111]

At times there is occasion to use impure or crude antigens with antiserum specific for one component. Knowledge of combining ratios of the "pure" system and the extinction of the antigen permits an estimate of antibody precipitated. The lower the antigen extinction and the higher Ab/Ag combining ratio, the smaller the error in such calculations.[112a]

If one is dealing with an antigen containing a chromophore group such as an azo protein or a DNP protein, it is possible to estimate its contribution to the specific precipitate by measuring absorption at the specific wavelength in the visible region. Karush and Marks[113] have detected the concentration of azo groups in the dissolved precipitates (0.1 N NaOH) by reading the absorption at 445 mμ. Farah et al.[114] have shown how reading the absorption at 360 mμ (DNP groups) and 278 mμ (antigen and antibody) allows a calculation for both antigen and antibody. After correction for antigen and antibody blanks, the absorbance at 278 mμ was corrected for the antigen contribution. The latter correction was based on the absorbance of DNP-BGG at 360 mμ and at 278 mμ. Another correction was made for the contribution of antibody to the 360 mμ absorbance. The formula was employed as follows:

$$B = \frac{V}{E_B}(a - R[b - f(a - Rb)]) \text{ and } G = \frac{V}{E_G}(b - f[a - Rb])$$

where B is antibody, G is antigen, V is volume (ml), E_G is the extinction coefficient of antigen at 278 mμ, E_B is extinction coefficient of antibody at 360 mμ, a is absorbance at 278 mμ, b is absorbance at 360 mμ, R is ratio of absorbancies for antigen at 278 mμ/360 mμ, and f is ratio of absorbancies for antibody at 360 mμ/278 mμ. With maximally substituted DNP-BGG, $R = 0.58$ to 0.60, $f = 0.01$ at neutral pH and 0.05 in 0.25 M acetic acid. This formula was used to obtain the data in Table XIII.

A general discussion of spectrophotometry and a table of extinctions is given in Vol. II. Chap. 10.A, 12.A.9, and Appendix I.

(d) *Folin-Ciocalteau.* With several modifications, this colorimetric method can measure 2 to 30 μg of N with an error of ± 1 μg of N (see Vol. II, Chap. 12.A.7). In the original method developed by Heidelberger and MacPherson[115] for analysis of human antisera, the precipitate is dissolved in NaOH and the volume adjusted to 2.5 ml. To 2.0 ml aliquots are added Na_2CO_3–$CuSO_4$ solution and then the Folin reagent, the final volume being 10 ml. Other modifications entail dissolving

[112a] A. S. Hafleigh and C. A. Williams, *Science* **151**, 1530 (1966).
[113] F. Karush and R. Marks, *J. Immunol.* **78**, 296 (1957).
[114] F. S. Farah, M. Kern, and H. N. Eisen, *J. Exptl. Med.* **112**, 1195 (1960).
[115] M. Heidelberger and C. F. C. MacPherson, *Science* **97**, 405; **98**, 63 (1943).

TABLE XIII

SPECIFIC PRECIPITATION OF PURIFIED ANTIBODY[a, b]

Antigen added[c] (μg)	Absorbance				Antibody precipitated[d]		Antigen precipitated[d]	
	Supernatants		Precipitates					
	278 mμ	360 mμ	278 mμ	360 mμ	mg	%	μg	%
None	1.591	0.013	0.003	0.001	—	—	—	—
85.5	0.383	0.013	0.374	0.148	0.89	76	84	98
143	0.163	0.012	0.480	0.245	1.06	91	142	99
171	0.151	0.016	0.520	0.296	1.07	91	169	99
200	0.142	0.020	0.534	0.338	1.08	92	197	99
256	0.153	0.037	0.584	0.434	1.07	91	251	98
114[e]	0.422	0.720	0.001	0.001	—	—	—	—
200[e]	0.760	1.312	0.001	0.000	—	—	—	—

[a] From Farah et al.[114]

[b] 1.19 mg of antibody protein was added to each tube. Total volume in each vessel was 1.0 ml. Supernatants were read without dilution. Precipitates were washed once with 0.15 M NaCl, air-dried, and dissolved in 4.0 ml 0.25 M acetic acid.

[c] DNP–BGG about 60 moles DNP per 160,000 gm of BGG.

[d] Based on supernatant analyses. Indistinguishable results were obtained by analyses of 0.25 M acetic acid solutions of washed precipitates, providing the assumption is made that in these solutions the antibody absorbance at 360 mμ is 5% of its absorbance at 278 mμ (rather than 1% as used in the corresponding supernatant analyses).

[e] Antigen controls (no antibody added). The "supernatant" absorbances in these tubes provide two of the constants required for calculating the amounts of antigen and of antibody: (a) the ratio of absorbances 278 mμ/360 mμ is 0.58; (b) $E_{1\ cm}^{1\ \%}$ for the antigen at 360 mμ is 65.

the specific precipitate in the calibrated tube and adding the Na_2CO_3, $CuSO_4$, and Folin reagent directly in the tube.[116] Final volumes as small as 1.0 or 2.0 ml have been employed.[117] In the author's laboratory, a micromethod for analysis of 2 to 30 μg of AbN has been employed. Five milliliter centrifuge tubes calibrated at the 1.00-ml mark and micro-cuvettes (0.5 ml) are used for these small amounts of antibody measured with microliter pipets. With standard reagent concentrations, 2 to 10 μg AbN can be determined, and with a 2 to 5 dilution of the Folin reagent up to 30 μg of Ab N can be analyzed. A blank of about 2 μg of N is consistently found by materials present in all sera. Centrifugation of sera at 20,000 g for 1 hour reduces this value slightly. After development of

[116] R. C. Krueger and M. Heidelberger, J. Lab. Clin. Med. **38**, 157 (1951).
[117] E. A. Kabat and G. Schiffman, J. Immunol. **88**, 782 (1962).

the blue color, absorbancy is read at 750 mμ. (If a slight turbidity develops, the solutions are centrifuged before being read in the spectrophotometer.) The color is due mainly to the reaction of the tyrosine and tryptophan and, to a limited extent, of reducing groups such as SH. This means that, when the antigens are polysaccharides or gelatin or synthetic polymers containing amino acids, such as glutamic acid, alanine, or lysine, there is little contribution to the color by the antigen and the absorbancy at 750 mμ is therefore given by the antibody alone. Appropriate calibration curves are needed for the different reaction volumes. Also, if the absorbancy (optical density) of the reaction mixture does not fall on the linear portion of the plot of absorbancy (optical density) vs. micrograms of γ-globulin N, the solution may be diluted 1:2 or even 1:5 with the reagents employed (reagent blank). However, appropriate calibration curves of the dilutions are necessary for determination of the antibody values. This method allows an extension of the amount of γ-globulin that can be analyzed [Table XII and footnote in Section 13.A.3.b.ii.(b)].

(e) *Ninhydrin and Micro Ninhydrin.* This method, as applied to proteins, depends on the development of a purple color when the ninhydrin reagent reacts with the terminal α-amino groups and ϵ-amino groups of lysine in the protein (see Vol. II, Chap. 12.A.8 for additional technical methods). As each γ-globulin and protein may have different amounts of lysine and different extinction coefficients, known solutions of the specific antibody and protein antigen should be included in the analysis [see Table XII and footnote in Section 13.A.3.6.ii(b)]. In the micro ninhydrin method, the washed precipitate in the centrifuge tube is first treated with a Kjeldahl digestion mixture. Superoxol is also included at a later stage of digestion to help convert all the N to $(NH_4)_2SO_4$. After digestion, the NH_3 is analyzed with ninhydrin by a modification of the procedure of Rosevear and Smith.[118] Development of the final color is done in a volumetric flask, and the color is read at 570 mμ. Standards in this analysis are ammonium sulfate. The sensitivity for these methods is of the order 1 to 20 μg of antibody N.

(f) *Dye Precipitation Method.* An ultramicromethod for analysis of microliter amounts of serum or fluid developed by Glick et al.[119] entails dissolving the specific precipitate in microliter amounts of NaOH, adding 50 to 150 μl of bromosulphalein reagent, and adjusting the final volume to 0.25 or 0.4 ml. The microtubes are centrifuged at room temperature to remove the precipitated protein dye complex, and the supernatants are

[118] J. W. Rosevear and E. L. Smith, *J. Biol. Chem.* **236**, 425 (1961).
[119] D. Glick, R. A. Good, L. J. Greenberg, J. Eddy, and N. K. Day, *Science* **128**, 1625 (1958).

decanted. Aliquots of the supernatants are reacted with NaOH, and the color is read at 580 mμ to determine the amount of dye remaining unreacted. Known amounts of γ-globulin are treated similarly to obtain calibration curves. In this micromethod, samples of as little as 1 ml of serum have been used for a complete analysis. It is necessary to incubate antigen–antibody reaction mixtures for at least a week in the cold and to employ microanalytical procedures for the washing of these tiny precipitates.

(g) *General Notes.* With all the colorimetric methods for determining antibody, it is possible that the sensitivity may be increased by using microcuvettes. This also permits the use of smaller amounts of precipitate. However, one of the main limiting factors will be the solubility of the antigen–antibody complex in the equivalence region.

When the complete precipitin curve from antibody excess through the equivalence and antigen excess regions is obtained, the serum, at the dilution employed, is said to be calibrated. The serum may be calibrated according to any of the methods above; i.e., the total amount of antigen–antibody aggregate precipitated may be expressed in terms of total N, or absorbancy at the specific wavelength of absorption, i.e., 277 or 287, 555, 750, or 570 mμ.

iii. Analysis of Supernatants

Testing the supernatants (Section 13.A.3.b.1 above) for excess antigen and antibody serves two main purposes: (1) determination of the equivalence zone (or the zone of slight antigen excess); (2) establishment of the homogeneity or heterogeneity of the antigen–antibody system under study. The supernatant of each tube may be divided into 2 unequal portions (1:2). To the smaller volume is added some undiluted serum (0.1 to 0.2 ml), and to the other aliquot additional antigen. There is no problem associated with adding too much antibody to detect antigen, for excess antigen and antigen–antibody complexes are usually precipitated. The major problem lies in testing for excess antibody in supernatants from which most of the antibody has been removed. Addition of too much antigen will lead to the formation of soluble complexes and may therefore indicate the absence of antibody even when excess antibody is present. The problem in detecting excess antibody by this technique increases as the amount of antibody being analyzed decreases, thus about 2 to 5 μg of antigen, in a very small volume, should be used to detect excess supernatant antibody by this procedure. Tubes are mixed and incubated as originally. After centrifugation, the bottom of each tube is tapped to observe precipitate formation. Other tests discussed in this chapter, such as the interfacial ring test and the agar diffusion techniques, have been used for supernatant analysis. If the antigen has some biological activity such as a specific toxic or enzymic activity or is trace labeled with isotope or other marker either internally or externally, the appropriate method of detection may be employed. Similarly, if the antibody has the ability to neutralize a toxin or enzyme, the appropriate biological assay may be employed. The agglutination test with red cells or latex particles coated with antigen (see Chap. 16.B,E) and the inhibition of hemagglutination of antigen-coated cells (see Chap. 16.C) can be used to detect traces of excess antibody and antigen, respectively.

4. PARTICULAR APPLICATIONS OF THE QUANTITATIVE PRECIPITIN REACTION

The use of the quantitative precipitin reaction for obtaining information discussed below constitutes a major portion of the excellent reference book "Experimental Immunochemistry."[15] Only brief examples in each area will be presented here.

a. CALCULATION OF ANTIBODY:ANTIGEN RATIOS

If the molecular weights of both the antigen and the specific antibody under study are known, and also the amount of each component in the precipitate, then it becomes possible to calculate the molecular ratio (composition) of the components in the specific precipitate. As discussed previously, the proportion of the two reactants changes in different parts of the precipitin curve. In the region of antibody excess, one can estimate the number of reactive areas (antigenic groupings or valences) existing on the antigen molecule. In the ovalbumin (Ea)–anti-Ea system, for example, the plot of $(AbN)/(EaN)$ vs. EaN added gives a straight line with an intercept (initial combining ratio) of about 20. When it is assumed that the respective molecular weights of the antibody and antigen are about 160,000 and 40,000, respectively, a molecular composition of Ea_1Ab_5 is obtained as follows: $20/160,000 \text{ gm/mole} \div 1/40,000 \text{ gm/mole} = 5$. (Since the percentage of N is the same in both antigen and antibody, the conversion of N to absolute weight is omitted.) The result indicates that ovalbumin (40,000 molecular weight) has a valence of 5; valence, however, increases with the size of the antigenic molecule. The Ab/Ag ratio decreases as one approaches the zones of equivalence and antigen excess. Such values are given in Table XIV for several antigens, it being assumed that the amount of antigen in the precipitate is known, i.e., all the added antigen is found precipitated in the region of antibody excess. In the region of extreme antigen excess where soluble complexes exist, it has been possible by similar calculations to determine the valence of antibody as 2. Here, however, the presence of small soluble complexes in the antigen excess region made it necessary to use agents capable of precipitating the complexes. The precipitation of the soluble complexes by active complement or anti-antibody (anti rabbit γ-globulin) and the use of ^{131}I-labeled antigens and antibodies allowed a calculation of the amount of antigen and antibody in the precipitates.[120] The values obtained in the rabbit anti-BSA and anti-BGG systems indicated a valence of 2 for rabbit antibody which agrees with published figures

TABLE XIV

MOLECULAR COMPOSITION OF SPECIFIC PRECIPITATES FROM RABBIT ANTISERA[a]

| | | Molecular ratio of antibody to antigen | | |
| | | | Equivalence zone | |
Antigen	Molecular weight	Extreme antibody excess zone	Antibody excess side	Antigen excess side
Bovine ribonuclease	13,400	2.8	1.55	1.45
Egg albumin	42,000	5	3	2.5
Horse serum albumin	67,000	6	4	3
Human γ-globulin	160,000	7	4.5	3.5
Horse apoferritin	465,000	26	14	7
Thyroglobulin	700,000	40	14	10
Keyhole limpet hemocyanin	6,630,000	—	120	83
Tomato bushy stunt virus	8,000,000	90	45	17
Tobacco mosaic virus	40,700,000	650–950	130	70

[a] From Kabat.[15]

obtained by other methods such as equilibrium dialysis (see Chap. 15.B) and fluorescence quenching (see Chap. 15.C).

b. DETECTION AND QUANTITATION OF ANTIGENS IN MIXTURES

Immunochemical techniques have also allowed the detection of a possible impurity or minor constituent in preparations of proteins and polysaccharides. If one has available a calibrated antiserum, whose course of precipitation with given amounts of antigen is known, then it is possible (1) to detect this antigen in a mixture and (2) to quantitate the amount of the substance. Because very small amounts of antigen are needed for any analysis and no fractionation is needed, this method has

[120] W. O. Weigle and P. H. Maurer, *J. Immunol.* **79**, 223 (1957).

been useful in many situations.[15] Of utmost importance is the fact that the reaction takes place in the region of antibody excess with respect to the specific material under study. The usual precautions mentioned above in running the precipitin reaction should be borne in mind. If at all possible, at least 2 to 3 points should be determined in antibody excess.

It has been possible to measure serum albumin[121] and γ-globulin[122] in various fluids, pneumococcal type-specific carbohydrate in broth cultures,[123] and ovalbumin in egg white.[15] As an example, the ovalbumin content of egg white can be estimated as follows. If addition of 0.06 mg of N of egg white to a calibrated anti-Ea serum leads to the precipitation of 0.30 mg of total N, which is known to correspond to the presence of 0.02 mg of Ea N, then the ovalbumin constitutes $(0.02/0.06) \times 100 = 33\%$ of the total proteins.

c. DETECTION OF HETEROGENEITY OF ANTIGEN AND ANTIBODY

Although this information is obtained more easily with agar diffusion techniques (see Chap. 14), the course and shape of the precipitin curve with any one antigen–antibody system can give information concerning the homogeneity of the system. This is predicted on the assumption that the impurity, when present, is antigenic.

The testing of supernatants for excess antigen and antibody is of paramount importance in establishing homogeneity of a system since in a complex system both "Ag" and "Ab" will appear to coexist. Also, the quantitative precipitin curve will be atypical in heterogeneous antigen–antibody reactions because the equivalence zones of two systems involving antigen A and antigen B usually do not occur in the same region of the curve. In the antigen-excess zone for antigen A, where diminished precipitation should occur, precipitation due to antigen B system may be rising and approaching equivalence. This could lead to a bimodal curve. In fact, it has been suggested that the precipitation behavior in *antigen* excess may be used as an indication of homogeneity of the system.[124] The shape of the precipitin curve can indicate the course of purification of a component. By progressive purification of crude diphtheria toxin and by absorption of impurities in antitoxin a progressively more regular precipitin curve was noted (Fig. 4).[31, 32] With most pure protein systems, the amount of antigen–antibody complex precipitated rapidly

[121] D. Gitlin and C. A. Janeway, *J. Clin. Invest.* **31**, 223 (1952).

[122] E. A. Kabat, D. F. Freedman, J. P. Murray, and V. Knaub, *Am. J. Med. Sci.* **219**, 55 (1950).

[123] O. T. Avery and M. Heidelberger, *J. Exptl. Med.* **38**, 81 (1923).

[124] M. Cohn, L. R. Wetter, and H. F. Deutsch, *J. Immunol.* **61**, 283 (1949).

falls nearly to zero at antigen concentrations about 5 to 10 times the equivalence concentration. It can be stated, therefore, that if a regular curve with marked inhibition is exhibited over a wide concentration of antigen added (up to 100 to 1000 times equivalence) then one may be dealing with a homogeneous system.

It is important to remember that inspection of the shape of the precipitin curve can indicate heterogeneity, yet plural reaction curves can at times be found superimposed. In well-suited systems such as those listed in Table XII, it would not be probable that an antigenic impurity would remain undetected.

There are other situations where homogeneity cannot be assumed, such as precipitin curves secured with high molecular weight polysaccharides, denatured proteins, and viral antigens. In these, broad equivalence zones are often noted (Fig. 2).

d. Determination of Coprecipitating (Nonprecipitating) Antibody

Sometimes, antibody synthesized early in the course of immunization does not precipitate with antigen. This type of antibody may be detectable by techniques such as passive cutaneous anaphylaxis or passive hemagglutination. (See Volume IV, Chapter 16.B.2.) However, it is possible to estimate accurately the amount of antibody present by determining the increment contributed by this antibody when *coprecipitating* with a known amount of precipitating antibody and specific antigen. The experimental setup has to ensure that the reactions take place in the equivalence zone where all the antigen is in the precipitate. As a specific volume of unknown serum is reacted with a known volume and amount of specific precipitating antibody, appropriate controls of normal serum plus antigen, saline, and serum, etc., have to be employed. The measurement of anti-BSA in an early bleeding of guinea pig serum serves as an example. A calibrated specific rabbit anti-BSA serum was employed. The guinea pig serum was first decomplemented by two additions of 100 μg of N-specific precipitate (Ea–anti-Ea) per milliliter of guinea pig serum. When 1.0 ml of the calibrated rabbit anti-BSA (100 μg of N/ml) was mixed with 2.0 ml of decomplemented normal guinea pig serum, 120 μg of total N was precipitated; when 2.0 ml of the guinea pig immune sera was used, instead, 140 μg of total N was precipitated. Accordingly, 20 μg of Ab N was present per 2 ml of serum, or 10 μg of Ab N per milliliter. Although this amount of antibody N serum should be capable of precipitating with antigen alone, there are other characteristics of the antibody which may mitigate against this. In fact, as much as 170 μg of nonprecipitable antibody N per milliliter of horse serum (anti-Ea) has been noted in an early bleeding.[25, 27]

e. Determination of Structural Relationships among Macromolecules

Cross reactions, wherein heterologous materials react with antibody produced against a homologous antigen, are due to structural similarities between the antigens under study. In the study of cross-reactions, it is a major concern to assure that a single reaction system is being investigated, that is, the heterologous antigen must be pure or the antiserum must be unispecific. It is also necessary to realize that the "cross-reacting" antibodies usually represent a fractional part of the total antibody population, only some of the antibody molecules usually possessing the ability to cross-react.

Since animals within any species may not necessarily react against the same determinants in an antigen, cross-reactions should be studied with several specimens of antisera. Sera should not be pooled until the behavior of each serum is known. With repeated immunization, animals may produce antibody against a larger area of the "antigenic patch" and possibly against more groupings in the antigen. From this, it follows that the extent of cross-reactions may increase with repeated immunizations. For example, the extent of cross reaction of hog thyroglobulin (Tg) with rabbit antihuman Tg sera was found to increase from 20% with "first-course" sera to 40% with third-course sera.[12]

Reciprocal cross reactions among 2 macromolecules (that is, A reacting with anti-B serum compared with B reacting with anti-A serum) can be unlike in extent, or "one-way" cross-reactions may be found. Different animal species may not produce antibody against the same configurations of the homologous antigen, hence different degrees of cross reaction may be noted depending on the species of animal being used for antibody production.

In the majority of cross reactions, the antigen added is incompletely precipitated. This complicates calculations for the extent of cross reaction in protein–antiprotein systems unless one can determine either the fraction of antigen present in the precipitate or remaining in the supernatant. The residual amount in the supernatant can be determined with an antiserum specific for the cross-reacting antigen. The problem, however, is that some or all of the cross-reacting antigen in the supernatant may be present as soluble Ag–Ab complexes with its reactive sites blocked. If the antigen added is labeled with an isotope or it has some specific grouping, such as hydroxyproline in gelatin, iodine in thyroglobulin, or iron in ferritin, the issue may be settled simply. With polysaccharide antigens, the problem is less serious as these antigens as a class do not contribute much N to the precipitate or affect the absorbancy in colorimetric analyses for antibody.

A rough indication of the relative number of cross-reacting groups in the antigens may be obtained from the amount of heterologous antigen relative to the amount of homologous antigen needed to achieve equivalence with the antibody. The more heterologous antigen needed, the fewer would be the number of the reactive groupings. This relationship would hold, however, only for antigens whose multiple reaction sites were all alike. The opposite would be true for antigens whose determinants were mostly different, a situation characteristic of proteins.

Quantitative studies of cross-reactions between mammalian albumins and between mammalian γ-globulins with rabbit antisera have been reported,[7, 125, 126, 126a] as well as cross-reactions between sheep, bovine, and human thyroglobulins.[12] With rabbit antisera, sheep and bovine Tg appeared closely related, whereas human Tg differed immunochemically from the sheep and beef Tg preparations.

The first quantitative cross reactions among the carbohydrates were performed with the types III and VIII pneumococcal polysaccharides and horse antisera.[127, 128] S III cross-reacted with an anti-S VIII serum to the extent of 33% while the reciprocal cross-reaction was 25%. The cross reactions were less when rabbit antisera were used; i.e., for S III–anti-S VIII, 21%; for S VIII–anti-S III, 17%.[129] These cross-reactions were not unexpected since both polysaccharides contain the same cellobiuronic acid as part of their structure.

Cross-reactions with various polysaccharide antigens and antibody against the pneumococcal polysaccharides are shown in Table XV. A considerable degree of cross-reaction of the dextrans with anti-type II and type XX sera is due to the high proportion of α-1,6 linkages joining the glucose residues. The bases for other cross reactions are discussed by Kabat.[15]

f. DETECTION OF ALTERATIONS OF MACROMOLECULES INDUCED BY CHEMICAL TREATMENTS

Chemical treatment or modification of protein and polysaccharide antigens has been employed in attempts to learn the *nature* of the reactive groupings in the *specific antigen*.[130] With proteins, limited information has been obtained from introduction or modification of the amino,

[125] M. E. Adair and J. Hamilton, *J. Hyg.* **39**, 170 (1939).
[126] L. R. Melcher, S. P. Masouredis, and R. Reed, *J. Immunol.* **70**, 125 (1953).
[126a] W. O. Weigle, *J. Immunol.* **87**, 599 (1961).
[127] M. Heidelberger, E. A. Kabat, and D. L. Shrivastava, *J. Exptl. Med.* **65**, 487 (1937).
[128] M. Heidelberger, E. A. Kabat, and M. Mayer, *J. Exptl. Med.* **75**, 35 (1942).
[129] A. G. Osler and M. Heidelberger, *J. Immunol.* **60**, 317 (1948).
[130] P. H. Maurer, *in* "Serological and Biochemical Comparisons of Proteins" (W. H. Cole, ed.), p. 56. Rutgers Univ. Press., New Brunswick, New Jersey, 1958.

TABLE XV

Cross-Reactions of Polyglucoses and Other Polysaccharides with Five Antipneumococcal Horse Sera, Amount of Polysaccharide Required, and Maximum Antibody N Precipitated from Type[a]

Polysaccharide	II Polysaccharide added (μg)	II Antibody N pptd. (μg)	IX Polysaccharide added (μg)	IX Antibody N pptd. (μg)	XII Polysaccharide added (μg)	XII Antibody N pptd. (μg)	XX Polysaccharide added (μg)	XX Antibody N pptd. (μg)	XXII Polysaccharide added (μg)	XXII Antibody N pptd. (μg)
Homologous specific polysaccharide	420	3600	340	1655	500	1820	140	468	180	847
Dextrans[b]										
B512 (24)	500	550	—	0	500	125	210	96	80	84
B-1355-S-4 (57)	3,450	605	1500	490	3000	455	1500	118	1500	234
B-1299-S-3 (50)	1,500	505	1750	345	1750	960	1070	113	980	206
Synthetic polyglucose A	—	—	5000	570[c]	5000	900[c]	2000	251[c]	3000	280[c]
Oyster glycogen	6,000	188	1000	283	1000	320[c]	1000	40	—	—
Phosphorylase limit dextrin, A_{Ib}	3,000	290	5000	264	—	—	1000	32, 42	—	—
Rabbit liver glycogen	10,000	162	5000	232	2000	61	2000	33	—	—
Rabbit liver phosphorylase limit dextrin	3,000	248	5000	205	500	87	500	43	—	—
Amylopectin (corn, alkali purified)	500	68	1000	38	1000	3	1000	8	1000	54, 36

[a] Data have been corrected back to original undiluted antiserum.
[b] Values in parentheses refer to percent α 1 → 6 linkages in dextran preparation.
[c] Anti-C not absorbed.

carboxyl, aliphatic, and aromatic hydroxyl groups. Interpretation of the immunochemical data obtained from such studies presents many problems. Just because the modification results in a change or loss of activity, it cannot be assumed that the modified group is actually participating in the antigen–antibody reaction. One must be sure that denaturation or

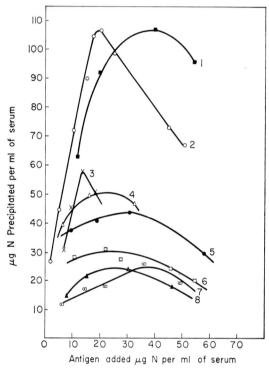

Fig. 16. Reactions of derivatives of BSA with an anti-BSA serum. Curves: *1*, guanidinated BSA; *2*, BSA; *3*, acetylated BSA (24-hour reaction with Ac_2O); *4*, acetylated BSA (1 hour reaction with Ac_2O); *5*, acetylated BSA (1 hour) heated for 2 hours; *6*, acetylated BSA (24 hours) heated for 2 hours; *7*, guanidinated derivative of heat denatured BSA; *8*, guanidinated BSA heated 2 hours. From Maurer *et al.*[131]

conformational change in structure of the antigen has not occurred. Also, the loss of *precipitating* ability may be a reflection of the change in solubility of the Ag–Ab complexes rather than loss in reactivity of antigen.

Effects on precipitation by modifying the amino groups of crystalline BSA is shown in Fig. 16 from Maurer *et al.*,[131] and quantitative data obtained in other reactions are listed in Table XVI. It appears that the

[131] P. H. Maurer, J. Sri Ram, and S. Ehrenpreis, *Arch. Biochem. Biophys.* **67**, 196 (1957).

amino groups of BSA are unimportant for reaction with antibody. The loss in precipitation noted with the succinylated and carboxymethylated protein was attributed to denaturation effects. Modification of more than 44% of the tyrosyl groups by O-acetylation left 30 to 40% of the original capacity for precipitation. This, and the observation that a completely

TABLE XVI

Effect of Chemical Modification of Bovine Serum Albumin on the Precipitation of Rabbit Antibodies[a]

Chemical modification or reagent employed	Groups modified and number as percent of original	Precipitin reaction with anti-BSA (%)
None	—	100
N-Acetylation	Amino 90	70
Guanidination	Amino 95	100
Deamination I	Amino 60 Tyrosyl 32	66
Deamination II	Amino 90 Tyrosyl 100	40
O-Acetylation	Tyrosyl 44 Aliphatic 8 Amino 5	30
Deacetylation of the O-acetyl derivative	—	40
Esterification I	Carboxyl 30	77
Esterification II	Carboxyl 42	32
Esterification III	Carboxyl 55	0
Deesterification of esterified derivative III	(a) 46% of COOH groups still blocked	18
	(b) 20% of COOH groups still blocked	60
S-Alkylation with iodoacetamide	The single-SH of BSA blocked	100
Succinylation	Amino 95	5
Polyglycylation	Amino 33	67
BrCH$_2$COOH	Amino 90	0

[a] From Sri Ram et al.[132]

nitrosated derivative still had considerable reactivity with antibody, indicated that the tyrosyl groups were not essential for reaction with antibodies. Similar arguments were advanced for the nonessential role of the carboxyl groups. The results of similar chemical modification of the groupings in many proteins have been summarized by Sri Ram et al.[132]

[132] J. Sri Ram, M. Bier, and P. H. Maurer, Advan. Enzymol. 24, 105 (1962).

Chemical modifications of polysaccharides have not been made extensively. Methylation of S III led to a product that precipitated about 66% of the specific horse antibody but none of the rabbit anti-S III.[3] Esterification of S III led to a loss in precipitation with horse antibody, and deesterification with alkali restored the precipitating ability.[133] Along similar lines, it was noted that hydrolytic products of S III (molecular weights 550 to 1800) precipitated with horse, but not with rabbit, anti-S III.

Synthetic polypeptides of average formula $poly(Glu^{59}Lys^{41})_n$ have been modified by guanidination, acetylation, and deamination of amino groups, and by esterification of carboxyl groups.[134] All these treatments reduced markedly or abolished the capacity to react, hence both the lysine and glutamic acid moieties in the polypeptide appear to be involved in the antigenic sites. However, unpublished observations from the author's laboratory[135] show that chemical modification of polymers of amino acids can also lead to increased cross-reactions (precipitation of more antibody with the heterologous system). When the polymer $poly(L\text{-}Glu^{60}\text{-}L\text{-}Ala^{30}\text{-}L\text{-}Tyr^{10})_n$ was completely O-acetylated a considerable amount of cross-reactivity with antibody produced in several sheep remained (50–80%). However, nitration of 10–15% of the tyrosine rings of the polymer using tetranitromethane led to a decrease with one antiserum and an increase of 120–150% in the cross-reactivity with two other antisera. Subsequent conversion of the nitro tyrosine to amino tyrosine residues restored cross-reactivity to the level obtained with the unmodified polymer.

[133] H. Markowitz and M. Heidelberger, *J. Am. Chem. Soc.* **76**, 1313 (1954).
[134] T. J. Gill, H. J. Gould, and H. W. Kunz, *J. Biol. Chem.* **239**, 3083 (1964).
[135] G. Odstrchel, and P. H. Maurer, Unpublished observations (1969).

B. Inhibition of Precipitation Reactions*

1. INTRODUCTION

This discussion will deal with protein–antiprotein reactions, but the principles and methods are more widely applicable. The inhibitory activity of protein fragments suggested that antigenic combining sites of proteins were limited regions of the whole antigen molecule long before either purified antibodies or homogeneous proteins were studied in immunological systems. In the 1930's Landsteiner and van der Scheer[1]

* Section 13.B was contributed by John J. Cebra.

[1] K. Landsteiner and J. van der Scheer *Proc. Soc. Exptl. Biol. Med.* **28**, 983 (1931).

enzymatically degraded coagulated serum proteins. The digest products obtained failed to inhibit the reactions between the native proteins and their antisera, but one class of large products ("heteroalbumose") was found to be capable of evoking an antibody response in its own right, if absorbed to blood charcoal.[2] Still smaller enzymatic digest products were isolated, and some of these were able to inhibit the reaction of the heteroalbumose with its own antiserum. Thus, fragments of an antigen were shown to retain certain antigenic determinants present in the parent molecule and to interact with antibody. Early studies on the cross-reactivity of various crystalline ovalbumins indicated the presence of more than one kind of antigenic determinant on a protein molecule.[3, 4] The clear demonstration, by immunoelectrophoresis, of the physical separation of sets of antigenic sites after proteolysis of native serum albumin[5] stimulated many analyses of the antigenic structures of homogeneous protein antigens (see review by Kaminski[6]).

At the present time, quantitative inhibition measurements are being used to estimate the size of antigenic determinants of proteins[7] and the proportion of an antiprotein antibody population which reacts with a particular set of antigenic sites present on a well defined fragment of the whole antigen.[8] Inhibition assays have more recently been employed for the elucidation of antibody structure. By measuring the inhibitory effect of various enzymatic digest products of antibody on the precipitation of antigen by intact antibody, the antibody combining site has been localized to part of the γ-globulin molecule.[9]

2. GENERAL APPLICATIONS

Measurement of inhibitory activity is still the principal assay, used along with degradative procedures, to characterize antigenic sites of proteins. Use of such an assay is indicated, along with chemical determination of the structure of antigen fragments, to define antigenic determinants, for comparison of the immunological properties of fragments obtained from related or cross-reacting proteins, for assessing the contribution of secondary-tertiary structure of protein molecules to the antigenic determinants, etc.

Although high molecular weight, synthetic copolymers of α-amino acids

[2] K. Landsteiner and M. W. Chase, *Proc. Soc. Exptl. Biol. Med.* **30,** 1413 (1933).

[3] S. B. Hooker and W. C. Boyd, *J. Immunol.* **26,** 469 (1934).

[4] S. B. Hooker and W. C. Boyd, *J. Immunol.* **30,** 41 (1936).

[5] C. Lapresle, M. Kaminski, and C. E. Tanner, *J. Immunol.* **82,** 94 (1959).

[6] M. Kaminski, *Progr. Allergy* **9,** 79 (1965).

[7] J. J. Cebra, *J. Immunol.* **86,** 205 (1961).

[8] E. M. Press and R. R. Porter, *Biochem. J.* **83,** 172 (1962).

[9] R. R. Porter, *Biochem. J.* **73,** 119 (1959).

are immunogenic and can serve as models for protein antigens, their amino acid sequence and size is somewhat variable. The contribution of particular amino acids or amino acids sequences to the immunogenicity of these complex copolymers can be assessed by using a series of simpler polymers of varied but known composition to inhibit the reaction of the immunogenic copolymer with its antiserum[10] (see Vol. I, Chap. 1.E.7).

Inhibition of the precipitation of antigen and intact antibody provides a simple method for the detection and semiquantitation of single antibody combining sites.

3. TECHNIQUES FOR OBTAINING ANTIGEN FRAGMENTS THAT RETAIN ANTIBODY BINDING PROPERTIES

a. PARTIAL PROTEOLYSIS

Relatively large fragments of proteins may be obtained by the following methods.

i. Digestion of "Native" Globular Proteins under Conditions Favoring Slow Proteolysis

Such conditions include low temperature, high substrate to enzyme ratio, or pH other than optimal for a particular enzyme. After limited proteolysis, mild reduction with cysteine or mercaptoethanol (0.05 M) may be necessary to release fragments from the whole molecule. An example of the use of proteolysis under suboptimal conditions to fragment a protein would be the digestion of γ-globulin at pH 4.5 using pepsin, followed by reduction[11] (see Vol. I, Chap. 5).

ii. Use of Insoluble Enzymes to Minimally Cleave Proteins[12, 13]

The insoluble enzymes can be efficiently and rapidly removed from the substrate protein by centrifugation or filtration after very brief periods of proteolysis. They can be employed at low substrate to enzyme ratios under suboptimal conditions for catalysis and still be completely removed from the solution of substrate.

iii. Simultaneous Enzymatic Digestion and Ultrafiltration

The reaction mixture, containing protein substrate and enzyme, is subjected to positive pressure in a dialysis sac during proteolysis (see Vol.

[10] S. Fuchs and M. Sela, *Biochem. J.* **87**, 70 (1963).
[11] A. Nisonoff, F. C. Wissler, and S. L. Woernley, *Arch. Biochem. Biophys.* **88**, 241 (1960).
[12] A. Bar-Eli and E. Katchalski, *J. Biol. Chem.* **238**, 1690 (1963).
[13] J. J. Cebra, D. Givol, H. I. Silman, and E. Katchalski, *J. Biol. Chem.* **236**, 1720 (1961).

II, Chap. 8). This procedure permits the separation of products small enough to pass through the membrane from the larger molecules in the reaction mixture. It also makes possible the isolation of intermediate products of digestion which can dialyze away from enzyme before further proteolysis can occur.[8, 14]

iv. Acid Hydrolysis under Conditions Not Resulting in Complete Conversion of Protein to Amino Acids

For instance, hydrolysis with 5.7 or 12 N HCl or with 50% (by volume) sulfuric acid at temperatures between 20 and 30° for from 4 hours to several days will usually result in the degradation of a protein to a wide variety of oligopeptides.[15]

v. Enzymatic Cleavage of All Susceptible Bonds after Performic Acid Oxidation or Carboxymethylation of Globular Proteins[16]

Usually a well defined set of oligopeptides can be obtained by this method. However, much of the conformation of the antigenic sites present in the original molecule may be lost.

b. CHARACTERIZATION OF PRODUCTS

The average chain length of a mixture of oligopeptides may be approximated by comparing the yield of either amino nitrogen (by Van Slyke's procedure)[17] or amino-terminal amino acid (by dinitrophenylation)[18] to the yield of total nitrogen determined by the Kjeldahl method (Vol. II, Chap. 12.A.3). Alternately, the ninhydrin color yield before and after basic hydrolysis can be used to estimate average peptide length.[19]

4. METHODS FOR QUANTITATIVE INHIBITION STUDIES

a. MATERIALS

i. Buffer

The immunoglobulins and antigens should be equilibrated with, and the peptide inhibitors made up in, either of the following buffers: (a)

---

[14] J. W. Goodman, *Biochemistry* **3**, 857 (1964).

[15] K. Landsteiner, *J. Exptl. Med.* **75**, 269 (1942).

[16] R. K. Brown, *J. Biol. Chem.* **237**, 1162 (1962).

[17] E. A. Kabat, *in* "Experimental Immunochemistry" (E. A. Kabat and M. M. Mayer, eds.), 2nd ed., p. 488. Thomas, Springfield, Illinois, 1961.

[18] E. A. Kabat, *in* "Experimental Immunochemistry" (E. A. Kabat and M. M. Mayer, eds.), 2nd ed., p. 599. Thomas, Springfield, Illinois, 1961.

[19] C. H. W. Hirs, S. Moore, and W. H. Stein, *J. Biol. Chem.* **219**, 623 (1956).

0.01 M sodium phosphate, 0.15 M sodium chloride buffer, pH 7.3* or (b) phosphate–borate buffer, pH 8.0.†

ii. Immunoglobulin Solution or Immune Serum

To minimize coprecipitation of nonantibody protein by the antigen–antibody aggregates, it is desirable to fractionate the serum and to prepare immunoglobulin for use in the test system. The method of Levy and Sober[20] (see Vol. I, Chap. 3.A.3) permits recovery of a sizable proportion of γG-antibody from human, rabbit, goat, and guinea pig serum free of contamination with other serum proteins. The immunoglobulin solution, after concentration by pressure dialysis against the appropriate buffer, should be passed through a Millipore filter (1.2 μ pore size) before use. An amount of immunoglobulin containing a defined quantity (2 to 4 mg) of antibody in a volume of 0.5 ml is used for each reaction tube.

iii. Solution of Homologous Antigen

A stock solution of antigen is prepared by dissolution of lyophylized protein and equilibration against the appropriate buffer. The final concentration of the protein can be determined from either optical density measurements, if the extinction coefficient is known (see Vol. II, Chap. 10.A) or from nitrogen determinations. Ordinarily, the concentration should be such that 0.1 to 0.2 ml of this solution contains the amount of antigen required to give maximal precipitation with the antibody present in 0.5 ml of the stock γ-globulin solution. Data for constructing a quantitative precipitin curve is obtained in advance (see Section 13.A.3) and usually indicates that maximal precipitation with a given amount of immunoglobulin occurs with an amount of antigen slightly greater than that required to precipitate all antibody. In certain instances it may be desirable to measure inhibition of a precipitating system containing a given amount of antibody and only one-half the quantity of antigen required to yield maximal precipitation. Such a precipitate, formed in the region of antibody excess, contains more antibody molecules relative to antigen than corresponding precipitates formed at "equivalence." Such precipitating systems may allow more sensitive measurement of the inhibitory effect of an antigen fragment to which only a small proportion of the antiprotein antibodies are directed. Precipitates, formed in anti-

---

* Phosphate-buffered saline, pH 7.3: 7.08 gm of Na_2HPO_4 (anhydrous), 1.40 gm of $NaH_2PO_4 \cdot H_2O$, and 52.8 gm of NaCl; make up to 6 liters.

† Borate buffer, pH 8.0: Mix 165 ml of a solution 0.16 M in NaOH with 1 liter of a solution of 0.2 M boric acid containing 0.16 M NaCl.

[20] H. B. Levy and H. A. Sober, *Proc. Soc. Exptl. Biol. Med.* **103,** 250 (1960).

body excess, are richer in those antibodies reactive with "weaker" antigenic determinants and hence are better suited to the measurement of these sites.

iv. Stock Solution of Inhibitor

A stock solution of the isolated fragment of antigen, mixture of oligopeptides from the antigen, or fragments of antibody containing single combining sites is prepared in the appropriate buffer. Ideally, the inhibitors should be salt free before dissolution, having been desalted by gel filtration or by freeze drying from a volatile buffer. The pH of the inhibitor solution should be checked after solution is complete and adjusted if necessary. Concentration of the inhibitor is determined from optical density, dry weight, or nitrogen measurements and expressed in terms of molarity when possible. The range of inhibitor concentrations to be used in the quantitative study may be approximated by setting up a preliminary, qualitative set of tests. Two drops of immune serum or immunoglobulin solution are added to a solution containing an optimal amount of antigen and a variable amount of inhibitor in a total volume of 0.25 ml. After the initial mixing, turbidity is graded visually at set intervals of time with respect to control mixtures containing no inhibitor. Amounts of inhibitor should be varied in 10-fold steps. Fragments of antigen still able to react with antibody can usually be detected by inhibition of turbidity when present at 10^0 to 10^3 times the molar concentration of intact antigen. If the inhibitor is a fragment of antibody then it usually produces a visible effect on precipitation when used at 2 to 20 times the molar concentration of intact antibody.

b. QUANTITATIVE INHIBITION ASSAY

i. Reaction Mixture

Known varying amounts of inhibitor solution and buffer are added to 0.5 ml of the immunoglobulin solution to give a final volume of 0.9 ml. Conical glass centrifuge tubes of 2.0 ml capacity are ideal for this assay. The mixtures are stirred and allowed to stand for 30 minutes at 37°. Then a predetermined, constant amount of intact antigen in 0.1 ml is added to each tube. The contents of the tubes are again mixed and the tubes are incubated for 1 hour at 37° and then allowed to stand at 3° to 5° for 3 days. Duplicate tests at each inhibitor concentration should be set up. In addition, duplicate controls should be set up containing (a) intact antigen and immunoglobulin in the absence of inhibitor and (b) immunoglobulin in the absence of both antigen and inhibitor. After incubation and standing, the amount of precipitate formed in each tube is

determined exactly as described for quantitative measurement of precipitation (Section 13.A.3) by nitrogen analysis, colorimetrically, or from
optical density measurements.

ii. Cautions, Limitations, and Special Controls

The above procedure applies to inhibitors which themselves are not
precipitated by antibody. A set of controls should initially be run using
mixtures of inhibitor and immunoglobulin to establish whether specific
or nonspecific precipitation occurs between these two components.
If larger fragments of antigen are themselves precipitated by antibody,
they may still be compared with intact antigen by using increasing
amounts of each to produce "antigen excess" inhibition of precipitation.
In some instances, inhibitor molecules may be coprecipitated along with
antigen and antibody even though they do not precipitate with antibody
alone. Ordinarily, the addition of coprecipitated inhibitor to the precipitate is negligible. However, the particular procedure used to measure the
amount of precipitate may exaggerate the coprecipitated inhibitor—for
instance, if the assay procedure is based on measurement of tyrosine
residue, and the inhibiting peptide is rich in tyrosine. If the supposed inhibitor appears instead to enhance precipitation, the use of radio-labeled
fragments or oligopeptides may be useful to indicate coprecipitation.

iii. Theoretical Treatment of Results

A series of direct plots of percent inhibition [1.0 − (amount of precipitate in presence of inhibitor/amount of precipitate in absence of
inhibitor)] × 100 vs. inhibitor concentration for several peptide inhibitors
of the silk fibroin–antisilk fibroin system are shown in Fig. 1. Such plots
allow a rough comparison of the effectiveness of members of a series of
inhibitors. If total inhibition is observed, for instance with a mixture of
unfractionated fragments derived from an antigen, it is probable that at
least parts of all antigenic determinants have survived proteolysis and
are capable of interacting with antibody. If the percentage of inhibition
is found to increase with inhibitor concentration up to a point and then
remain unchanged with further increase in inhibitor concentration, it is
possible that the fragment represents only one or some of the antigenic
determinants which have given rise to antibodies present in the test immunoglobulin. However, due to the heterogeneity of antibody combining
sites, a plot of percent inhibition vs. inhibitor concentration is seldom linear, even though total inhibition may be achieved (see Section 13.4.a.iv).
Relative association constants , K_0 (rel), may be calculated for a series
of inhibitors effecting the *same* antigen–antibody system (see Section
13.4.b.ii) by plotting percent inhibition vs. the logarithm of inhibitor concentration as shown in Fig. 2. The linear distance along the abscissa (the

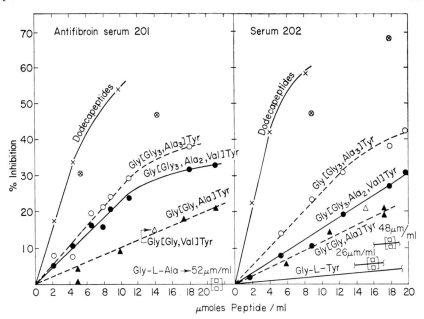

FIG. 1. Comparison of activity of peptide inhibitors in two fibroin–antifibroin systems. From Cebra.[7]

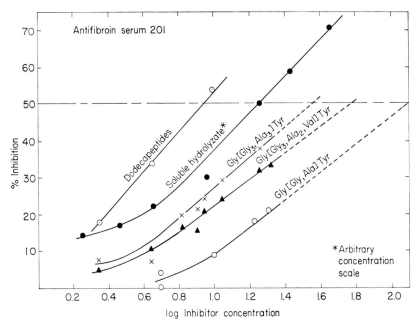

FIG. 2. Plots used to obtain relative average combining constants, K_0 (rel), of peptide inhibitors.

log inhibitor axis) between each curve and the curve for a standard inhibitor is then a relative measure of log K_0. One inhibitor is defined as a standard with $K_0 = 1$ and log $K_0 = 0$. The distance between each curve and the standard curve at 50% inhibition is then measured to obtain log K_0 (rel). Where necessary, the plots of data may be extrapolated to 50% inhibition to permit measurement of distance at this ordinate to minimize the effects of variation of antibody heterogeneity index with respect to the different inhibitors. The difference in change in standard free energy for the combination of two different peptides with antibody, $\Delta(\Delta F^\circ)$, can be calculated as described in Chapter 15.E.4.

iv. Alternate Procedures for Measuring Inhibition of Protein–Antiprotein Reactions

The delay in flocculation time[8] or the inhibition of complement fixation[21] caused by fragments of antigen added to intact antigen and antibody have been used to indicate activity of the fragments when amounts of material are limited.

[21] E. Benjamini, J. D. Young, M. Shimizer, and C. Y. Leung, *Biochemistry* **3**, 1115 (1964).

C. Ammonium Sulfate Precipitation of Soluble Antigen–Antibody Complexes

1. DETERMINATION OF ANTIGEN-BINDING CAPACITY*

a. PRINCIPLE

This test measures both precipitating and nonprecipitating antibody to bovine serum albumin (BSA). It is based on the principle that ^{131}I-labeled BSA (^{131}I-BSA) is soluble when mixed with buffered normal serum and treated with 50% saturated ammonium sulfate (SAS/2) whereas complexes of ^{131}I-BSA and antibody globulin are insoluble under the same conditions.[1] When a constant amount of ^{131}I-BSA is added to serial dilutions of anti-BSA, a point will be reached when antigen excess is achieved, spontaneous precipitation of ^{131}I-BSA-antibody aggregates cannot occur, and equilibrium in solution is established as represented in Eq. (1)

$$^{131}I\text{-}BSA + ab \underset{k_\text{d}}{\overset{k_\text{a}}{\rightleftharpoons}} {}^{131}I\text{-}BSA\text{-}ab \tag{1}$$

when $^{131}I\text{-}BSA$ represents one of several antigen sites on a given ^{131} I-BSA molecule, and ab represents one combining site on an antibody molecule.

* Section 13.C.1 was contributed by Richard S. Farr.

[1] R. S. Farr, *J. Infect. Diseases* **103**, 239 (1958).

Upon addition of SAS/2, the soluble ^{131}I-BSA-ab complexes are pre-cipitated, and ^{131}I-BSA not bound to antibody remains in the super-natant. This fractionation procedure does not appreciably alter the pro-portions of ^{131}I-BSA which were bound to antibody or free in solution prior to the addition of SAS/2, because SAS/2 markedly inhibits the formation and dissociation of ^{131}I-BSA antibody complexes.[1–3] The pre-cipitated radioactivity which this test measures is an indication of anti-gen-binding capacity (ABC) rather than the amount of antigen or anti-body spontaneously precipitated, and results are expressed as micrograms of ^{131}I-BSA N bound per milliliter of undiluted serum. A useful modifica-tion of the basic method will estimate the weight of precipitable antibody in an antiserum (Section 13.C.2).

b. APPLICATION

This technique accurately and reproducibly measures as little as 0.005 μg of precipitating antibody nitrogen. In addition, it measures bind-ing capacity in antiserum which contains no detectable precipitating anti-body. Although originally developed for use in the BSA-anti-BSA system, the method has also been used with varying degrees of success with other antigens: ten additional mammalian albumins[4, 4a]; egg albumin[5]; α-lac-talbumin[6]; type-specific streptococcal M proteins,[7] crude[8] and purified antigens[9] derived from ragweed pollens; somatic antigens from gram-negative bacteria,[10] and a protein fraction of rabbit spinal cord.[11] The specificity of any particular ^{131}I-antigen–antibody reaction studied with this method can be tested by adding an excess amount of unlabeled anti-gen to the serum prior to the addition of ^{131}I-antigen. Under these condi-tions, precipitation of specific ^{131}I-antigen–antibody complexes is com-pletely inhibited by unlabeled homologous antigen and precipitation is unaltered by the addition of non-cross-reacting antigens.

Modification of this method can also be used to: (a) study the rates of association and dissociation of ^{131}I-antigen–antibody complexes,[1–3] (b) detect the presence of circulating antigen–antibody complexes *in vivo*,[12]

[2] D. W. Talmage, *J. Infect. Diseases* **107**, 115 (1960).

[3] H. M. Grey, *J. Immunol.* **91**, 90 (1963).

[4] W. O. Weigle, *J. Immunol.* **87**, 599 (1961).

[4a] W. O. Weigle, *J. Immunol.* **88**, 9 (1962).

[5] W. O. Weigle and P. J. McConahey, *J. Immunol.* **88**, 121 (1962).

[6] R. Rothberg and R. S. Farr, *Pediatrics* **35**, 571 (1965).

[7] H. M. Grey, *J. Exptl. Med.* **115**, 671 (1962).

[8] D. Lidd and R. S. Farr, *J. Allergy* **33**, 45 (1962).

[9] D. Lidd and J. T. Connell, *J. Allergy* **35**, 289 (1964).

[10] R. Freter, *J. Infect. Diseases* **111**, 25 (1962).

[11] R. F. Kibler and A. E. Barnes, *J. Exptl. Med.* **116**, 807 (1962).

[12] F. J. Dixon, J. J. Vasquez, W. O. Weigle, and C. G. Cochrane, *A.M.A. Arch. Pathol.* **65**, 18 (1958).

(c) quantitate and discriminate between trace amounts of identical or cross-reacting antigenic groups present in purified protein solutions,[13] and in heterogeneous antigen mixtures, such as serum,[14] extracts of grass pollens,[15] and milk.[6]

c. Detailed Procedure

i. Reagents

Borate buffer, pH 8.3 to 8.5, ionic strength = 0.1: 6.184 gm of boric acid, 9.536 gm of borax (sodium tetraborate), 4.384 gm of sodium chloride; make up to 1 liter with distilled water.

Normal serum (1:10): Add 1 part normal serum to 9 parts borate buffer. *Use serum from the same species being tested for antibody.*

Normal serum (1:100): Add 1 part normal serum to 99 parts borate buffer.

Saturated ammonium sulfate (SAS): Store at 4° with crystals remaining in the flask to prevent the solution from becoming supersaturated. Filter before using.

50% Saturated ammonium sulfate: Add one part of SAS to one part borate buffer.

Stock ^{131}I-BSA solution: Prepare trace-labeled ^{131}I-BSA containing less than 1 molecule of iodine per molecule of albumin and having a specific activity of 2 to 3 mCi per microgram of nitrogen. The nitrogen content of the stock ^{131}I-BSA should be carefully determined and will contain 90 to 100 μg of ^{131}I-BSA N/ml when prepared as previously described.[1]

Specific activity counting standards: Using volumetric glassware, dilute an aliquot of the stock ^{131}I-BSA with normal serum (1:100) to the desired concentration in the range to be used for the test antigen. Pipet 1 ml aliquots of this carefully diluted stock antigen into 7 ml Wasserman tubes and mark the nitrogen content per milliliter on the label.

Test Antigen: Dilute another aliquot of the stock ^{131}I-BSA solution with normal serum (1:100) to the exact concentration desired for the test antigen. This is usually between 0.02 and 2.0 μg of nitrogen per milliliter.

Trichloroacetic acid (TCA), 20% aqueous solution.

ii. Antiserum Dilutions and Experimental Tubes

First dilution: Add 1 part antiserum to 9 parts borate buffer to make a 1:10 dilution. In practice, this is usually 0.5 ml of antiserum added to 4.5 ml of borate buffer.

[13] W. D. Linscott, *Science* **142,** 1170 (1963).
[14] R. S. Farr, W. Dickinson, and K. Smith, *Federation Proc.* **19,** 199 (abstr.) (1960).
[15] D. Lidd and R. S. Farr, *J. Allergy* **34,** 1 (1963).

Subsequent dilutions: Make serial 1:3 or 1:5 dilutions with normal serum (1:10); e.g., add 1.0 ml of previous dilution to 2.0 or 4.0 ml of normal serum (1:10). Use separate volumetric pipets for each dilution.

Experimental tubes: Pipet duplicate 0.5 ml aliquots from each dilution into 7 ml Wasserman tubes. A single volumetric pipet may be used for each serum by starting with the most dilute solution and rinsing the pipet in the next highest concentration.

iii. Controls for Each Experiment

Normal serum controls: To each of four tubes add 0.5 ml aliquots of normal serum (1:10). These tubes will receive both ^{131}I-antigen and SAS.

Protein-bound ^{131}I-controls: To two tubes add 0.5 ml aliquots of normal serum (1:10). These tubes will receive TCA, but not SAS.

Antigen-added controls: Four tubes will be used to receive antigen only. These tubes will not receive serum, or SAS, but will be used as counting standards.

iv. Addition of Antigen

Pipet 0.5 ml of labeled antigen to all experimental and control tubes. Mix the tubes well and incubate overnight at 4°. If incubation is carried out for a longer period of time, significant evaporation occurs and the tubes must be stoppered.

v. Precipitation of ^{131}I-BSA-Antibody Complexes with Ammonium Sulfate

Keep all reagents and tubes at 4°. Add 1.0 ml SAS to all experimental tubes and the normal serum control tubes only. Mix immediately. No more than 1 to 2 minutes should elapse between the addition of SAS and mixing of the tube. SAS has a greater specific gravity than the other reactants and will settle to the bottom of the tube unless vigorous agitation is used. Until satisfied that complete mixing is being routinely attained, check for schlieren (wavy) lines in each tube. *Improper mixing following the addition of SAS is the most common source of error encountered with this method.* After addition of SAS, incubate at 4° for 30 minutes. Centrifuge for 30 minutes at 4° in an International PR-2 centrifuge at 2000 rpm.

Decant and discard the supernatants. Blot the tubes on absorbent towels to take up the remaining drops on the edges of the tubes. Wash these precipitates by adding 3 ml of 50% SAS. Shake tubes if necessary to resuspend the precipitates. Centrifuge tubes immediately at 4° for 30 minutes at 2000 rpm. Decant and blot as previously.

Add 1.0 ml of 20% TCA to the two protein-bound ^{131}I control tubes. Centrifuge for 30 minutes at 2000 rpm; decant, and discard the supernatant.

vi. Counting and Calculating Procedure

Using a γ-ray detector, determine the counts per minute (cpm) in the specific activity counting standards (Std.), the antigen-added control tubes (Ag-add), the normal serum control precipitate tubes (NsPpt), the protein-bound ^{131}I control (TCAPpt), and the experimental precipitate tubes (ExPpt). Repeat a given set of tubes if the counts per minute in one of the duplicates differs more than $\pm 5\%$ of the other.

Average the data, subtract background and make the following calculations:

$$\% \text{ Protein-bound }^{131}\text{I} = \frac{\text{cpm in TCAPpt}}{\text{cpm in Ag-add}} \times 100 \qquad (2)$$

The antigen should be used only if this value is greater than 97%. Calculate the μg ^{131}I-BSA N in the antigen-added control as follows:

$$\frac{\text{Cpm in Ag-add}}{\text{Cpm in Std.}} \mu\text{g }^{131}\text{I-BSA N in Std.} = \mu\text{g }^{131}\text{I-BSA N in Ag-add} = \text{AgN} \quad (3)$$

The total amount of ^{131}I-BSA in the precipitate is partly antibody bound and partly non-antibody bound. The small amount of non-antibody-bound ^{131}I-BSA that is nonspecifically precipitated by ammonium sulfate in either normal serum or in an antiserum must be accounted for in each individual determination. *This amount is proportional to the amount of ^{131}I-BSA in the supernatant which is entirely non-antibody bound; it is not proportional to the total amount of test antigen added.* Accordingly, correction for the non-antibody-bound ^{131}I-BSA in a given experimental precipitate cannot be accomplished merely by subtracting the amount of ^{131}I-BSA in the control normal serum precipitate. Instead, the data may be readily corrected in a manner which has been previously described in detail.[1]

More recently, another method for calculating data has been proposed and is recommended because of its greater simplicity. This method is also based on the fact that ^{131}I-BSA in the supernatant is directly proportional to the total amount of non-antibody-bound ^{131}I-BSA in a given mixture.* The simplified stepwise procedure may be carried out as follows:

Step 1. To obtain the counts per minute of the normal serum supernatant (NsSup), subtract the cpm in the NsPpt from the cpm of the Ag-add.

---

* The author wishes to thank Dr. James H. Day, Department of Medicine, Queen's University, Kingston, Ontario, Canada, for this valuable simplification, which was

Step 2. To obtain the cpm in the experimental supernatant (ExSup), subtract the cpm in the ExPpt from the cpm of the Ag-add.

Step 3. Divide the cpm in the ExSup by the cpm in the NsSup and multiply by 100 to obtain the % cpm non-antibody bound. This is the percentage of Ag-add in the supernatant (%S), and the method of calculation has automatically corrected this value for the amount of non-antibody-labeled antigen nonspecifically present, i.e., not antibody-bound in each experimental precipitate.

Step 4. Subtract the %S from 100 to obtain the % Ag-add in the precipitate (%P) or the % Ag-add which is specifically bound to antibody.

Plot the percent antigen precipitated versus the reciprocal of the dilution of that tube on semilogarithmic paper. The percentage antigen precipitated is plotted on the linear axis, and the reciprocal of the antiserum dilution is plotted on the logarithmic axis. From these plots, determine the reciprocal dilution of antiserum which would have precipitated exactly 33% of the antigen added. Designate this dilution as the ABC-33 end point.

Since 0.5 ml of the antiserum dilution designated as the ABC-33 end point specifically precipitated 33% of the ^{131}I-BSA N used for the test, the ABC-33 value is calculated as follows:

(2)(ABC-33 end point)(0.33)(AgN)
= ^{131}IBSA N bound/ml undiluted serum at the antigen concentration employed   (4)

For example, if 0.5 ml of a 1:50 dilution of antiserum bound 33% of 0.02 μg ^{131}I-BSA N, the ABC-33 is $2 \times 50 \times 0.33 \times 0.02 = 0.66$ μg ^{131}I-BSA N bound per milliliter of undiluted serum. Also, for reasons described below, the concentration of antigen used for a given test should be indicated by a subscript such as: ABC-33$_{0.02\,\mu g}$ = 0.66 μg ^{131}I-BSA N/ml.

---

derived as follows:

$$\frac{\text{Cpm of (Ag-add)}}{\text{Cpm of (NsSup)}} = \frac{\text{Total non-antibody bound cpm in ExPpt}}{\text{cpm of (ExSup)}}$$

$$\text{Total non-antibody bound cpm in ExPpt} = (\text{ExSup})\frac{(\text{Ag-add})}{(\text{NsSup})}$$

$$= \text{cpm of ExSup, adjusted}$$

$$\% \text{ Ag-added in adjusted supernatant} = \frac{[(\text{ExSup})(\text{Ag-add})]/\text{NsSup}}{\text{Ag-add}} \times 100$$

$$= \frac{\text{ExSup}}{\text{NsSup}} \times 100 = \%S$$

$$100 - \%S = \%P \text{ or } \% \text{ Ag-add specifically bound to antibody}$$

The 33% precipitation end point was arbitrarily selected because spontaneous precipitation does not occur at this degree of antigen excess but enough of the ^{131}I activity is in the precipitate to permit accurate counting procedures. Using the 33% end point, multiple tests performed with the same antigen on a single antiserum are highly reproducible. The average percentage of the antigen-added in the precipitate should have a standard deviation of the mean of less than 3%. Because of spontaneous precipitation, end points with more than 33% of the antigen in the precipitate are not recommended. End points with 20 or 25% of the antigen in the precipitate are satisfactory, but should be designated as ABC-20 or ABC-25.

d. Analysis of Data

The ABC-33 represents the amount of iodine-labeled antigen bound to antibody at the time the ammonium sulfate was added, but this value does not reflect the number of unoccupied antibody sites in equilibrium with the antigen–antibody complexes when the reaction is stopped by the fractionation procedure. Similar to equilibrium dialysis, ABC determinations may be performed with more than one concentration of test antigen to detect the presence or absence of unoccupied antibody sites in solution at the ABC-33 end point. If most of the available antibody sites are bound to antigen at an ABC-33 end point, an increase in the concentration of test antigen will not increase the ABC-33. On the other hand, if many antibody sites are unoccupied and dissociated from the antigen–antibody complexes at an ABC-33 end point, an increase in the concentration of test antigen will increase the ABC-33. In practice, the ABC-33 is usually greater, but never less, when the concentration of test antigen is increased. As a general rule, a marked discrepancy between ABC-33$_{0.02 \mu g}$ and ABC-33$_{0.2 \mu g}$ indicates the presence of a large proportion of "nonavid" antibody. This is evidenced by rapid half dissociation times of the iodine-labeled BSA–antibody complexes when studied by appropriate methods.[1-3]

Limitations

Before applying this procedure to new antigens, a few important limitations must be considered. The following criteria must be met when using ammonium sulfate fractionation to accurately *quantitate* antigen-binding capacity: (1) The labeled antigen must be a homogeneous population of molecules, immunologically unaltered by the isotope labeling procedure. (2) The labeled antigen must be soluble in 40 to 50% saturated ammonium sulfate. (3) It must be determined that the fractionation procedure has no appreciable effect upon the equilibrium that had been established between free and antibody-bound antigen prior to the addition of SAS/2. (4) It is desirable, but not necessary, that the isotope employed emit γ-radiation because the counting procedure for other isotopes, such as ^{35}S and ^{14}C, is more time consuming.

The criteria set forth represent the ideal circumstances as exemplified by the use of iodine-labeled BSA as the test antigen. On the other hand, the method can sometimes yield useful information even when these criteria cannot be met. Under such circumstances, the limitations involved when using the antigen in question should be recognized and the data should not be calculated and interpreted in the manner described above.[7, 9]

2. WEIGHT ESTIMATES OF ANTIBODY BASED ON ANTIGEN BINDING CAPACITY*

The method described by Farr in Section 13.C.1, which is capable of yielding comparative values of the antigen-binding capacity (ABC) of immune sera, has been modified to yield antibody weight estimates at the microgram level. In studies of the biological activities of antibodies there is need for an analytic method that will register all antibody molecules, regardless of their aggregating capabilities. Conventional methods based on chemical analyses of washed specific precipitates are applicable only to those immunoglobulins capable of forming immune aggregates of relatively low solubility.

In the Farr procedure, the presence of radiolabeled albumin in the proteins precipitated at SAS/2 serves as an index for antibody globulins capable of binding this antigen. The dilution of antiserum is determined at which one-third of the labeled albumin is thus precipitated. The results are expressed as ABC-33, the micrograms of iodinated BSA bound per milliliter of undiluted antiserum.

Despite its great utility for antibody detection, the method is subject to error when applied to comparative estimates of antibody content. The major difficulty arises from the fact that the affinity of immunoglobulins for antigen may vary by several orders of magnitude, even for the antibody molecules in a single serum specimen. As a result, extrapolation of the observed values to undiluted serum may be misleading. To meet this problem, the Farr technique is often carried out with two levels of antigen, e.g., 0.02 and 0.2 μg N. Since this stratagem yields only relative estimates of overall "avidity" the antibody estimates are not rectified.

A simple modification of the Farr technique termed mABC or modified antigen-binding capacity, has been introduced to render the procedure suitable for measurements of antibody on a weight basis. The modifica-

* Section 13.C.2 was contributed by Abraham G. Osler.

tion involves the use of large quantities of antigen in order to achieve a molecular ratio of antigen to antibody in the resulting immune complex of 2:1 with respect to the 7 S immunoglobulins. On this basis it is possible to calculate the molar concentration of antibody from measurements of radio-labeled albumin in the proteins precipitated by ammonium sulfate.

a. MATERIALS AND METHODS

i. Buffers

Isotonic barbital buffer (Buffer 6 B, Vol. II, Appendix II) was used as diluent for all reagents unless otherwise specified. Ethylenediaminetetraacetic acid disodium salt (EDTA)-barbital buffer was prepared by adding 1 volume of an aqueous solution of 0.1 M EDTA, pH 7.4, to 7 volumes of isotonic barbital, to yield a final concentration of 0.0125 M with respect to EDTA. A phosphate buffer (0.1 M), pH 7.8, was used for the iodination of proteins.

ii. Ammonium Sulfate

Saturated ammonium sulfate (SAS) was prepared at room temperature, then kept at 4° until 24 hours before use, when it was placed at 0° in an ethylene glycol–water bath. Immediately before use an aliquot was adjusted to pH 6.8 with 10 N NaOH. Half-saturated ammonium sulfate (SAS/2) was prepared by mixing equal volumes of the unadjusted SAS and isotonic barbital buffer, both at 0°. The pH of the SAS/2 was 6.8.

iii. Antigens

Human serum albumin (HSA) was purchased from Behringwerke AG, Marburg-Lahn, Germany. At concentrations approximating 100 μg of N/ml, only a single line of precipitation was observed in microimmunoelectrophoretic assays with a potent rabbit antiserum to whole human serum. In view of polymerization of serum albumin[1] calculations are based on an "average molecular weight," which was estimated as follows:

Approximately 50 mg of ^{125}I·HSA were applied to a column of Sephadex G-200 (2.54 cm × 40.2 cm). Fractions of 1 ml, collected by elution with phosphate-buffered saline, pH 7.0, were assayed for ^{125}I·HSA activity in

[1] J. Sponar, I. Fric, S. Stokrova, and J. Kovarikova, *Collection Czech. Chem. Commun.* **28,** 1831 (1963).

a well-type scintillation counter. The percentages of polymer and mono-mer were calculated assuming that the polymer existed only in the dime-rized state, and that the molecular weight of the monomer was 66,000.[2] The average molecular weights obtained in this fashion were 85,700 for one lot and 83,400 for another lot.

iv. Iodination

Labeling has been carried out as described by Masouredis et al.[3] with minor modifications (see also Section 4.A.2, Vol. I). The carrier-free iodine (ca. 1 mCi in a volume of less than 0.1 ml) was diluted with 2.0 ml of iodination buffer and 0.2 ml of a 0.05 M solution of iodine in 0.1 M potassium iodide. The resulting iodine solution was added slowly to the previously cooled (4°) protein solution (250 mg in 40 ml of iodination buffer), with constant mixing at room temperature until the characteristic iodine color disappeared. After 30 to 35 minutes the labeled protein solution was passed through an anion exchange column (PBI Rezikit, E. R. Squibb and Sons, New Brunswick, New Jersey), previously washed with iodination buffer and then dialyzed exhaustively with 0.15 N NaCl at 4°. Generally, the HSA preparations contained 8 to 16% of the total ^{125}I input, with specific activities in the range of 4000 to 8000 cpm/μg N. This corresponded to approximately 0.5 atom of iodine per molecule of HSA. More than 99% of the isotope was precipitable with 10% tri-chloroacetic acid and with rabbit antibody in the region of antibody excess. Protein concentrations were determined by optical density meas-urements at $\lambda = 278$ mμ, (Chapter 10, Volume II). Replicate analyses by the micro-Kjeldahl procedure yielded an average conversion factor of 0.0035 OD unit/μg HSA-N/ml. Iodinated and noniodinated prepara-tions yielded identical quantitative precipitin curves.

v. Sera

(a) Normal Rabbit Serum. Although several pools of normal rabbit serum were found to be equally suitable for these analyses, all determina-tions for the accompanying tables were carried out with a single large, sterile pool, obtained commercially. This serum pool was heated at 56° for 45 minutes, centrifuged in the cold at 13,000 g for 60 minutes at 2°, and added to the reaction medium in a final concentration of 10%.

(b) Hyperimmune Rabbit Anti-HSA. Male albino rabbits (3 to 4 kg) received weekly intramuscular injections of 30 mg of HSA in complete

[2] J. T. Edsall, J. Polymer Sci. **12**, 252 (1954).
[3] S. P. Masouredis, L. R. Melcher, and D. C. Koblock, J. Immunol. **66**, 297 (1951).

Freund's adjuvant (Difco). Each animal received a total of 100 to 300 mg of protein and was bled by cardiac puncture at weekly intervals, beginning 7 days after the third inoculation. The sera obtained from the individual bleedings were pooled and stored at $-20°$. The sera were then thawed, heated at $56°$ for 45 minutes and absorbed six times with commercial preparations of human α, β-, and γ-globulins, and stored at $-20°$. Immunoelectrophoretic analyses of such serum pools with undiluted whole human serum yielded only a single line of precipitation with a mobility corresponding to serum albumin. Ouchterlony analyses confirmed the presence of a single band of precipitate. Immediately before use in precipitin and antigen-binding assays, an aliquot of the serum was clarified by centrifugation at 13,000 g for 60 minutes at $2°$.

vi. Antibody-Nitrogen Estimations

(a) *Specific Precipitation.* Precipitin analyses were set up in duplicate, using Pyrex test tubes (13 by 100 mm), previously calibrated at 4.0 ml. The reaction mixtures were generally restricted to an antibody nitrogen content of 30 to 75 μg and to a volume of 0.7 ml to minimize solubility effects. The reaction medium contained EDTA at a final concentration of 0.005 M to minimize the inclusion of complement components with the specific precipitate. After addition of the antigen to the antiserum, the contents were carefully mixed; the tubes were stoppered and incubated at $37°$ for 60 minutes, then at $0°$ for at least 7 days. The tubes were then centrifuged, the precipitates were washed twice with 1.5 ml of cold 0.15 N NaCl, and dissolved in 4.0 ml of 0.25 N acetic acid. Assays for antibody content of the precipitates were carried out spectrophotometrically.

(b) *Modified Antigen-Binding Capacity (mABC) Technique.* (1) *Serum dilution.* To maintain the uniform serum concentration required for this assay, antisera were initially diluted 1:5 (1.0 ml serum + 4.0 ml diluent) in isotonic barbital buffer. When necessary, further dilutions were prepared in normal rabbit serum (NRS) which had also been diluted 1:5 in the same buffer.

(2) *Antigen dilution.* The radiolabeled HSA (^{125}I·HSA) was diluted in a solution of unlabeled HSA in isotonic barbital buffer to yield a final concentration of about 600 μg of N per milliliter or more as desired. Subsequent dilutions were prepared in the same buffer. The labeled HSA constituted less than 5% of the total antigen so that the specific activity of the HSA ranged from 200 to 400 cpm per microgram of N.

(3) *Procedure.* The antigen and antiserum dilutions were equilibrated at $4°$ before use. Exactly 1.0 ml of the trace-labeled HSA was added to 13- by 100-mm Lusteroid tubes (International Equipment Co., Boston, Massachusetts, Catalog No. 655), in duplicate. The antiserum dilutions

were then added in a volume of 1.0 ml as the contents of the tubes were being thoroughly mixed. Control tubes containing 1.0 ml of each trace-labeled antigen dilution plus 1.0 ml of NRS 1:5 were included, as were tubes containing 1.0 ml of the trace-labeled antigen alone. The tubes were generally incubated at 4° for several days. After this time, exactly 2.0 ml of cold SAS were added to all the tubes, except to those containing the antigen alone. The additions of SAS were always made while the contents of the tubes were being rapidly mixed. It is of utmost importance that the mixing be rapid and thorough. The tubes, now containing the precipitated globulins, were placed in an ethylene glycol–water bath at 0° for 30 min or longer, and then centrifuged at 2° for 45 minutes at a speed of 2500 g (International Equipment Co., Boston, Massachusetts, Centrifuge Angle Head No. 845). The supernatant fluid was carefully decanted, and the inverted tubes were allowed to drain. The lips of the tubes were wiped with absorbent paper strips, and the precipitates were homogenized by vigorous tapping, care being taken to avoid spattering on the sides of the tubes. The precipitates were then washed with 2.0 ml of cold SAS/2. After thorough mixing on the stirrer, the tubes were held at 0° for 30 minutes, and recentrifuged at 2500 g at 2° for 45 minutes. The precipitates were washed twice in this manner, and then assayed for [125]I·HSA. The total amount of antigen bound with the precipitated globulins was determined by dividing the average counts per minute obtained from the duplicate tubes by the specific activity of the antigen. The weight of antigen bound specifically to antibody was obtained by subtracting the number of micrograms of HSA-N bound in the NRS controls from the total weight of HSA in the precipitate. This value was used to calculate the weight of antibody in the sample, assuming that the molecular configuration of the immune complex in extreme antigen excess takes the limiting form, Ag_2Ab, and that the molecular weight of the rabbit antibody in the hyperimmune serum approximates 160,000. Thus

$$\mu g \text{ anti-HSA in test sample} = Ab/2\ Ag = \frac{160,000}{(2) \times (83,400)}$$
$$\times\ \mu g \text{ of HSA-N bound specifically}$$

A representative experiment is described in Table I.

b. RESULTS

Many of the conditions governing precipitation of the immune complexes by ammonium sulfate were explored in the original studies reported by Farr. These were checked for their applicability to the present modification. Thus, a final concentration of 50% SAS was found optimal for

TABLE I

WEIGHT ESTIMATES OF RABBIT ANTI-HSA^a-N BY MEANS OF THE MODIFIED ANTIGEN-BINDING CAPACITY PROCEDURE

Tube	Rabbit anti-HSA^b		NRS^a 1:5 (ml)	HSA added in 1.0 ml (μg)	^{125}I in washed precipitate (cpm)	Total HSA in precipitate^c (μg N)	Specifically bound HSA in precipitate^d (μg N)	Anti-HSA precipitated^e (μg N)
	Dilution	μg Ab-N in 1.9 ml						
1	1:1200	1.1	0	272	2414	8.1	1.3	0.9
2	1:1200	1.1	0	544	3561	12.0	0.6	
3	1:576	2.3	0	272	2686	9.0	2.2	2.1
4	1:576	2.3	0	544	4000	13.5	2.1	
5	1:384	3.5	0	272	3216	10.8	4.0	3.5
6	1:384	3.5	0	544	4358	14.7	3.3	
7	1:240	5.6	0	272	3892	13.1	6.3	5.5
8	1:240	5.6	0	544	4917	16.6	5.2	
9	1:80	16.7	0	272	7233	24.4	17.6	16.3
10	1:80	16.7	0	544	8242	27.8	16.4	

11	1:40	33.3	0	272	11919	40.1	33.3	31.0
12	1:40	33.3	0	544	12656	42.6	33.2	—
13	None added	0	1.0	272	2008	6.8	—	—
14	None added	0	1.0	544	3386	11.4	—	—

[a] HSA = human serum albumin; NRS = normal rabbit serum.

[b] The particular pool contained 1.330 mg of precipitable antihuman serum albumin (HSA)-N/ml. The diluent for the antiserum levels in tubes 1 to 12 was 1:5 normal rabbit serum (NRS) in isotonic-barbital buffer. Upon addition of the antigen, the final serum concentration was 10%.

[c] Specific activity of ^{125}I-HSA for this preparation = 297 cpm/μg HSA-N.

[d] The value obtained in the NRS controls, tubes 13 and 14, was subtracted from the corresponding values in the test system; e.g., for tube 1, 8.1 minus 6.8 = 1.3; for tube 2, 12.0 minus 11.4 = 0.6.

[e] $160,000/[(2)(83,400)] \times$ average specifically-bound HSA in precipitate = μg antibody N precipitated, e.g., for tubes 1 and 2, $(160,000)/[(2)(83,400)] \times (1.3 + 0.6)/2 = 0.91$ μg anti-HSA N. The mean difference between duplicate measurements of the amount of antigen precipitated at half-saturated ammonium sulfate (SAS/2) with NRS in 13 experiments was 0.30 ± 0.27 μg N.

antibody recovery in a reaction medium containing either a 5, 10, or 20% final concentration of NRS, and a reaction temperature of either 0° or 25°.

i. Effect of Varying Antigen Concentration

The basic assumption in the design of this procedure, and in the calculation, is that all the molecular complexes formed have the composition Ag_2Ab. The evidence for verifying this assumption is admittedly indirect and rests on the following rationale and experimental findings. The original concept as outlined by Farr was that the union of antigen with antibody would not be altered appreciably by precipitation of the globulins in SAS/2. With a constant antibody level, it can be anticipated that the weight of antigen in the precipitate will reach a maximum when the concentration of antigen is increased to the point where all the antibody-combining sites have reacted with antigen. The amount of antigen required to attain this peak value will vary with the amount and affinity of the antibody. Beyond this critical quantity of antigen input, the amount of HSA in the SAS/2 precipitate should be invariant over a wide range of antigen concentrations. A typical experiment designed to test this hypothesis is described in Fig. 1. As indicated in the figure, four assays were undertaken, each with a constant level of antibody. Each level of antibody was allowed to react with increasing amounts of HSA, ranging from 50 to 800 μg N. The final serum concentration was maintained at 10%. The results plotted in Fig. 1 indicate that beyond a certain antigen level, the amount of specifically bound HSA remains quite constant, as predicted. The minimal quantity of HSA required to attain each of the plateau values increases with the antibody input and is difficult to define by a single point. The latter finding is most likely due to the multivalency of the antigen and antibody which results in the formation of complexes with varying antigen:antibody ratios. With a sufficient excess of antigen, the limiting configuration of Ag_2Ab is achieved. Beyond this point, further increases in the HSA input, even up to 800 μg N, do not augment the weight of HSA in the precipitate, suggesting that equilibrium conditions have been established between the immune reactants. There was no evidence of aggregation in these reaction mixtures, as judged by the absence of opalescence or sedimentation.

The data obtained for the experiment described in Fig. 1 are plotted in Fig. 2 in terms of antibody input and recovery. The individual points represent the plateau values of Fig. 1 multiplied by the weight-ratio factor (0.93 for this HSA preparation). The values plotted in Fig. 2 show that 2.8, 5.8, 11.0, and 21.4 μg of anti-HSA N were recovered for antibody inputs of 2.6, 5.2, 10.3, and 20.5 μg of anti-HSA N, respectively.

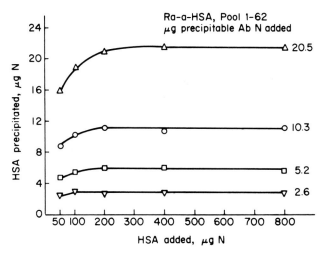

FIG. 1. The effect of increasing HSA concentration on the amount of HSA specifically precipitated with various concentrations of rabbit anti-HSA in the presence of half-saturated ammonium sulfate. Ra-a-HSA = rabbit anti-HSA.

The line in Fig. 2 was drawn with a slope of 1, through the origin, to illustrate the close correspondence observed with this serum pool between the precipitable antibody N values and those obtained by the mABC technique. Entirely concordant results have also been obtained with other hyperimmune sera. In other instances, as detailed below, antibody estimations by the mABC technique often exceeded those obtained in

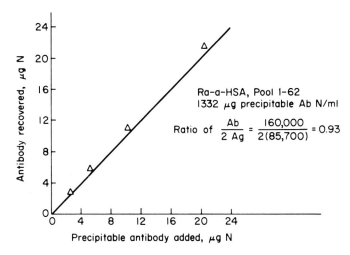

FIG. 2. The recovery of rabbit anti-HSA by means of the mABC technique.

quantitative precipitin studies, particularly with serum obtained early during the course of immunization.

ii. Effect of EDTA

A potential source of error in quantitative precipitin analyses of low antibody levels emerges from the possible incorporation of compounds that may interact with the antigen–antibody aggregates. Among these may be mentioned rheumatoid factor-like substances, the components of the complement system, and conglutinin. In the mABC technique, the likelihood of interaction with complement is relatively small due to the conditions of great antigen excess.[4] This was verified in assays with freshly obtained and unheated rabbit anti-HSA sera carried out with and without EDTA. The latter compound was used to chelate divalent cations, thereby minimizing those interactions involving complement and conglutinin.

iii. Solubility of Immune Complexes in Ammonium Sulfate

In several experiments the precipitates formed at SAS/2 were washed four times, each with 2.0 ml of SAS/2. Assays of the precipitates, performed after each wash, showed that they were soluble to an extent not exceeding 0.2 μg of anti-HSA-N/ml of SAS/2. In one experiment, 12.2 μg and 11.3 μg of anti-HSA N were recovered after the first and fourth washes, respectively, for an antibody input of 12.7 μg of precipitable anti-HSA-N. Similarly, the same pool yielded 14.2 and 12.5 μg of anti-HSA-N after the first and fourth washes for an antibody input of 12.6 μg of precipitable anti-HSA-N.

iv. Length of Incubation

The amount of specifically-bound ^{125}I·HSA precipitable at SAS/2 after interaction with anti-HSA did not vary by more than 0.5 μg when the specific reactants were incubated at 0° for periods ranging from 0.5 to 144 hours.

v. Effect of pH

Precipitation of the immune complexes with equal volumes of SAS adjusted to pH 4.4 or 6.8 yielded comparable recovery values.

vi. Verification of mABC Estimates by Precipitation of Soluble Complexes with Sheep Anti-Rabbit γ-Globulin Serum

Rabbit anti-HSA sera (2 pools were tested) were diluted 1:5 in isotonic barbital buffer, and then in 1:5 NRS. Soluble complexes were formed in

[4] A. G. Osler, M. M. Mayer, and M. Heidelberger, *J. Immunol.* **60**, 205 (1948).

antigen excess in duplicate, for each serum dilution. One set of reaction mixtures was analyzed by the usual mABC procedure. To an aliquot of each tube of the second set was added 0.5 ml of a sheep anti-rabbit γ-globulin serum, a quantity sufficient to precipitate all the rabbit γ-globulins in the assay mixture. After incubation at 0° for 7 days, the precipitates were washed twice with cold saline and analyzed for $^{125}I\cdot HSA$ activity. The values thus obtained were used for calculating the anti-HSA content of the soluble complexes. Precipitation of the complexes at SAS/2 yielded slightly higher results than those obtained with the sheep anti-rabbit γ-globulin reagent.

vii. Specificity Studies

Significant quantities of $^{125}I\cdot HSA$ could not be precipitated if this protein were added to rabbit antisera prepared against a variety of other antigens.

The data in Table II illustrate one application of the mABC procedure. The findings indicate that relatively large quantities of 7 S antibody are present in the sera of rabbits during the first 18 days after immunization. Since these immunoglobulins have feeble if any hemagglutinating or precipitating ability, they were not detected in studies which claim that 19 S antibodies are produced earlier than those of the 7 S class. In some instances, such as in the serum of rabbit 501 taken 18 days after immunization, there were no detectable 19 S antibodies (≤ 2 μg Ab N) and 192 μg N of the 7 S variety.

The mABC procedure differs from the technique described by Farr in several respects. Unlike the original method, the antibody concentration is maintained at a constant level, and the amount of antigen is vastly increased in order to form soluble immune complexes of the configuration Ag_2Ab. The quantity of antigen used in the original Farr technique was fixed at 0.2 or 0.02 μg N, and the reaction end point was determined by the dilution of serum required to precipitate 33% of the radio-labeled albumin antigen. This antibody:antigen ratio corresponds to moderate antigen excess, a region in which the molecular composition of the immune complexes is variable. This circumstance, coupled with the well known variations in antigen-combining ratios of immunoglobulins in different, or even in the same serum, precluded the use of the original procedure for absolute antibody weight estimations. The use of a large excess of antigen and the resulting uniformity in molecular composition of the immune complexes provides a relatively sensitive method for precise antibody estimations which is independent of the aggregating abilities of the immunoglobulins.

One of the assumptions incorporated in the calculations of antibody

TABLE II
COMPARATIVE PRECIPITIN, MODIFIED ANTIGEN-BINDING CAPACITY (mABC), AND HEMAGGLUTININ ASSAYS ON INDIVIDUAL RABBIT ANTI-HUMAN SERUM ALBUMIN (HSA) SERA OBTAINED AFTER A SINGLE INJECTION OF HSA

Rabbit anti-HSA serum No.	Days after injection	Whole serum					
		μg Ab N/ml by		HA		PCA	
		Pptn	mABC	Pre	Post[a]	Serum diln[b]	Diameter (mm)
500[c]	8	24	21	270	0	7	13.8
						21	9.0
500[c]	18	60	58	810	810	18	16.1
						54	11.8
501[c]	8	21	18	270	50	6	10.4
						18	6.8
501[c]	18	56	71	810	810	24	13.6
						72	10.2

Rabbit anti-HSA serum No.	Days after injection	Peak I (19 S) effluents					
		μg Ab N by mABC		HA		PCA	
		Per ml	Total	Pre	Post[a]	Diln[b]	Diameter (mm)
500[c]	8	0	—	30	0	1	0
500[c]	18	1.8	24	90	0	1	0.4
501[c]	8	0.6	7	90	0	1	0
501[c]	18	0	—	270	0	1	2.2

weight in the mABC procedure concerns the molecular composition of the immune complexes which are formed. The calculations that have been made are based upon a weight ratio involving only the complex Ag_2Ab, and this assumption was justified by experiments such as the one shown in Fig. 1. The attainment of plateau values at molar ratios of antigen to antibody of about 100 is most simply interpreted by the formation of only one type of complex, namely, Ag_2Ab. However, recent findings of Lapresle and Webb[5,6] have provided substantial evidence as to the heterogeneity of the determinants on the HSA molecule. On this basis, a single anti-serum could theoretically contain at least two types of antibodies, with

[5] C. Lapresle and T. Webb, *Biochem. J.* **95**, 245 (1965).
[6] T. Webb and C. Lapresle, *Biochem. J.* **91**, 24 (1964).

TABLE II (*Continued*)

Rabbit anti-HSA serum No.	Days after injection	Peak II (7 S) effluents					
		μg Ab N by mABC		HA		PCA	
		Per ml	Total	Pre	Post[a]	Diln[b]	Diameter
500[c]	8	2.5	57	5	5	1	13.7
						2.5	9.6
500[c]	18	5.6	160	30	30	1.8	15.8
						5.4	11.1
501[c]	8	2.0	60	0	5	1	10.2
						2	7.4
501[c]	18	5.6	192	30	30	1.8	13.4
						5.4	10.1

[a] Before and after treatment with 2-ME and iodoacetamide. The numbers refer to the reciprocals of the serum dilution titers.
[b] Reciprocal of serum or column effluent dilution; 0.1 ml used in the passive cutaneous anaphylaxis test.
[c] HSA, 1 mg, in toe pads.

specificities directed toward HSA, but to different determinants on the same molecule. A consequence of this finding is that the limiting complex in extreme antigen excess could be Ag_3Ab_2, not Ag_2Ab. However, studies of this question by Webb and Lapresle have diminished the likelihood that the form Ag_3Ab_2 occurs to any significant degree with molar ratios of antigen:antibody exceeding 13.5.[6]

A second assumption of critical importance for the validity of the mABC procedure concerns the molecular weights of the immunoglobulins. For the hyperimmune serum pools a molecular weight of 160,000 was assumed, and this assumption was validated in gel filtration experiments with Sephadex G-200. Recoveries of 94.7, 88.9, and 94.1% of the applied antibody nitrogen have been obtained, and these were associated entirely with the 7 S immunoglobulins from hyperimmune serum pools. However, in studies with "early" anti-HSA sera, the 19 S and 7 S character of the immunoglobulins must be investigated further, particularly in regard to the molecular weights and number of antigen-binding sites.

It was expected that the mABC procedure would be applicable to a variety of immune systems, particularly those involving haptens, carbohydrates, nucleotides and other antigens that are soluble at high concentrations of ammonium sulfate. In addition, the choice of precipitants other than SAS/2 may permit an extension of this procedure to still different immune systems.

D. Turbidimetric Analysis of Precipitation Reactions* †

1. INTRODUCTION

Turbidimetric analysis of precipitin systems is a reliable and relatively simple method, allowing quantitation in terms of protein nitrogen in the antigen and in the precipitate. The primary immunological data are plotted as modal curves on rectilinear paper, or, when the range of antigen concentrations is great, on semilogarithmic paper (Chap. 10.B., Fig. 3 in Vol. II). Familiarity with such curves permits judgments regarding the relative concentrations and the qualitative similarities of the antigens and/or the antisera being studied or compared. Techniques are given in Vol. II, Chap. 10.B.

Turbidimetry offers some special advantages. It is possible to make immunologic measurements in solutions of extremely high concentrations of test antigens (6 to 65 mg of protein per milliliter) without the hazard of multiple handlings and washings of the precipitates. It is easy also to determine the quantity and quality of specific antigens in complex solutions and to compare the precipitin qualities of antisera. Examples of the method presented here were selected to illustrate some of the capabilities of turbidimeters for studying antigens and antisera.

2. COMPARISON OF ANTIGENS

a. NATIVE ANTIGENS

The earliest applications of the method were in making comparisons of corresponding, naturally occurring (native) proteins from living organisms.[1-4] An example is shown in Fig. 1. The method is also used to study the immunological properties of chemically altered proteins.[5,6] The α-pre-

* Section 13.D was contributed by Charles A. Leone.

† The work reported in this paper was supported, in part, by contract AT(11-1)-1073 with the Atomic Energy Commission and by grant RH00063-08 from the United States Public Health Service.
[1] A. A. Boyden, *Physiol. Zool.* **15**, 109 (1942).
[2] A. A. Boyden, *in* "Serological Approaches to Studies of Protein Metabolism" (W. H. Cole, ed.), p. 74. Rutgers Univ. Press, New Brunswick, New Jersey, 1954.
[3] A. A. Boyden, *in* "Serological and Biochemical Comparisons of Proteins" (W. H. Cole, ed.), p. 3. Rutgers Univ. Press, New Brunswick, New Jersey, 1958.
[4] C. A. Leone, ed., "Taxonomic Biochemistry and Serology." Ronald Press, New York, 1964.
[5] C. A. Leone, *J. Immunol.* **70**, 386 (1958).
[6] C. A. Leone, *in* "Ionizing Radiations and Immune Processes" (C. A. Leone, ed.), p. 115. Science Publ., Inc., New York, 1962.

cipitin procedure (constant antiserum and varying amounts of antigen) is employed regularly to analyze antigens.[7] In performing a test, a range of antigen dilutions is chosen, so far as this is possible, to provide "whole curves" for comparison.[2, 8] Accordingly, the entire range of combining proportions is covered, and the total precipitating capacity of an antiserum for a given antigen is indicated in the resulting curves. In Fig. 1,

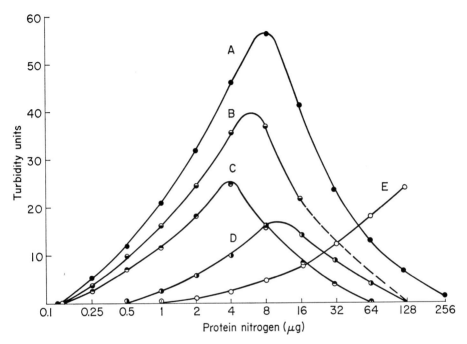

Fig. 1. Immunological comparisons of γ-globulins in serum of three species (beef, sheep, pig) with rabbit antibovine γ-globulin, and cross-reactions with the γ-globulins of horse and goat. The total protein in the starting concentration of the dilution sequence was the same (256 μg of protein N/ml) for all the antigens. The displacements of the curves for horse and goat result from the presence of nonreactive protein. ●, Bovine γ-globulin; ◖, sheep γ-globulin; ◗, pig γ-globulin; ◑, horse serum; ○, goat serum.

curves A, B, and C show typical results obtained when the amounts of reacting antigen in each system are known and accordingly plotted. The shift of the peak in curves B and C toward a lesser concentration of antigen is normally found with cross-reacting native proteins. Curve B illus-

[7] W. C. Boyd, "Fundamentals of Immunology," 4th ed., p. 362. Wiley (Interscience), New York, 1966.
[8] A. A. Boyden and R. S. DeFalco, *Physiol. Zool.* **16**, 229 (1943).

trates a partial curve, the consequence of having available only a limited amount of antigen, the curve being completed as a reasonable estimate (dashed line). Curve D exemplifies how a curve is displaced if the amount of reactive protein is less than the total protein, as determined by micro-Kjeldahl tests, which is present in the antigen solution. The same situation exists for curve E excepting that the reactive protein in the antigen solution is considerably less and the displacement is greater.

It is customary to study the quality of the antigens by measuring the areas under the curves, comparing values found in the cross-reacting systems with that of the reference system, curve A (the maximum reaction possible under the conditions of testing). In actual practice, the readings obtained in the turbidimeter for a test are summed and taken as a value proportional to the area of the curve.[8] The advantages of comparing "whole curves" are obvious in the case of curve D. Its displacement is of no immunological consequence because the area would not change regardless of its location on the antigen axis.

Curve E, plotted as protein nitrogen of whole serum, is shifted far to the right. As shown, only a portion of the postzone is present. The reacting molecules may exist in the test solution in very low concentration, or the antigen reacting in curve E may represent interaction between a non-γ-globulin in the test antigen with unsuspected antibody in the antiserum. The obvious control is to react the antiserum with whole bovine serum and see whether a curve similar to curve A is obtained.

Let it be assumed, for an illustration, that all the curves in Fig. 1 are caused by analogous antigen molecules. Curve E is obviously not as usable as curves B through D for comparison with curve A. When the peak region of the curve is not present, it is difficult to estimate how much of the postzone is depicted. Some curve-matching of the postzone of curve E with those of the other curves may be possible, based upon the extrinsic knowledge concerning the antigen. Comparisons of only the postzone of the several curves will yield useful but more restricted information than that obtained from whole curves. Sometimes the realities of carrying out a series of experiments may require comparison of only the corresponding portions of postzones in order to measure immunological similarities and differences.

b. Altered Antigens

Turbidimetric analyses have been used extensively to study the structural degradation of proteins by ionizing radiations.[9-11] In Fig. 2 the loss

[9] H. Fricke, C. A. Leone, and W. Landmann, *Nature* **180**, 1423 (1957).
[10] C. A. Leone, *J. Immunol.* **85**, 107, 112, and 268 (1960).
[11] G. H. Sweet and C. A. Leone, *Bull. Serol. Museum* No. 37, 1 (1967).

of reactive protein is revealed by shift of the precipitin curves toward the region of high antigen concentration. Fricke and co-workers showed that the immunological activity of irradiated protein, relative to that of native protein, could be indicated by a measurement they termed the "ratios of the peaks."[9] In these measurements, the amount of antigen-nitrogen required to obtain the maximum precipitate, with use of a constant amount of antibody, is accurately determined. A factor is established by dividing into the quantity representing the native protein (N) the quantity representing the irradiated protein (I). This fraction, converted to its

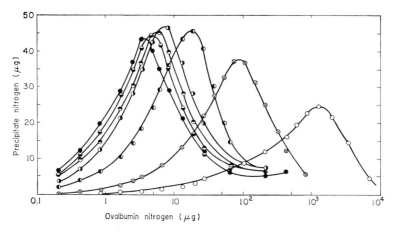

Fig. 2. A semilogarithmic plot of reactions of anti-native ovalbumin with native ovalbumin and γ-irradiated, lyophilized ovalbumin. As the radiation dosage is increased, the precipitin curve becomes displaced to the right in the direction of increased antigen concentration, which indicates destruction of reactive protein. At the higher dosages there is, in addition, reduction in the height of the curve indicating; the occurrence of qualitative change in the reacting antigen. ●, Native ovalbumin; ◕, 30 electron volts absorbed per molecule of ovalbumin (ev/mole); ◔, 63 ev/mole; ◑, 143 ev/mole; ◐, 300 ev/mole; ⊗, 478 ev/mole; ○, 878 ev/mole.

decimal form, indicates the relative immunological activity of irradiated protein to native protein. The N/I values proved to have general usefulness in studying the effects of γ-rays on proteins representing a wide range of molecular weights (Fig. 3).[6] For small proteins such as ovalbumin, immunological activity decreased exponentially as the dose of radiation increased, denoting "single hit" destruction of a molecule. As sizes of the proteins increased, the curves depicting loss of activity became increasingly sigmoid, denoting a "multiple hit" requirement for destruction of a molecule.

Besides N/I measurements, other kinds of comparative measures may be made on the data shown in Fig. 2. The amount of measured precipitate, for example, obtained at any value of antigen up to 4 μg P-N/ml would give an indication of loss of reactivity in relation to radiation dose. Similarly, for a given amount of turbidity (20 μg of precipitate P-N/ml, for example) the displacement of the postzone curve along the antigen axis can be correlated with radiation dosage and radiation damage.[12] The areas under the curves are not, in these tests, useful values for measuring radiation damage. In fact, for γ-ray dosages up to 3.2×10^6 rads (15

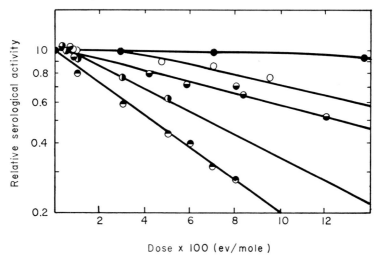

Dose x 100 (ev/mole)

FIG. 3. The relative immunological activity of irradiated, 1%, aerated solutions of proteins of different molecular weight classes, using N/I values of the peak reactions as the measure of activity. ●, *Limulus polyphemus* hemocyanin, M.W. 1,740,000; ○, *Callinectes sapidus* hemocyanin, M.W. 692,000; ◓, *Cancer magister* hemocyanin, M.W. 631,000; ◑ human serum γ-globulin, M.W. 160,000; ◔, chicken ovalbumin, M.W. 45,000. The curves become increasingly sigmoid as the molecular weight increases.

electron volts absorbed per molecule of lyophilized ovalbumin) the areas of curves for native and irradiated ovalbumin are the same and for larger dosages, up to 300 electron volts per molecule the areas of the curves of the irradiated ovalbumins exceed that of native ovalbumin. For larger molecules, such as human γ-globulin and hemocyanin, the absorbed dosages are much larger before the areas under the curves show detectable differences.

The increases in the peak turbidities of the samples absorbing between 32 and 300 electron volts per molecule indicate the presence of soluble

[12] H. Fricke, W. Landmann, C. A. Leone, and J. Vincent, *J. Phys. Chem.* **63,** 932 (1959).

aggregates of protein that are being precipitated by the anti-native anti-bodies.[11] The depression of the peaks of the curves representing oval-bumin receiving 300 and 478 electron volts per molecule indicate that the available reactive sites on the antigen have been qualitatively changed.[6]

Thermal augmentation of radiation damage to protein molecules was studied readily in the turbidimeter (Fig. 4). Samples of irradiated HGG heated at 30° to 56° for 30 minutes to 120 minutes developed immunologi-cally active, soluble aggregates (supermolecules) that were precipitable

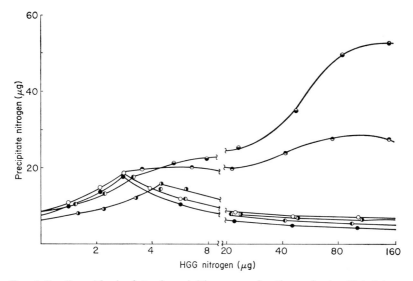

FIG. 4. Semilogarithmic plots of precipitin curves of native and γ-irradiated, human γ-globulin preparations tested with anti-native human γ-globulin antibodies. γ-Ray dosages are expressed as electron volts absorbed per protein molecule (ev/mole). ●, Native; ○, native heated at 55° for 120 minutes; ◑, 32 ev/mole; ◐, 32 ev/mole heated at 55° for 120 minutes; ◑, 50 ev/mole; ◑, 50 ev/mole heated at 55° for 120 minutes.

at much lowered antibody-to-antigen ratios.[11] There was a direct relation between increase in temperature of heating and the amounts of aggregate created in a given irradiated sample, and a direct relation between radia-tion dosages and the amounts of aggregate formed by heating at a given temperature.

3. COMPARISONS OF ANTISERA

The increase in the precipitating capacity of an antiserum during the course of immunization is readily measured in turbidimeters.[13] Figure 5

[13] C. A. Leone, *J. Immunol.* **69**, 285 (1952).

shows the changes occurring in the antiserum of a rabbit as detected in 3 partial bleedings during a course of immunization. Two effects are most noteworthy. The amount of precipitate increased, indicating greater concentration of antibody, and the specificity of the antiserum decreased, indicating the appearance of antibodies against more kinds of antigenic

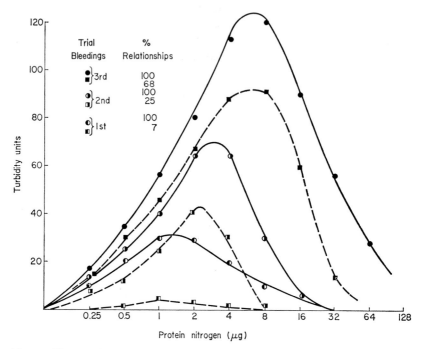

Fig. 5. Changes in an antiserum during the course of immunization with bovine γ-globulin, showing increase in reactivity and decrease in specificity. Reference reactions are shown in circles connected by solid lines; cross-reactions are shown in squares connected by dashed lines. Total precipitate increased in the second and third partial bleedings. The relative amount of cross-reaction increased from 7% to 68% of the reference reaction. O, Bovine γ-globulin; □, sheep γ-globulin.

sites. (In the fourth and fifth bleedings, the amounts of precipitable antibody increased only slightly and the extent of cross-reactivity remained constant.)

After prolonged immunization with ovalbumin[10] or hemocyanins,[13] a rabbit may reach a hyperimmune state in which the antibody level (approximately 2000 μg PN/ml) remains relatively constant and the specificity of the antiserum is minimal and constant.

Irradiated human γ-globulin (HGG) has proved to be useful, when used in conjunction with a turbidimeter, to detect qualitative changes in the precipitin properties of antisera.[13] Figure 6 illustrates such changes in an early (first) bleeding and late (tenth) bleeding from a single rabbit undergoing injections with native HGG. In the early antiserum, the curves for the irradiated samples of HGG shifted predictably to the right

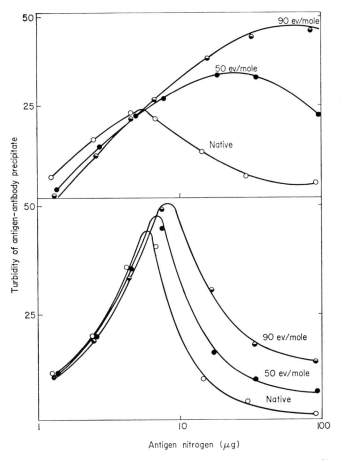

Fig. 6. Semilogarithmic plots of precipitin curves of native and γ-irradiated HGG preparations tested with early anti-native HGG antiserum (upper curves) and with hyperimmune anti-native HGG antiserum (lower curves) from the same rabbit. O, Native HGG; ●, 50 ev/mole; ◑, 90 ev/mole.

and also, predictably, exceeded the reference curve obtained with native HGG. Before the late antiserum was tested, it was diluted so that maximum precipitation was approximately equal to that of the early antiserum. Because the same antigens were used in testing the early and late antisera, the differences observed in the shapes of the precipitin curves were attributable to the differing precipitating qualities of the antisera. Three notable differences were (1) the requirement, in the early antiserum, for higher concentrations of antigen to obtain the maximum amount of precipitate, (2) the broader zone of equivalence in the early antiserum, and (3) the relatively greater amount of precipitate obtained with native HGG in the hyperimmune serum. The results are those to be expected from an early highly specific antiserum which contained antibodies directed against only one or two kinds of antigenic sites, and from a less specific, hyperimmune antiserum containing antibodies directed against numerous kinds of antigenic sites.

Light-transmission instruments such as the B & L Spectronic 20 or the Leitz colorimeter can be adapted to function as light-reflection instruments.[14] In general, instruments so modified have a lower sensitivity and smaller range of measurement, but, with appropriate dilutions of antisera and careful selection of antigen systems, essentially the same kinds of immunological data can be obtained as with a regular turbidimeter.

[14] J. G. Baier, *Bull. Serol. Museum* No. 21, 5 (1959).

E. Estimation of Antigen Concentration in Complex Mixtures by Optical Density of Turbid Suspensions*

1. INTRODUCTION

It is often desirable to assay rapidly an antigenic substance in the presence of other antigens or other contaminants of the same type. One example is a routine estimation of a serum component; another might be a means to distinguish between the loss of activity of an enzyme and the loss of protein in tissue extracts. As with any precipitation test for an impure antigen in liquid medium, satisfactory results with turbidimetry depend upon the availability of monospecific antiserum and strict adherence to predetermined procedures. The turbidimetric method for the determination of immune precipitates, while quantitative only in relative terms, offers the advantages of simple manipulation and speed.

Measurement of deflected light by the photronreflectometer has been discussed in Section 13.D of this volume and in Chap. 10.B, Vol. II. Although that instrument is effective for turbidity assays,[1] it is not readily available in most laboratories. The procedure described here is therefore designed to be employed with colorimeters or spectrophotometers

* Section 13.E was contributed by I. W. Li and Curtis A. Williams.

[1] J. G. Baier, Jr., *Physiol. Zool.* **20**, 172 (1947).

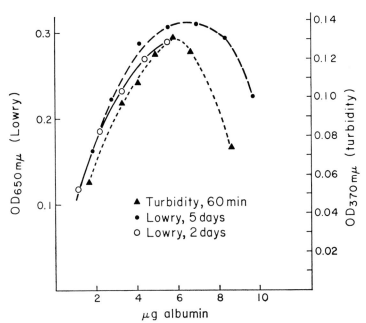

FIG. 1. Comparison of turbidity curve with quantitative precipitin curves of mouse serum albumin and a constant amount of rabbit anti-mouse albumin serum. Reaction mixtures for turbidity assay were made with 35 μl of antiserum in 1-ml volumes, incubated for 60 minutes at 37°; quantitative analysis by the Lowry method of precipitates from 250 μl of antiserum in 2.5-ml volumes, incubated at 37° for 60 minutes and then 2 days or 5 days at 4°.

that measure transmitted light, i.e., the light that is not deflected from a straight path by particles in suspension.

Since the relationship between turbidity and concentration of suspended particles is very complex and almost never linear,* in practice, it

---

* The approximate relationship between turbidity (T) and concentration (c) is shown by the equation of Wells[2]:

$$T = k \frac{cld^3}{d^4 + \alpha\lambda^4}$$

in which, k is a constant depending both on the medium and on the method of measurement, α is a constant for the method only, l is the thickness of the layer of medium, d is the average diameter of the suspended particles, and λ is the wavelength of the illumination. The great effect of wavelength on turbidity is evident, and the equation also implies that for dilute suspensions Beer's proportions should hold; i.e., with two suspensions of the same kind, when $T = T_1$, $c/c_1 = l_1/l$. However, this simple proportion is not valid for the majority of nephelometric or turbidimetric determinations, even when monochromatic light is used.[3]

[2] P. V. Wells, *Chem. Rev.* **3**, 331 (1927).

is necessary (1) to determine whether the suspension of reaction products and the medium have suitable optical properties; (2) to establish the optimum conditions and to adhere rigidly to them; and (3) to construct an empirically determined calibration curve for each system and set of conditions.[3]

It may be seen in Fig. 1 that turbidities of antigen–antibody precipitates measured with a Zeiss PMQ II spectrophotometer at 370 mμ show good correlation with the standard quantitative precipitin results of an identical system assayed by the Lowry method (see Section 13.A.3.b.ii). Difference in the rate of formation of the equilibrium complex at various antigen–antibody ratios may be responsible for the different shapes of the three curves assayed after different periods of incubation. Turbidimetry, of course, does not measure protein or precipitate *per se*, but rather the amount of light deflected from a defined path. Since this will vary with the number and size of particles in suspension, incubation time is also expected to affect this parameter differently in the equivalence and the antibody excess regions.

2. PROCEDURE

a. SELECTION OF WAVELENGTH

It is well known that turbidity values are progressively reduced with the increase in wavelength of the incident light (see Vol. II, Chap. 10.B.4). When economical use of antiserum becomes a dominant consideration, as in routine assay of a large number of samples, it is of clear advantage to run the test at a shorter wavelength. That wavelength must be determined empirically, however, to avoid bands of high absorption by soluble substances contained in either the antiserum or the antigen solution. A method for selecting a wavelength is illustrated in Fig. 2, which compares spectral analyses of identical amounts of antiserum alone and when incubated with antigen. The differences between the optical density values of the reaction mixture and the serum blank represent readings of a constant amount of precipitate at different wavelengths.

Antisera differ not only in antibody content, but also in the amount of solutes absorbing light in the visible range. Hemoglobin, for instance, has a very strong absorption band between 400 and 420 mμ and a weaker one at 540 mμ. Turbidity measurements should be made outside these ranges. If conservation of antiserum is a minor consideration, 500 mμ would be a good choice. If it is necessary to use a short wavelength in order to obtain sufficiently high optical density values in more dilute systems, the 320 to

[3] T. R. P. Gibb, Jr., "Optical Methods of Chemical Analysis." McGraw-Hill, New York, 1942.

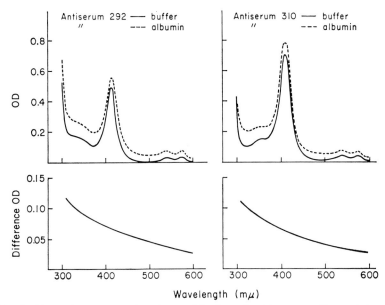

F. 2. Absorption spectra of antiserum blanks and antiserum–antigen mixtures in 1-ml volumes incubated for 60 minutes at 37°. See text for explanation.

380 mμ region may be considered, the precise wavelength depending on other minor absorption peaks. For example, 325 mμ might be suitable for antiserum No. 310 but 370 mμ is a better choice for antiserum No. 292. (See Fig. 2.)

b. Specificity of Antiserum

Monospecific antisera are available for relatively few antigens. The antigen to be assayed is referred to here as the *principal antigen*. It is important to detect antibodies to any secondary antigens other than the one of interest and to remove them by absorption with the appropriate antigen.

If purified secondary antigen is not available or if absorption with a mixture of antigens results in too great a loss of the desired principal antibody, it must then be determined what contribution the contaminating precipitate would make to the overall error. This latter procedure requires absorption of the antiserum with purified principal antigen so that only the unwanted antibodies remain for titration. A quantitative precipitin curve or a turbidimetric curve is then determined using this absorbed antiserum and mixture of antigens similar to those which will be present in the contemplated routine tests. If the curves indicate that a reaction with the contaminating antibody can be expected in the antibody excess region of the routine tests, a control reaction with antiserum absorbed by the principal antigen is required in each test to give a correction value. Such corrections are feasible only for very minor heterogeneities, however, and if there is any doubt of their validity, another assay method, such as a diffusion technique, should be employed (see Chapter 14).

c. STANDARD TURBIDITY CURVE

A standard turbidity curve with varying amounts of antigen and a constant amount of antibody is prepared under conditions identical to the routine test to be used.

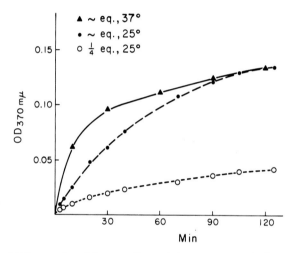

FIG. 3. Turbidity produced by reaction mixtures near equivalence plotted as a function of incubation time at 37°(▲) or 25°(●); antibody excess reaction made with approximately one-fourth of the equivalence amount antigen, at 25°(○). All tubes contained equal amounts of antiserum to which indicated amounts of antigen were added.

In this laboratory the immune system is incubated for 1 hour at 37°, but adequate results could be obtained also at 25° after a longer period of incubation. Constant temperature is important, however. Although the optical density continues to rise after a 1-hour period at 37°, the rate of increase is greatly reduced so that reading a test 2 to 3 minutes early or late would introduce errors of only 1% (see Fig. 3).

The standard curve is prepared with an antigen mixture similar to the intended unknowns. The principal antigen content of this standard mixture may be determined by quantitative precipitation with the antiserum after standardization with purified antigen (see Section 13.A.3.b). Antigen concentration can then be plotted against turbidity values. Inclusion of two or more tests with different amounts of the standard antigen sample in each routine series of unknowns serves as a control on conditions of the test in relation to the standard curve. And if necessary, the new standard values can be used to adjust the standard curve for a particular test series.

Turbidity curves determined with both a purified antigen and the same antigen in a complex mixture reacted with identical amounts of antiserum, are shown in Fig. 4. From the shape of the curve and the absor-

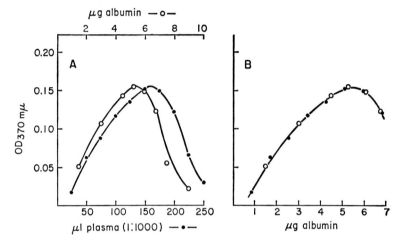

FIG. 4. Construction of a standard turbidity curve of an immune precipitation system of mouse plasma and rabbit antiserum to mouse serum albumin. (A) Comparison of turbidity curves of 1000 times diluted mouse plasma (●) added in increments and of purified mouse serum albumin, (○) added in known amounts to identical aliquots of antiserum. (B) Turbidity curve of normal mouse plasma replotted according to its albumin content derived by equating the point of maximum precipitation to that obtained with the purified mouse serum albumin.

bency values it is clear that only a certain range of antigen concentrations will provide a useful test when these are added to the antibody. If the curve is too steep, as in the lower range, the test is too sensitive to procedural imprecision and optical contaminants. If the curve is too flat, such as when approaching equivalence proportion, the test may be insufficiently sensitive to differences in antigen concentrations.

d. TEST PROCEDURE

Generally the particular antigen–antibody system to be assayed will determine the test procedure within the framework of the principles discussed above. The detailed procedure given here is an example of a system where the monospecific antiserum is relatively weak and in short supply. The test is designed, therefore, for maximum conservation of reagents consistent with acceptable precision. Specifically, it is designed for testing a rabbit antibody made against mouse serum albumin. All figures shown here represent tests with this system.

Step 1. Only clear antiserum should be used.* Dilutions are made in buffered saline (0.01 M Na_2HPO_4-NaH_2PO_4, 0.15 M NaCl, pH 7.2) so that, mixed with an equivalence quantity of antigen contained in an equal volume, an OD of about 0.2 would be read in 1 hour. As a guide, antiserum should be diluted to provide between 30 and 40 μg of antibody protein per milliliter, to which is added an equal volume of the antigen solution. The amount of antibody employed in the test should not be so great as to produce sedimenting aggregates during the period of incubation and optical measurement. The diluted antiserum and the antigen solutions are warmed in a 37° water bath before mixing.

Step 2. Dilute the antigen in buffered saline so that, on an equal volume basis, it would contain between one-fourth and three-fourths of the amount required for equivalence with the antibody dilution used. In this case, mouse plasma containing 30 to 40 mg albumin per ml is diluted some 5000 times.

Step 3. Tubes with 0.5 ml of antigen dilutions are warmed for 10 minutes in 37° water bath before 0.5 ml of diluted antiserum is added to each tube; mix thoroughly. The reaction mixtures are returned to 37° and incubated for 1 hour. Add the antiserum to successive tubes at intervals of time in order to allow unhurried reading of OD on the optical instrument to be used. Larger reaction volumes must be prepared if the colorimeter is not adaptable to 1-ml curvettes (2 mm × 10 mm light path). Baier[4] has worked out procedures for using the Bausch and Lomb Spectronic 20.

Step 4. Controls:

(a) *Standard reaction.* A sample of known antigen content should be mixed with antiserum in the same manner as the unknowns. This serves to allow any needed adjustment of the standard curve for each test series.

(b) *Antiserum blank.* An antiserum blank is made by mixing and in-

---

* Turbidity of serum specimens, which often is greater in samples that have been frozen, can be lessened markedly by centrifugation at 12,500 g for 30 minutes. If excess fat or lipid rises to the surface because of centrifugation, the clearer lower layer can be removed by capillary pipet and passed one or more times through Millipore filters which have been prewetted with saline and sucked free of excess moisture.

[4] J. G. Baier, *Bull. Serol. Museum* No. 21 (1959).

cubating equal volumes of the antiserum dilution and buffered saline in place of the antigen.

(c) *Contaminant reaction*. The test antigen sample is mixed with a similar dilution of antiserum which has been absorbed with the principal antigen. This control is employed only under special circumstances described above (Section 2.b); the OD values of this reaction are to be subtracted from the values of the reaction with unabsorbed antiserum.

Step 5. Transfer incubated reactions to suitable cuvettes and, at the appropriate time intervals, read against the antiserum blank at 370 mμ or another wavelength selected to avoid exceptional absorption bands of soluble substances in the antiserum.

TABLE I

Turbidity Assay for Albumin Concentrations of Mouse Plasmas[a]

Plasma sample	OD at 370 mμ	MSA in test[b] (μg)	Corrected MSA[c] (μg)	MSA (mg/ml plasma)[d]
Standard	0.118	3.42	3.25	34.0
Test 1	0.115	3.32	3.16	33.0
2	0.114	3.28	3.12	32.6
3	0.127	3.77	3.58	37.4
4	0.124	3.65	3.47	36.3
5	0.111	3.18	3.02	31.6
6	0.113	3.25	3.09	32.3
7	0.107	3.05	2.90	30.3
8	0.086	2.43	2.31	24.2
9	0.110	3.15	3.00	31.4
10	0.096	2.72	2.59	27.1
11	0.112	3.21	3.05	31.9
12	0.130	3.88	3.69	38.6
13	0.120	3.48	3.31	34.6
14	0.105	3.00	2.85	29.8
15	0.067	1.95	1.85	19.4

[a] $OD_{370mμ}$ values were obtained by using 0.5 ml of 1:15 ml of 1:5226 dilution of plasma and 0.5 ml of 1:15 dilution of rabbit antimouse albumin serum incubated for 60 minutes at 37°.

[b] Mouse serum albumin (MSA), micrograms per 0.5 ml test volume of plasma dilution read from the turbidity curve for calibrated normal mouse plasma in Fig. 4B.

[c] MSA values corrected to conform to the standard plasma known to contain 3.25 μg of albumin in 0.5 ml of a 1:5226 dilution (dilutions made by adding 25 μl of plasma to 5 ml of diluent, thence 0.2 ml to 5 ml).

[d] Corrected micrograms of MSA multiplied by dilution and volume factor:

$$\frac{5226}{0.5 \times 1000} = 10.5$$

e. EXAMPLE

A group of mouse plasma samples were assayed for their albumin concentrations by the use of the turbidity curve for normal mouse plasma shown in Fig. 4B.

In this test each plasma sample (including the standard plasma which had been used in making the standard turbidity curve and was known to contain 34 mg of albumin per milliliter) was diluted 5226 times with buffered saline. The OD values developed by incubating 0.5 ml of each plasma dilution with an equal volume of 1 : 15 dilution of antiserum No. 310 were read on a Zeiss spectrophotometer at 370 mμ against the antiserum blank. The results may be seen in Table I.

CHAPTER 14

Precipitation Analysis by Diffusion in Gels

A. Introduction

1. CHARACTERISTICS OF ANTIGEN–ANTIBODY REACTIONS IN GELS*

a. GENERAL CONSIDERATIONS

Antigen–antibody precipitation in gels was first employed in 1905 in order to study the Liesegang phenomenon supposed then to occur in this reaction.[1] Although practical applications to the identification of bacterial strains growing on agar plates had been introduced in 1932, multiple precipitation zones in the gel were still considered to be Liesegang rings.[2] Analysis of antigen mixtures by diffusion and specific precipitation in gels was introduced in 1946, using agar tubes. Its validity was based on the demonstration that, under suitable conditions, the reaction of a single antigen with its corresponding antibodies gave rise to a single precipitation zone; and it was further demonstrated that the precipitation zones due to distinct antigens were developed independently of each other.[3] The ever broadening range of applications for diffusion in gels depends on these principles.

Immunochemical techniques described prior to the development of gel-diffusion methods did not provide for a critical analysis of antigen mixtures. They were designed primarily for the quantitative estimation of a single antigen or antibody. Reactions in gels are also capable of furnishing quantitative information, but it should be emphasized that any immunochemical study in gels must begin with a qualitative analysis. First, the number of distinct precipitating antigens must be determined. Second, the antigens must be identified. Finally antigen may be titered and specific antibodies assayed.

It is important to remember, however, that even in qualitative analyses

---

* Section 14.A.1 was contributed by Jacques Oudin and Curtis A. Williams.

[1] H. Bechhold, *Z. Physik. Chem.* **52,** 185 (1905).

[2] G. F. Petrie, *Brit. J. Exptl. Pathol.* **13,** 380 (1932).

[3] J. Oudin, *Compt. Rend.* **222,** 115 (1946).

quantitative aspects must be considered. It is obvious that no antigen can be detected unless there is a sufficient concentration of specific precipitating antibody in the antiserum. It follows, therefore, that immunochemical analysis cannot demonstrate the purity of an antigen. Impurities, on the other hand, even minor ones, may often be revealed by a multispecific antiserum. Another important quantitative consideration is the relative amounts of reactants present. With some techniques, appreciable quantities of one reactant may fail to give a satisfactory reaction if the other is in great excess.

b. VARIETY OF METHODS

Although there are many apparently different methods for the analysis of antigen–antibody reactions in gelified media,[4] the same basic principles apply to all. There is no evidence that precipitates are formed in gels in a manner different from those obtained by mixing the reactants in liquid media. Thus, whatever advantages are to be expected from the use of gels depend as much or more on the physical properties of the system as on the immunochemical properties. In fact, it may be of greater interest to compare gel-diffusion techniques to purely physicochemical rather than to other immunochemical methods. The advantages of immunochemical analyses in gels over many physicochemical methods employed for similar purposes derive from their significantly higher sensitivity and their generally greater resolving power.

Other advantages include the frequent possibility of determining directly the chemical nature of the precipitated antigens, or of detecting the presence of antigenic components with specific biochemical activities. This is achieved by the use of dyes or color reactions many of which were originally devised for histochemical analysis (Section 14.E.1). In addition, information may be obtained concerning physical properties such as diffusion coefficients (Section 14.C.1) and electrophoretic mobilities of the reactants (14.D).

The main differences among the various techniques concern modifications affecting the diffusion patterns of the reactants and the scale of the method. Such modifications must be chosen with great care, however, since they will determine the type and quality of information which may be obtained.

Gel-diffusion techniques are customarily classified as simple diffusion or double diffusion. Simple-diffusion techniques are those in which one reactant, generally in liquid solution, is permitted to diffuse into a gelified solution of the complementary reactant (Section 14.B.1). In the case of double diffusion, the antigen solution and the antibody solution are

[4] O. Ouchterlony, *Progr. Allergy* **5**, 1 (1958).

separated initially by a zone of gel into which both reactants diffuse (Sections 14.B.2 and 3).

If the reservoirs containing the reactants are arranged so that diffusion is along a single axis, the method is called one-dimensional. Such would be the case for all reactions in tubes and certain kinds of cells (Section 14.B.4), although it is possible to devise plates for one-dimensional diffusion. Diffusion in two dimensions occurs when the reactant reservoirs are surrounded by gel and diffusion is radial, or when the diffusion of two reactants is not on the same axis.

Immunoelectrophoretic analysis is an example of a combined technique in which an additional physical parameter is added to that of diffusion. Electrophoresis of one reactant solution may be performed in the gel to be used for development of the precipitate pattern, or the electrophoretic separation may be carried out in some other medium first and transferred to a gel suitable for development by double diffusion.

c. CHOICE OF METHOD

In view of the variety of techniques available to the investigator, it is necessary to discuss the relative merits of the general types of techniques.

Other considerations being equal, diffusion in tubes offers greater sensitivity than two-dimensional techniques in plates, and single diffusion makes possible the precise measurements favorable to quantitative applications. Double diffusion has the greater ability to detect and study antigens in low concentration, but single diffusion is more reliable for the enumeration of antigens if they are present in sufficient excess, since the causes of artifacts are well known in single-diffusion tubes.

If comparative information concerning antigenic composition of different solutions is desired, double-diffusion techniques in plates should receive first consideration since the comparison may be made directly on the same plate. By the use of diffusion cells (Section 14.B.4), both single and double diffusion in one dimension may be also extended to allow the comparative study of two or more antigen solutions or antisera in the same vessel. Subsequent analysis of the precipitated antigens by characteristic color reactions or autoradiography (Section 14.E.4) may be carried out most conveniently on double-diffusion plates.

Techniques which combine electrophoresis and immunochemical analysis require somewhat more elaborate equipment and are not among the most sensitive. They do have the greatest resolving power, however, since they make use of distinct and unrelated properties of the reactants. In addition, of course, immunoelectrophoretic analysis furnishes information on the electrophoretic mobility of antigens or antibodies.

In view of the foregoing discussion, it may be unnecessary to state that no single gel-diffusion technique, nor even a judiciously selected combination of them, is likely to provide satisfactory information without equally critical attention to the preparation of materials and to the interpretation of experimental results in immunochemical terms. In the descriptions of methods in this chapter, a particular effort has been made to offer guidelines in these regards.

d. Sources of Error

In gel-diffusion analysis, as with any analytical method, precautions must be taken in order to avoid certain errors in the determination of the number of the detected constituents. In addition to precipitation reactions due to nonantigenic substances, several artifacts of known cause have been described. They are due to changes in temperature, and therefore in rate of diffusion, or to changes in the concentration of the reactants following certain manipulations (see Section 14.B.1.c). These artifacts are the traces left behind by a moving precipitation zone, and a feature common to them is that the artifacts themselves do not move.[5] It seems that other artifacts of as yet undetermined origin occur with certain techniques. To eliminate most of the known artifacts, and probably to decrease the frequency of others, care should be taken to avoid changes in temperature, changes in concentration of the reagents in their reservoirs during diffusion, and desiccation of the gel; care should also be taken to ensure the adherence of the gel to the walls of the vessel or plate.

It has been reported that, in the reaction of certain systems involving antibodies against simple haptens in double-diffusion plates, two precipitation zones might be observed, one of which does not appear if the immune serum has been deprived of the $C'1$ component of complement.[6]

It was stated in Section a above that, under properly controlled conditions, a single antigen gives rise to a single precipitation zone. The occasional observation of two or more zones formed with presumed single antigens has led to the proposal of contrary hypotheses. One is that several precipitation zones might be formed by antibodies specific for different antigenic determinants reacting with the same antigen molecule. It should be kept in mind that no experimental example could be considered as supporting this opinion unless two conditions are fulfilled: (1) artifacts should either be avoided or recognized with certainty, and (2) the antibodies supposed to be responsible for the distinct precipitation zones should react with the same and conclusively single, antigen.

The latter condition explains why the multiple precipitation zones

[5] J. Oudin, *Proc. 4th Intern. Congr. Allergol., New York, 1961*, pp. 319–338. Macmillan, New York, 1962.

[6] W. E. Paul and B. Benacerraf, *J. Immunol.* **95**, 1067 (1965).

which have been observed in the reaction of the immunoglobulin G by several groups of authors (e.g., Williams and Grabar[7] and Edelman et al.[8]) have not been attributed in the papers quoted to the reaction of a single antigen except as a hypothesis discussed together with the possibility of multiple antigens. At that time the complexity of the IgG was not yet known to be as great as it is now known to be (see, for example, Mannik and Kunkel[9]). Moreover, the IgG's have since then been shown to split slowly in serum without any added enzyme.[10] Two precipitation zones always observed together in the reaction of certain rabbit anti-allotypic sera with the IgG's of certain rabbits were definitely attributed to two distinct antigens, the existence of which was then unexplained.[11] With the knowledge gained since then, they could be logically attributed to subclasses of rabbit IgG heavy or light chains, similar to those demonstrated in man and mouse with the help of myeloma proteins, carrying different but linked genetic markers. This example illustrates that the absence of a precise explanation of two precipitation zones in the reactions of a material which is not definitely known to be a single antigen is not sufficient evidence for the attribution of the multiple zones to the multiplicity of the antibodies alone.

The hypothesis that several antibodies against distinct determinant groups of the same antigen give rise to several precipitation zones does not seem compatible with the reaction of protein antigens. Protein antigens usually possess a number of distinct antigenic determinants. Therefore, according to the discussed hypothesis, several precipitation zones might be expected to be observed in the reaction of a single protein antigen with the homologous antiserum, instead of the single zone which is observed. This shows that the above hypothesis should not be considered correct unless a positive and definite experimental demonstration is provided. On the contrary, several pieces of evidence show that antibodies against several distinct specific groups of the same antigen do not give rise to several precipitation zones in gels. The molecule of human serum albumin was split enzymatically into three antigenically distinct fragments. The three precipitation zones given by the reaction of a preparation of the degraded protein coalesced into the single zone of the native albumin reacting next to it with the same antiserum.[12]

[7] C. A. Williams and P. Grabar, *J. Immunol.* **74**, 158 (1955).
[8] G. M. Edelman, J. Heremans, M. T. Heremans, and H. G. Kunkel, *J. Exptl. Med.* **112**, 203 (1960).
[9] M. Mannik and H. G. Kunkel, *J. Exptl. Med.* **117**, 213 (1965).
[10] F. Skvaril, *Nature* **185**, 475 (1960).
[11] J. Oudin, *J. Exptl. Med.* **112**, 107 (1960).
[12] C. Lapresle, *Ann. Inst. Pasteur* **89**, 654 (1965).

Moreover, attempts have been made to observe two precipitation zones which would have been generated by the reaction of two distinct haptenic groups attached to the same molecule with the homologous antibodies. These attempts resulted in single zones in simple diffusion[13] and in double diffusion[14] although in the double diffusion Fujio *et al.* had purposely varied the proportions of the two antisera in the reacting mixture in order to try to include the conditions eventually favorable to the appearance of two zones.

It is of course conceivable that a cause of multiple precipitation zones, of a still undescribed kind or undemonstrated mechanism, may be encountered. But it follows from experience acquired to date that its manifestation would be very exceptional.

[13] M. Richter, B. Rose, and A. H. Sehon, *Can. J. Biochem. Physiol.* **36**, 1105 (1958).
[14] H. Fujio, Y. Noma, and T. Amano, *Biken's J.* **2**, 35 (1959).

2. DIFFUSION THEORY FOR ANTIGEN–ANTIBODY REACTIONS IN GELS*

a. GENERAL

The basic hypothesis of the theory of diffusion is that the rate of transfer of diffusing material across an infinitesimally small element of area is proportional to the concentration gradient of the material in the direction perpendicular to the area. This may be expressed as

$$F = -D \frac{\partial C}{\partial n} \tag{1}$$

where F is the flux, i.e., the rate of transfer of diffusing material per unit area of the plane per unit time, C is the concentration of diffusing material (a function of position and time), $\partial C/\partial n$ is the concentration gradient at n, where n denotes the direction perpendicular to the element of area, and D is a proportionality constant called the diffusion coefficient. In general, the value of D for a given material will vary somewhat with temperature and concentration. In cases of low concentration, if the temperature is constant and the medium isotropic (i.e., there is no preferential direction of diffusion), D may be considered a constant for a given diffusing substance in a given medium, and it will be considered as such in this section. The negative sign in Eq. (1) indicates that diffusion occurs in the direction opposite to that of concentration increase.

We note from Eq. (1) that the amount of substance crossing a given infinitesimally small area in an infinitesimally small interval of time

* Section 14.A.2 was contributed by Frederick Aladjem.

is proportional to the area and to the concentration gradient. This may be expressed as

$$dM = -DA \frac{\partial C}{\partial n} dt \tag{2a}$$

where dM is the amount of material which crosses area A in time interval dt. The amount of material transferred across area A after time t is

$$M = - \int_0^t DA \frac{\partial C}{\partial n} dt \tag{2b}$$

b. The Diffusion Equation

We now derive the equation for one-dimensional diffusion, which includes all cases of diffusion in which, for reasons of symmetry or otherwise, the distribution of diffusing material varies along only one of the coordinates of three-dimensional space. Diffusion is considered to take place along the x-coordinate. We examine first the processes which take place during a small interval of time dt in the volume bounded by cross-sectional areas at x and some small distance away at $x + dx$. If we call dM the amount of material which enters at x, then the amount of mate-

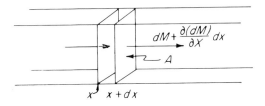

rial which leaves at $x + dx$ is to a first-degree approximation $dM + [\partial(dM)/\partial x]\, dx$. By the law of conservation of matter, the amount of material which accumulates in the time interval dt between x and $x + dx$ is

$$dM - \left(dM + \frac{\partial(dM)}{\partial x} dx \right) = - \frac{\partial(dM)}{\partial x} dx \tag{3}$$

The concentration of material which accumulates in the small volume $A\, dx$ is

$$- \frac{1}{A\, dx} \frac{\partial(dM)}{\partial x} dx$$

We may rewrite Eq. (3) in terms of concentration to obtain

$$\frac{\partial C}{\partial t} dt = - \frac{1}{A} \frac{\partial(dM)}{\partial x} \tag{4}$$

Differentiating Eq. (2a) we have

$$\frac{\partial(dM)}{\partial x} = -DA \frac{\partial^2 C}{\partial x^2} dt \tag{5}$$

Now, from Eqs. (4) and (5) we obtain

$$\frac{\partial C}{\partial t} = D \frac{\partial^2 C}{\partial x^2} \tag{6a}$$

which is the diffusion equation for one-dimensional diffusion in an isotropic medium with the diffusion coefficient constant.

By analogous reasoning[1] the equation for two-dimensional diffusion is found to be

$$\frac{\partial C}{\partial t} = D \left[\frac{\partial^2 C}{\partial x^2} + \frac{\partial^2 C}{\partial y^2} \right] \tag{6b}$$

and for diffusion in three dimensions it is

$$\frac{\partial C}{\partial t} = D \left[\frac{\partial^2 C}{\partial x^2} + \frac{\partial^2 C}{\partial y^2} + \frac{\partial^2 C}{\partial z^2} \right] \tag{6c}$$

c. Solutions of the Diffusion Equation

i. One-Dimensional Diffusion

Let us first consider the simplest case: a long tube of unit cross-sectional area at time $t = 0$ contains material in an infinitely thin plane at $x = 0$, where x is distance measured along the axis of the tube. At time $t > 0$ diffusion occurs in the positive and negative x-direction. For these conditions the solution of Eq. (6a) is

$$C(x, t) = \frac{M_0}{(4\pi Dt)^{1/2}} e^{-x^2/4Dt} \tag{7a}$$

where $C(x, t)$ is the concentration distribution of diffusing material at $t > 0$, i.e., the concentration of material at any point x, at any time t, and M_0 is the amount of material which was initially deposited in the plane at $x = 0$. This expression describes mathematically the familiar bell-shaped or "Gaussian" concentration profile, which originates as an abrupt peak and spreads as time progresses. Equation (7a) may be derived and

[1] J. Crank, "The Mathematics of Diffusion," Chapter 1. Oxford Univ. Press, London and New York, 1956.

shown to be a unique solution of Eq. (6a) by several methods,[2,3] but the matter is best left to mathematicians.

The usual geometric arrangement in tubes is the following: the bottom half of a tube is filled with antibody incorporated in agar; the top half is filled with antigen. We shall assume that antigen and antibody diffuse independently of each other and describe diffusion of antibody; diffusion of antigen would be described in an entirely analogous manner. We consider a rectangular coordinate system and locate the origin $x = 0$ of the coordinate system at the interface between antigen and antibody.

At the beginning of the experiment, $t = 0$, we have $C = C_0$, $x < x_0$; $C = 0$, $x > x_0$, where C is the amount of material per unit cross-sectional area at x, $-\infty < x < +\infty$. We divide the region $x < 0$ into infinitesimal intervals of width $d\xi$, where ξ represents the distance from the origin $x = 0$ to the interval $d\xi$. Diffusion in the system for $t > 0$ can be viewed as the composite of diffusion from all such intervals. We consider diffusion from an interval $d\xi$ to be approximated by the one-dimensional diffusion from a point source containing the same amount of material $C_0\, d\xi$ located at $x = \xi$

According to Eq. (7a), diffusion from such a point source will yield concentration

$$C_{d\xi}(x, t) = \frac{C_0\, d\xi}{(4\pi Dt)^{\frac{1}{2}}}\, e^{-(x-\xi)^2/4Dt} \tag{8}$$

at x. The contribution at x from all such point sources is obtained by superimposing all the individual contributions* to give

$$C(x, t) = \frac{C_0}{2}\left(1 - \frac{2}{\pi^{\frac{1}{2}}} \int_0^y e^{-y^2}\, dy\right) \tag{9a}$$

[2] J. Crank, "The Mathematics of Diffusion," Chapter 2. Oxford Univ. Press, London and New York, 1956.

[3] T. Mathews and R. L. Walker, "Mathematical Theory of Physics," Chapter 8. Benjamin, New York, 1965.

*

$$C(x, t) = \int_{-\infty}^0 C_{d\xi}(x, t) = \frac{C_0}{(4\pi Dt)^{\frac{1}{2}}} \int_{-\infty}^0 e^{-(x-\xi)^2/4Dt}\, d\xi = \frac{C_0}{\pi^{\frac{1}{2}}} \int_{x/(4Dt)^{\frac{1}{2}}}^{\infty} e^{-\eta^2}\, d\eta$$

where $\eta = (x - \xi)/(4Dt)^{\frac{1}{2}}$. Simplifying, we obtain

$$C(x, t) = \frac{C_0}{\pi^{\frac{1}{2}}} \int_y^{\infty} e^{-y^2}\, dy = \frac{C_0}{\pi^{\frac{1}{2}}} \int_0^{\infty} e^{-y^2}\, dy - \frac{C_0}{\pi^{\frac{1}{2}}} \int_0^y e^{-y^2}\, dy$$

$$= \frac{C_0}{2} - \frac{C_0}{\pi^{\frac{1}{2}}} \int_0^y e^{-y^2}\, dy = \frac{C_0}{2}\left(1 - \frac{2}{\pi^{\frac{1}{2}}} \int_0^y e^{-y^2}\, dy\right) \tag{9a}$$

where $y = x/(\pi Dt)^{1/2}$. If the concentration at the interface is maintained at the constant value C_0, then Eq. (9a) becomes

$$C(x, t) = C_0 \left(1 - \frac{2}{\pi^{1/2}} \int_0^y e^{-y^2}\, dy\right) \tag{9b}$$

Equations (9) are the basic equations that are used to describe immuno-diffusion in tubes.[4]

ii. Two-Dimensional Diffusion

We consider antigen and antibody to be placed into cylindrical wells of radius s in a diffusion plate, and we consider a cartesian coordinate system such that the center of the antigen well lies at $x = y = 0$ and the center of the antibody well lies at $x = a$, $y = 0$. We assume that antigen and antibody are deposited isotropically and that the height of the wells is identical to the height of the plate. The concentration distribution of material as a consequence of diffusion into the x-y plane can then be considered as a two-dimensional problem, namely diffusion from a disk-shaped source into the plane, rather than the more cumbersome diffusion from a cylindrical source into a volume.[5]

To apply the diffusion equation we must make certain assumptions about the reactive properties of the system. We will first assume that interactions between antigen and antibody before the initial zone of precipitation forms are so small as to be negligible, i.e., that diffusion of antigen and antibody are independent of each other. The boundary conditions for the solution of the diffusion equation then are

1. $C(r, 0) = M_0/\pi s^2$ when $r < s$
   $C(r, 0) = 0$ when $r > s$
2. $C(r, t) \to 0$ as $r \to \infty$, $t > 0$

where $r^2 = x^2 + y^2$, $C(r, t) =$ concentration (mass per unit area) of diffusing antigen or antibody at time t at distance r from the center of the well in which amount M_0 grams material was initially deposited.

For these conditions, the solution of the diffusion equation is given by Crank[6]

$$C(r, t) = \frac{M_0}{4\pi Dt} e^{-r^2/4Dt} \left[\frac{2}{s^2} \int_0^s e^{-s^2/4Dt} I_0\left(\frac{rs}{2Dt}\right) s\, ds\right] \tag{10}$$

where I_0 is the modified Bessel function of the first kind of order zero.*

[4] E. L. Becker, *Arch. Biochem. Biophys.* **93**, 617 (1961).
[5] F. Aladjem, *J. Immunol.* **93**, 682 (1964).
[6] J. Crank, "The Mathematics of Diffusion, Chapter 3. Oxford Univ. Press, London and New York, 1956.

* This expression may be derived by a superposition method resembling that of the previous footnote. Situations involving circular symmetry commonly give rise to Bessel functions.

The right side of Eq. (10) is the product of two terms. The first term, the term outside the square bracket, gives the concentration distribution that would occur as a consequence of diffusion from a point source. The second term, the term within the square brackets, gives the effect of the finite area of the well on the concentration distribution.

$C(r, t)$ as a function of r for several values of Dt for diffusion from a point source as well as from several area sources of interest ($s = 0.1$, 0.3, and 0.5 cm) is given in Figs. 1 through 4.

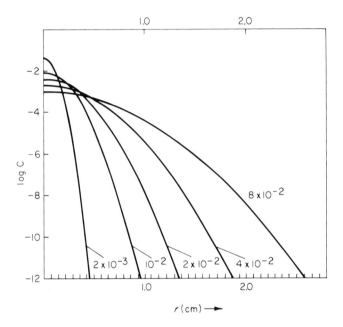

Fig. 1. The concentration distribution of diffusing material. Ordinate: concentration, abscissa: distance. The curves are for indicated values of Dt. $M_0 = 1$ mg; $s = 0$ (point source). Equation (10) was used for these calculations.

These graphs are meant primarily to convey a visual picture of the relation of concentration of diffusing material as a function of time and distance of diffusion. On the ordinate the logarithm of the concentration is plotted rather than the concentration to show the behavior of concentration distribution over a wide range of concentrations. It is to be noted from Eq. (10) that $C(r, t)$ is directly proportional to M_0, that there exists no simple relationship between $C(r, t)$ and D, t, r, or s, and that the diffusion coefficient and the time of diffusion always occur as the product Dt.

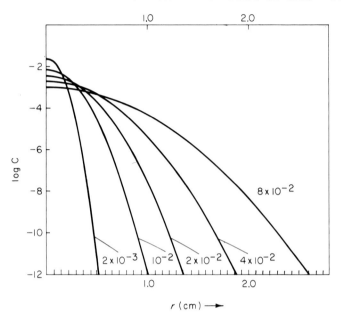

FIG. 2. Same as Fig. 1, except $s = 0.1$ cm (area source).

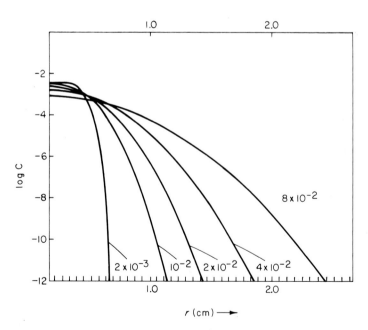

FIG. 3. Same as Fig. 1, except $s = 0.3$ cm (area source).

Figures 1 through 4 may also be used as an aid in deciding whether or not an observed precipitation line could indeed be due to the antigen–antibody system to which it is ascribed. The reasoning for this type of analysis is as follows: from experience with the quantitative precipitin reaction it is known that at least of the order of 1 μg/ml antigen–antibody precipitate is required for visible precipitation. The ratio of antibody to antigen in the precipitate varies over relatively narrow limits. For the egg albumin–rabbit anti-egg albumin system, for instance, mole ratios between approximately 5 and 2 (antibody excess–antigen excess) have

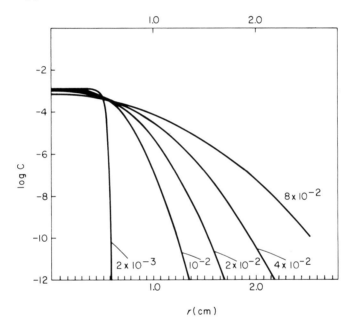

FIG. 4. Same as Fig. 1, except $s = 0.5$ cm (area source).

been observed; for human serum albumin–rabbit antiserum, mole ratios in the precipitates vary between approximately 7 and 2. Grossly, then, for such systems of the order of 0.1 μg of antigen and 1 μg of antibody have to be present at the location where the initial zone of precipitation becomes visible, at the time the zone becomes visible.

Suppose we perform an immunodiffusion experiment with 1 mg of human serum albumin and 1 mg of rabbit antibody, each placed into cylindrical wells of 0.5 cm radius; let the distance from the center of the wells be 2.5 cm. We may expect to observe the initial zone of precipitation about 1.4 cm from the center of the antigen well, 1.1 cm from the center of the antibody well, at about 6×10^4 sec.[7] Diffusion coefficient for human serum albumin (D_A) is about 6×10^{-7} cm²/sec, that for antibody (D_{AB}) about 4×10^{-7} cm²/sec; hence $D_A t = 0.036$ cm² and $D_{AB} t = 0.024$ cm². From Fig. 4 we see that for $Dt = 0.036$, $C(r, t) \simeq 2.5 \times 10^{-7}$ gm/cm² and for $Dt = 0.024$, $C(r, t) \simeq 2.5 \times 10^{-6}$ gm/cm², i.e., reasonable values. Suppose, now, that we had observed the initial zone of precipitation at the same time but 3 mm closer to the antigen well, i.e., 1.1 cm from the antigen well and 1.4 cm from the antibody well. The calculated values of $C(r, t)$ would then be approximately reversed: the antigen concentration would be 1×10^{-5} gm/cm², the antibody concentration 1.4×10^{-8} gm/cm²; i.e., we would have apparently an antigen–antibody mole ratio of 1600 in the initial zone of precipitation—an absurd result from the point of view of the precipitin reaction. Since this is much too large an error to be accounted for by the imperfection of immunodiffusion theory, we would suspect either an enormous error in M_0 and/or an error in Dt. An error in Dt would usually be due to an error in D because the appearance of the initial zone of precipitation can usually be established to within 15 to 30 minutes, i.e., within an error of a few percent. Both a very large error in M_0 and an error in D would cause us to doubt whether the material which gave rise to the zone of precipitation is indeed the material it was assumed to be.

An aid to such an analysis will be the curvature of the zone of precipitation as the zone develops. If $D_{AB} > D_A$ the zone will usually be curved convex toward the antigen well; if $D_{AB} < D_A$ it will usually be convex toward the antibody well; and if $D_{AB} = D_A$ it will usually have the form of a straight line.[7, 8]

So far we have only considered free diffusion. A first approximation which allows us to take into account antigen–antibody interaction is to assume that antigen–antibody complex formation occurs only at the location where the initial zone of precipitation will eventually form. If antigen and antibody arrive at that location at rates which lead to participation of all antigen and antibody molecules in complex formation, then the boundary condition for antigen and antibody will be $C(r, t) = 0$ at $r > r_p$, $t > 0$, where r_p is the distance from the center of the respective antigen or antibody wells to the location of the initial zone of precipitation. This location has been called the "sink."

M sink/cm, the amount of material which accumulates per unit length

[7] F. Aladjem, R. W. Jaross, R. L. Paldino, and J. A. Lackner, *J. Immunol.* **83**, 221 (1959).

[8] L. Korngold and G. van Leeuwen, *J. Immunol.* **78**, 172 (1957).

at r_p, is approximately

$$M \text{ sink/cm} = \frac{M_0}{2\pi r_p s^2 Dt} \int_{r_p}^{\infty} e^{-r^2/4Dt} \int_0^s e^{-s^2/4Dt} I_0 \left(\frac{rs}{2Dt} \right) s \, ds \, r \, dr \quad (11)$$

The reason this equation is approximate is that it does not take into account the increased rate of diffusion over free diffusion which results as a consequence of the condition $C = 0$ at r_p. This increased rate of diffusion was termed "sink effect"[9]; it can best be visualized by the analogy of a river (diffusion), a waterfall (the sink), and the rapids (the sink effect).

An exact solution of the diffusion equation for the boundary condition

   1. $C(r, 0) = M_0/\pi s^2$,
   2. $C(r, t) = 0$ when $r > r_p$, $t > 0$

has been shown[5] to be

$$M \text{ sink/cm} = \frac{2M_0}{\pi r_p^2 s} \sum_{n=1}^{\infty} \frac{J_1(s\alpha_n)}{\alpha_n^2 J_1(r_p \alpha_n)} (1 - e^{-D\alpha_n^2 t}) \quad (12)$$

where J_0 and J_1 are the Bessel function of order zero and one, respectively, and α_n is the nth positive root of $J_0(\alpha r_p)$.

Comparative computations based upon Eqs. (9), (10), and (11) have been reported.[5]

It should be pointed out that whenever it is intended to analyze immunodiffusion reactions by the methods just described, it is advisable to perform experiments with sufficiently large initial amounts of antigen and antibody to obtain sharp zones of precipitation. If either reagent is present in very low concentration, then the time required for precipitate formation may become significant compared to the time required for diffusion and error would be introduced in that way.

The mathematical treatment of immunoelectrophoresis is essentially identical to that of double diffusion in gels.[9]

We would like to conclude on an optimistic note. While we cannot expect to have exact expressions for analysis by diffusion in gels as long as we cannot describe accurately the processes of antigen–antibody combination and precipitation, we may confidently expect that the development of high speed computers will allow us to analyze precipitin and diffusion data with successively better approximations, that such analyses should lead to new and more incisive experiments, and hence a more rigorous understanding of immunochemical reactions.[5, 10]

[9] F. Aladjem, H. Klostergard, and R. W. Taylor, *J. Theoret. Biol.* **3**, 134 (1962).
[10] F. Aladjem, M. T. Palmiter, and Fu-Wu Chang, *Immunochemistry* **3**, 419 (1966).

B. Qualitative Analysis of Antigen–Antibody Reactions in Gels

1. SIMPLE DIFFUSION IN TUBES*

The term "simple diffusion" designates the system in which solutions of antigens and of antibodies are placed in two contiguous layers or regions, in contrast with "double diffusion," in which the two reactants diffuse toward each other through a zone of gel which initially separates the two solutions[1] (see Section 14.A.1).

The techniques of simple diffusion and the principle of immunochemical analysis in gels were described first in 1946.[2] Such analyses are nearly always carried out in tubes or in cells with parallel walls. Cells adaptable to simple and double diffusion are described in Section 14.B.4.

a. Techniques

i. Preparation of Tubes

The tubes used in the author's laboratory are usually of 1.5 to 2 mm internal diameter, with walls 0.2 to 0.5 mm thick, and about 10 cm long. This internal diameter is small enough to conserve reactants and large enough so that the solutions can be introduced into the tubes without difficulty. Narrower tubes (1 mm i.d. or even less) may be used if necessary to conserve precious reagents.

Glass tubing of uniform diameter is cut into segments 10 cm long. The tubes are cleaned with sulfochromic acid, rinsed with tap water and then with distilled water, dried, and sealed with a flame at one end.

Agar gel normally does not adhere to the glass. To prevent the reagents from seeping between the gel and the glass, the internal walls of the tubes are coated with agar and dried.[3] The tubes are placed in water at 60° to 70° with 1 to 3 cm above water level. Each tube is filled with 0.2% agar solution at 60° to 70° using a drawn Pasteur pipet which reaches the bottom of the tube and is controlled by a rubber mouth tube. The tube is immediately emptied with the same pipet and placed in an ice bath to solidify the thin layer of agar. This layer is then dried by putting the tube in a vacuum desiccator over phosphorus pentoxide. If the agar solution contains salt, the tube will have a moiré appearance that will disappear as soon as the reagents are placed in the tube.

* Section 14.B.1 was contributed by Jacques Oudin.

[1] J. Oudin, *Methods Med. Res.* **5**, 335–378 (1952).
[2] J. Oudin, *Compt. Rend.* **222**, 115–116 (1946).
[3] J. Oudin, *Ann. Inst. Pasteur* **75**, Part 1, 30–51; Part 2, 109–129 (1948).

ii. Introduction of the Reagents

The first layer to be introduced, which is always a gel, usually contains the antibodies. The immune serum (or the antibody solution), diluted if necessary, is placed in a water bath at a temperature between 45° and 50°. The agar solution, which should be perfectly clear, is rapidly melted in boiling water and placed in the same bath. These two solutions, containing some suitable antiseptic (e.g., Merthiolate 1:5000 or sodium azide 1:2500) are mixed in proportions calculated to bring both the antibodies and the agar to the desired final concentration. The optimal concentration of agar varies according to the preparation and source of agar. In the author's laboratory, Difco Agar Noble is now used at the final concentration of 0.2%. A higher concentration increases the opalescence of the gel and decreases the rate of migration of the precipitation zones. If one wishes to remove the plug of agar from the glass tube, however, a higher concentration must be used. When the aim of the experiment is essentially qualitative and the antigen concentration sufficiently large, the dilution of immune serum in the gel is usually between 1:4 and 3:4. The agar mixture for the lower layer is distributed in the tubes (avoiding bubbles), with a Pasteur pipet whose delivery is controlled by a mouth tube. This layer is usually 35 to 45 mm high.

Tubes may be used as soon as the agar solidifies, but they may also be stored for up to several weeks or months at 0° to 4° under conditions that avoid drying.[4]

The upper layer (usually containing antigens) is distributed to a height approximately uniform in all the tubes to be compared. This height is usually about 35 mm, although it can be as low as 10 mm to spare the solutions. The layer of antigen solution is nearly always liquid. Sometimes this layer too is a gel—for example, when the reaction of antibodies of the flocculating type (e.g., horse antitoxin) diffusing from the lower layer is to be observed. The interface is often difficult to see when both layers are gels.

The tubes must be hermetically sealed. In the author's laboratory, a mixture of beeswax and vacuum seal (Mastic P, Compagnie Générale de Radiologie, Paris) is used. Other materials—for example, modeling clay—may also be used.

iii. Conditions for Development, Observation, and Photography of the Reactions

It is advisable not to subject the tubes in which reactions are in progress to changes in temperature, especially to sharp changes, because of the

[4] H. M. Rubinstein, *J. Immunol.* **73**, 322–330 (1954).

artifacts that may be provoked. A constant temperature bath would probably provide ideal conditions for keeping the tubes except that it is difficult to observe and photograph the tubes without taking them out of the bath. In the author's laboratory, a special room is used, in which the temperature is maintained sufficiently constant by successive heatings and coolings close enough to each other so that the possible artifacts are usually not apparent. The average temperature is 20°, but other temperatures might be as suitable. An incubator cabinet at 37° would not be satisfactory because of temperature falls each time the door is opened. Accurate results may be obtained with tubes left in the laboratory, as long as one remembers that the artifacts due to changes in temperature have a characteristic appearance and are immobile (see Section 14.A.1.d).

It is very convenient to photograph the tubes, preferably after a constant time and at a constant enlargement enabling one to measure and compare the appearances of tubes on the photographs, even for reactions performed at different times. In the author's laboratory, the enlargement chosen is 2×, which allows 15 tubes to be photographed side by side (placed on a suitable frame built for this purpose) on a 9 by 12 cm photographic plate. For convenience of scheduling, the time of reaction chosen for photography is 7 days. Often, however, the tubes are observed and the results read after much shorter times, sometimes after a few hours. The tubes are illuminated from behind (below and above) by two horizontal fluorescent tubes and are observed or photographed against a background of black velvet. The angle of incidence of the light is important for the photography. Generally speaking, a small angle gives a greater sensitivity, and a wider angle probably gives better resolution.

Instruments have been devised, or adapted, for the measurement of the density of precipitate at the various levels of the tubes.[5]

b. Development of the Reaction

i. Appearance of Reaction

Development of the reaction will be described for the case of a protein antigen diffusing into a gel containing rabbit antibodies. It will be supposed that the antigen and the antibodies have the same diffusion coefficient and that the antigen is in excess of the antibodies, i.e., that the ratio of the initial concentrations of antigen and antibodies is greater than the equivalence ratio. Precipitation occurs rapidly (usually within a few minutes, rarely in a few hours) in the lower layer near the interface. Initially, the moving front of precipitate retains the curvature of the

---

[5] W. G. Glenn and A. C. Garner, *J. Immunol.* **78**, 395–400 (1957).

interface, but as the precipitation zone* moves downward its leading edge tends to flatten into a plane perpendicular to the axis of the tube (see Fig. 1). The leading edge is usually sharp when the antigen is a protein, although it may be less discrete depending on the antibodies, or even diffuse with certain immune sera. Some of the various kinds of precipitation zones that may be observed are shown in Fig. 3. Maximal density of precipitate is found close to the sharp leading edge; above this level the precipitate is more or less dissolved by the antigen in excess. The precipitation zone is shortened as the antigen excess is increased. Thus, a large excess of antigen is always advantageous, in contrast with certain double-diffusion techniques, for which the best ratio of the initial concentrations is equivalence.

ii. Principles of the Reaction

Many experimental results and conclusions, important even from a purely qualitative standpoint, are obtained from the comparison of several tubes. Thus, to interpret correctly the difference between the tubes under comparison, one has to avoid those differences which are due to unrecognized or uncontrolled variables. For the theoretical treatment of the development of the reactions, see Spiers and Augustin,[6] and Section 14.A.2.

(a) *Simple Precipitating Systems.* A single antigen takes part in the reaction, giving a single precipitation zone. The precipitation zone moves away from the interface into the antibody layer when the antigen is in excess. The distance h between the interface and the leading edge of the precipitation zone is often called *penetration* of the zone.

(1) *Variation of penetration with time and reagent concentrations.* The distance between the interface (or rather between a virtual origin often located a few tenths of a millimeter above the interface because of its convex shape) and the leading edge of the zone is proportional to the square root of time t (Fig. 1).

An increase in the initial antigen concentration causes an increase of the ratio $h/\sqrt{t}$. An increase in the initial antibody concentration causes a decrease of the ratio $h/\sqrt{t}$.

Within a fairly wide range of the antigen and antibody concentrations, the ratio $h/\sqrt{t}$ is essentially a linear function of the logarithm of the initial concentrations of antigen if the concentration of antibody is kept

---

* The term "precipitation zone" has been chosen instead of "zone of precipitate" in order to emphasize the fact that the movement of the zone is due to new precipitation at the leading edge, and dissolution (in most cases) at the trailing edge. The precipitate itself does not move.

[6] J. A. Spiers and R. Augustin, *Trans. Faraday Soc.* **54**, 287–295 (1958).

constant (Fig. 2A), or of the initial concentration of antibody if the antigen is constant (Fig. 2B).[7]

The slope of the straight line which represents the variation of $h/\sqrt{t}$ with respect to the logarithm of the antigen concentration is approximately proportional to the square root of the diffusion coefficient of the antigen.[8] Another relationship has been derived, which applies to the case when antigen concentration is very large and antibody concentration

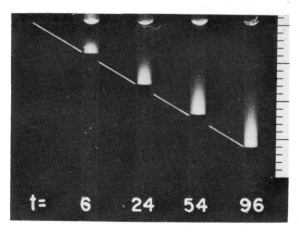

FIG. 1. Time course of the reaction of a simple precipitating system, demonstrating the law $h/\sqrt{t}$ = constant. The liquid antigen solution (human serum albumin, 4 mg of N per milliliter) and lower layer of rabbit anti-human serum albumin serum with agar were identical for all four tubes. The reaction was started (i.e., the antigen solution introduced) in the 4 tubes at, respectively, 6, 24, 54, and 96 hours before the photograph was taken. Since the square roots of the reaction times form an arithmetic progression and the space between two neighboring tubes is approximately uniform, the leading edges of the precipitation zones lie on a straight line, as indicated by the white dashes. An artifact due to a change in temperature is visible above the leading edge of the first tube from the left. A scale graduated in millimeters (small divisions) is shown on the right.

small. Under these conditions, h^2/t instead of $h/\sqrt{t}$ becomes a linear function of the logarithm of the antigen concentration.[9]

When the two layers of reagents are gels, the ratio $h/\sqrt{t}$ approaches 0 when the ratio of antigen concentration to antibody concentration is close to the equivalence ratio. If the diffusion coefficients of the antigen, D_G, and of the antibody, D_A, are different, $h/\sqrt{t}$ approaches 0 when the ratio of

[7] J. Oudin, *Compt. Rend.* **228**, 1890–1892 (1949).

[8] J. C. Neff and E. L. Becker, *J. Immunol.* **78**, 5–10 (1957).

[9] E. L. Becker, J. Munoz, C. Lapresle, and L. Lebeau, *J. Immunol.* **67**, 501–511 (1951).

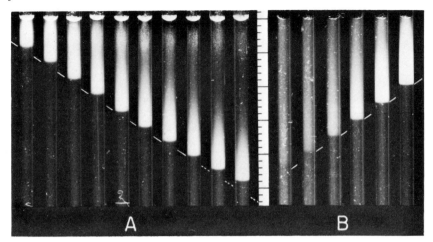

FIG. 2. (A) Reaction of a constant concentration of antibody with progressively increasing concentrations of antigen, photographed after 7 days. The lower (agar) layer in each tube contains a 1:16 dilution of antiserum albumin immune serum in agar. The upper (liquid) layer contains serum albumin in doubling concentrations from 4 μg of N per milliliter in the first tube on the extreme left. The penetration, h, in the first 8 tubes can be seen to vary linearly as the logarithm of the antigen concentration. Also it should be noted that the maximum density of precipitate of the zone is approximately the same in all but the first tube. Care was taken that the total density of the upper layer in all tubes was definitely greater than that of the diluted immune serum of the lower layer. For this purpose, the antigen dilutions were made in normal rabbit serum.

(B) Same reagents as in A. Reaction of a constant concentration of antigen (0.25 mg of N per milliliter) with progressively increasing concentrations of antibody in a geometrical progression of ratio 2 (photograph taken after 7 days). The dilutions of the immune serum in the lower (gel) layer (from left to right, 1:128 to 1:4) were obtained by mixing 0.4% agar with equal volumes of 2-fold dilutions of the immune serum in normal rabbit serum. The values of penetrations vary linearly as the logarithm of the antibody concentration, decreasing as the antibody concentration increases. The maximum density of the zone increases with the increasing antibody concentration.

antigen and antibody concentrations equals the equivalence ratio multiplied by $\sqrt{D_A/D_G}$.[6]

(2) *Other variables influencing penetration.* For one antibody concentration in the lower layer (gel) and one antigen concentration in the upper layer (liquid), two widely different values of h may be observed according to the total concentration of the substances dissolved in these layers, including the diffusible substances that are neither antigen nor antibodies.[10] The higher value of h is obtained for a density of the upper layer

[10] J. Oudin, *Discussions Faraday Soc.* **18,** 351–357 (1954).

greater than that in the lower layer. When both layers are gels, the value of h is the same as the lower value of h when the antigen solution is liquid. These differences have been explained as effects of convection phenomena, in keeping with the fact that they are not observed when both layers are gels.[11] As long as suitable precautions are taken it is not necessary, as it is sometimes stated, to use agar in both layers in order to avoid uncontrolled effects on penetration of the zones. In all the reactions shown in the accompanying figures, the antigen solutions were liquid. When the antigen solution is liquid, however, care should be taken that the density of this layer is either greater in all tubes to be compared, or lower in all tubes, than the density of the solution in the gel layer (the latter density being that which would be realized if this solution contained all the water and diffusible substances of the layer, but not the agar). An example of such a precaution is described in the legend to Fig. 2.

Substances other than antibody, in solution in the layer where the precipitation zone moves, may still modify the penetration of the zone through a modification of viscosity. The slope of the curve of $h/\sqrt{t}$ versus the logarithm of the initial antigen concentration is inversely proportional to the square root of the viscosity of the antibody solution.[8]

(3) *Density of precipitate.* The maximum density of the precipitation zone is essentially a function of only the antibody concentration, when the antigen is in sufficient excess. The maximum density is then almost independent of the antigen concentration and of time. When the antigen excess is small and particularly when the ratio is close to equivalence, the density of precipitate increases with time. It is easily understood that, when the conditions are such that the precipitation zone does not move, the precipitate accumulates at the level of the zone because of the continuous arrival of antigen and antibody.

Certain aspects of the reaction may change with the nature and precise origin of the reagents. The leading edge of the precipitation zone of one given antigen may be sharp or indistinct depending on the antibodies: a larger proportion of nonprecipitating antibodies seems to produce a less sharp leading edge (Fig. 3, C and D). In contrast with the leading edges of the precipitation zones of proteins (usually but not always sharp; see Fig. 7), those of polysaccharides are usually indistinct (Fig. 3, G). In the reaction of a given antigen with a given immune serum, the larger the antigen excess the narrower is the precipitation zone (Fig. 2). In addition, for a given antigen, a given value of the antigen excess, and a given antibody concentration, the extent of the zone in height may vary with the type of immunization and the species of the animal which produced

[11] J. R. Preer, Jr. and W. H. Telfer, *J. Immunol.* **79**, 288–293 (1957).

the antibodies (Fig. 3, A, B and E, F). The extent of the zone is sometimes smaller when the antibodies are of the horse antitoxin (flocculating)
type rather than of the rabbit (precipitating) type.

When antibodies in sufficient excess are layered above, they diffuse

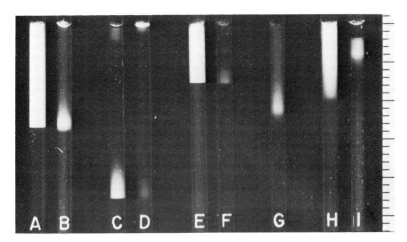

Fig. 3. Appearance of the precipitation zones from the reaction of various simple
precipitating systems. Tubes A to D. Reaction of protein antigens with rabbit immune
sera. Tubes A and B: Ovalbumin at the same concentration reacting with two immune
sera obtained from two rabbits immunized by different routes. The extent to which
the specific precipitate is dissolved by a similar antigen excess is different in the two
immune sera, despite their similar penetrations. Tubes C and D: Horse serum albumin, at the same concentration in both tubes, reacting with the same rabbit immune
serum; in tube D, the immune serum has been partially absorbed by the antigen; in
tube C, the immune serum is diluted in normal rabbit serum to permit a penetration
similar to that in tube D; the appearance of the zone is quite different in the two tubes
(note particularly the diffuse leading edge and the low density in tube D) because
of the larger proportion of nonprecipitating antibodies in tube D. Tubes E and F:
Reaction of human γ-globulin with two horse anti-γ-globulin immune sera showing
the great variation in appearance which can be encountered among the reactions of
various immune sera. Tube G: Reaction of the polysaccharide of the typhoid O antigen
with a rabbit immune serum. The diffuse leading edge is usual for reactions involving
polysaccharide antigens. Tubes H and I: Reactions of antibodies diffusing from the
upper layer into a gel layer containing the homologous antigen; in tube H, rabbit
antibody reacting with ovalbumin; in tube I, horse antibody reacting with human
γ-globulin. Photograph taken after 7 days, except for tubes C and D (6 days).

into the lower gel layer containing the antigen. If the antibodies are of the
horse flocculating type, the precipitation zone in the antigen layer is
separated from the interface by a region where the gel medium is quite
clear because the precipitate has been completely dissolved by the antibodies in excess (Fig. 3, I). If the antibodies are of the rabbit type, then

there is no clear region between the zone and the interface, whatever the antibody excess, but rather the density increases continuously from the leading edge to the interface (Fig. 3, H).

The sensitivity of the reaction in simple diffusion tubes, defined as the smallest concentration of precipitating antibody in the gel layer compatible with a visible precipitation zone when an excess of antigen is used, is of the same order of magnitude, or slightly less, than for the "ring test." This sensitivity may be considerably increased by a modified technique.[12] After the reaction has developed for a suitable time (usually a few hours), the solution containing the antigens is replaced by normal saline. The penetration of the precipitation zones becomes progressively slower (more

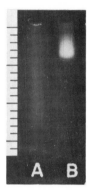

FIG. 4. Photograph, taken after 7 days, of two tubes started with the same reagents: human serum albumin (in large excess) and a poor rabbit homologous immune serum. Three hours after the antigen solution was added, it was replaced by normal saline in tube B but not in tube A. Note that the maximum density of precipitate is considerably greater in tube B than in tube A.

so than it would under normal circumstances), while their density increases with time because of the increase of the amount of antibody which takes part in the reaction (Fig. 4). It has been seen above that the minimal antigen concentration which makes a precipitation zone appear in the antibody layer becomes smaller as the antibody concentration is decreased. The antigen concentration needed can therefore be reduced if the antibody is diluted within the limit below which the precipitation zone would no longer be visible. An antigen whose concentration is too small to make a precipitation zone appear in the antibody layer can also manifest itself by a precipitation zone in the antigen layer if the antigen layer is a clear gel, or by the appearance of a precipitate sedimenting on the interface if the antigen layer is liquid and clear.

[12] J. Oudin, Ann. Inst. Pasteur **85**, 336–347 (1953).

(b) *Multiple Precipitating Systems.* When several precipitation zones appear in a tube, the distances between them remain proportional, since the distance of each of them to the interface is proportional to the square root of time. Furthermore, the maximum density of each changes only slightly unless their rate of migration is very small (Fig. 5). The resolution of the zones increases with time. It is sometimes sufficient to observe the tubes after a few hours; it is rarely necessary to observe them after more than a few days, and a single observation or photograph is nearly always enough.

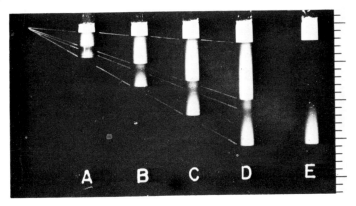

Fig. 5. Tubes A to D: Development of the reaction of a precipitating system with multiple precipitation zones. The reactions were started 6, 24, 54, and 96 hours, respectively, before photographs were made. Since the penetration h for each zone is proportional to $\sqrt{t}$, the respective penetrations of the zones for each component antigen in each tube and the distances between their leading edges remain proportional to each other. The maximal density of precipitate of each zone remains approximately constant. Tube E: Photograph after the same time as that of tube D, of a tube differing from tube D in that the same immune serum had been absorbed with the antigens responsible for two zones. Comparison of tubes D and E shows that non cross-reacting antigens react with specific antibodies independently of one another.

For each of the various distinct antigens which do not cross-react with the same antibodies in the system, a precipitation zone develops independently, each antigen reacting as if it were alone[2] (cf. Fig. 5, D and E). Thus each of the principles mentioned above in Section ii (a) for the simple precipitating systems is valid for each of these zones. Such multiple systems appear therefore as a superposition of the simple systems in which each of the antigens would react separately.

(c) *Complex Precipitating Systems.* If two antigens in a system cross-react with the antibodies, i.e., if some of the antibodies may be precipitated by either antigen (complex system), the penetration and density of the zone of one of these antigens may be influenced by the concentration of the other antigen. The simplest case is that in which the antigen solution contains two antigens cross-reacting with an immune serum homologous with one of them. If the reaction in the tube gives rise to two precipitation zones, the one farther from the interface is that of the heterologous antigen.[3] The distance between the leading edges of the two zones is mainly a function of the ratio of the initial concentrations of the two antigens.[13] Measurement of this distance and comparison with a calibration curve can lead to quantitative conclusions concerning this ratio.[14]

c. Application of Simple Diffusion to Immunochemical Analysis

Only qualitative immunochemical analysis by simple diffusion will be considered here, in its two steps: enumeration and identification of antigens in unknown mixtures. Quantitative analysis is treated in other sections (14.C.5 and 14.C.8) as is the determination of diffusion coefficients of antigens (Section 14.C.1).

i. Enumeration of Antigens

According to the main general principle of immunochemical analysis in gels (Section 14.A.1), the number of precipitation zones is smaller than or equal to the number of the precipitating antigens. The application of this principle, however, requires some test designed to distinguish the actual precipitation zones due to distinct antigens from that which might look like them. In the case of simple diffusion in tubes, this is nearly always very simple.

Precipitations which are not due to specific interaction of antigen with its antibody rarely resemble antigen–antibody precipitations. In addition, such precipitations would probably occur also in control tubes, for example, in which the immune serum would have been replaced in the lower layer by the serum of an unimmunized animal.

Rapid changes in temperature may sharply modify the density of the precipitation zones at the precise level at which antigen is combining with free antibody, i.e., at the leading edge. In case of a rise of temperature at the moment of the change, the density becomes abruptly greater for a short distance than it would have been if the temperature had remained constant (Fig. 6). Conversely, a sharp decrease in temperature causes a narrow band of decreased density in the precipitation zone. This phenomenon is explained by the increase in the number of the molecules of antigen and antibody coming initially into contact when temperature

[13] D. J. Buchanan-Davidson and J. Oudin, *J. Immunol.* **81**, 484–491 (1958).
[14] P. Bornstein and J. Oudin, *J. Exptl. Med.* **120**, 655–676 (1964).

is raised, and by a decrease in collisions when temperature is decreased. Of course, the position of the temperature-induced change in density does not migrate with time since formed precipitate itself does not move.[3] This effect of temperature fluctuations does not involve any property unique to antigen or antibodies, as it also may be observed with inorganic reagents[15] (Fig. 6, D). The appearance of these changes in density is rarely similar to that of precipitation zones. Moreover, because their

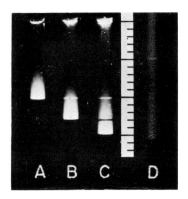

FIG. 6. Effect of sharp changes in temperature on the appearance of a precipitation zone. Photographs A, B, and C, taken at three successive times, show a tube in which hen ovalbumin (upper layer) was reacted with a homologous rabbit immune serum (gel layer). The tube was incubated at 20° for 49 hours and photographed (A). Immediately after photography, the tube was transferred at 37°. Twenty-three hours later, the tube was brought back to the room at 20° and immediately photographed again (B). Photograph C, taken 24 hours later, shows that the two striae due to changes in temperature remained at the level where the leading edge was when they appeared. Photograph D shows the lower part of a tube where ammonium sulfate was diffusing into a gel containing barium chloride. Changes in temperature, similar to those above, caused the same two kinds of striae.

immobility contrasts with the regular migration of the specific precipitation zones, errors of interpretation due to this cause are nearly always easy to avoid.

These two sources of error in simple diffusion in tubes, nonspecific precipitation and temperature effects, are the only ones that have been met in the author's laboratory. Nothing has ever been observed that might suggest a useful correlation with a phenomenon of the Liesegang type. As far as the author is aware, no unequivocal example of a Liesegang phenomenon in such reactions has yet been reported.[15]

[15] J. Oudin, *Proc. 4th Intern. Congr. Allergol., New York, 1961* pp. 319–338. Macmillan, New York, 1962.

ii. Identification of Antigens

The problem of associating a given antigen with a particular precipitation zone may be solved in several ways. In practice, there is no problem for two tubes with no difference other than the time of reaction (see Fig. 5). Also, there is usually no problem if it is known that the only difference between the tubes to be compared is that one of the two solutions of reagents is more dilute in one tube than in the other. However, the dilution of one antigen solution or of an antiserum may alter the order of the precipitation zones if the diffusion coefficients of the corresponding antigens are sufficiently different. Upon serial dilution of the antiserum used in the lower gel layer the zones with the smallest density will necessarily disappear before the others.

The main problem of identification consists in recognizing the zone of the same antigen in two or more tubes in which the antigen solutions (or possibly the antisera) are not the same. The means for solving such a problem may be classified into the four following categories.[16]

(*a*) *Identification of the Precipitation Zones by Their Appearance.* If different antigen solutions are added to several tubes containing the same immune serum at the same concentration, the mere appearances of the precipitation zones may be enough for the identification. In all tubes in which the only difference is the antigen concentration, the precipitation zone of a given antigen will have approximately the same appearance, e.g., the same maximum density and the same kind of leading edge. If these features are sufficiently different among the various zones, they will make identification of these zones possible (Fig. 7). The only differences will involve those features which vary with antigen concentration, namely the penetration and height of the zone.

(*b*) *Identification by Specific Modification of the Reaction.* The techniques of this category consist of making appropriate mixtures of two antigen or antibody solutions whose reactions are to be compared, and then studying the resulting modifications in the appearance of the reaction.

Absorption is the most frequently used technique to determine which antigens in one solution, S_1, are also detectable with a given immune serum in another solution, S_2. The immune serum is absorbed with S_2 and then the reaction, with S_1, of this absorbed immune serum is compared with that of the unabsorbed serum. If the absorption were complete (which is easy to ascertain by a ring test—see Chapter 13, Section A.3.d.i), the zones of all antigens contained in S_2 would disappear while the zones of the antigens present in S_1 and absent from S_2 would persist. However, if the

[16] J. Oudin, *Ann. Inst. Pasteur* **89**, 531–555 (1955).

viscosity of the immune serum were appreciably increased by the solution used for absorption, the penetrations of the remaining zones might be decreased.

Absorption does not necessarily have to be complete. Identification may be achieved by mixing with the immune serum an arbitrarily chosen

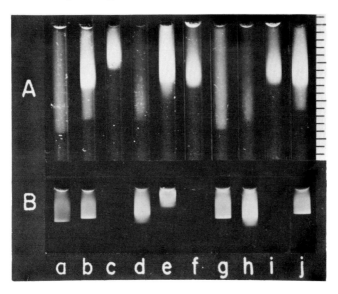

FIG. 7. Example of the identification of precipitation zones by their appearance. Ten antigen solutions were reacted with one immune serum in row A and with another immune serum in row B. Three types of precipitation zones can easily be recognized in all the tubes where they occur in row A. Type 1. A fairly faint zone with a sharp leading edge is visible in tubes a, b, g, and j. A very dense zone with a sharp leading edge may be seen in the corresponding tubes of row B, where the same antigen solutions react with another immune serum. Type 2. A faint zone with a diffuse leading edge is visible in tubes d, e, and h. Reactions with characteristic and uniform appearance are seen in the corresponding tubes of row B. Type 3. A dense zone is visible in 6 tubes (b, c, e, f, i, and j) of row A, either alone or with one of the above two, and does not correspond to any visible zone in the tubes of row B. Each of the three recognizable zones is related to an allotypic specificity carried by rabbit γ-globulins and detected by rabbit immune sera. Photograph was taken after 7 days.

amount of antigen solution. This is a useful means for comparing the antigenic contents of several solutions (Fig. 8). If several amounts of each antigen solution are used, the relative amounts of the various solutions needed for making the zone of one given antigen disappear supply information about the relative concentrations of this antigen in the different mixtures.

When the antigen solution used for absorption contains several antigens precipitable by the immune serum, it is often possible to proceed in such a way that the absorption suppresses the zone of only one of them. Serial dilutions of the antigen solution are mixed with a constant volume of immune serum, the resulting dilution of the immune serum being uniform. After standing overnight, the mixtures are centrifuged. The absorbed supernatants are then reacted with the antigen solution and their reaction is compared with that of the unabsorbed serum (Fig. 9). The

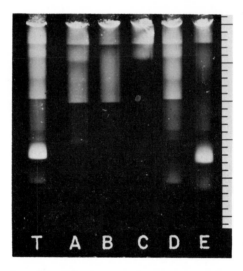

Fig. 8. Identification of precipitation zones by absorption of the immune serum. In all tubes, the reacting antigen solution is the same (a human serum globulin fraction). The rabbit immune serum is also the same except that, in tubes A through E, respectively, the serum had previously been absorbed by a uniform amount of 6 different subfractions of human γ-globulin.[12] It may be seen that one to six zones are lacking in tubes A to E as compared with tube T, and that the missing zones are not exactly the same in each case. Thus most of the zones may be characterized by the subfractions which make them disappear. Photograph was taken after 7 days.

various precipitation zones usually do not disappear simultaneously in these progressive absorptions, because the equivalence is not likely to be obtained for the various antigens at the same proportion of antigen solution and immune serum. The antigen whose zone disappears first is usually that responsible for the first zone (farthest from the interface). However, this may not be so if the diffusion coefficient of the antigen responsible for the first zone is sufficiently larger than that of another reacting antigen. Upon progressive absorption of an antiserum by increasing amounts of an antigen, the density of the affected zone successively decreases, while the penetration of the zone increases. It has been observed with such absorptions that, if the amounts of antigen added to the antiserum are plotted against the penetration of the precipitation zone, a straight line is obtained.[17] A technique for titrating the antigen has been derived from this observation.[18]

A definite advantage of the method of identification by absorption is that the reaction is simplified by the disappearance of certain zones. In practice, however, the technique is applicable only to the comparison of solutions (usually antigens) which contain a reactant in excess. In general,

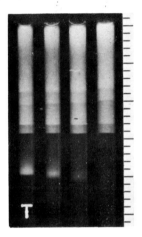

Fig. 9. The gel layer in tube T contains unabsorbed immune serum. The other tubes contain the immune serum absorbed with increasing amounts of the antigen mixture. A point is reached (last tube) with a suitable amount, at which antibodies against one antigen are absorbed, leaving the other antibodies almost unabsorbed. Photograph was taken after 7 days.

it cannot be used to compare the reactions of several immune sera with one given antigen solution.

Mixtures of antibody solutions may be used to establish the correspondence of the precipitation zones due to the same antigens in reactions of a given antigen solution with two different immune sera. Mixtures of immune sera, IS_1 and IS_2, in proportions such as $4:0$, $3:1$, $2:2$, $1:3$, $0:4$ are reacted with the antigen solution and the results are compared.[3, 17] It is usually possible to follow the zone due to a given antigen from one tube to the next. The antigens whose antibodies are present in only one of the

[17] W. H. Telfer and C. M. Williams, *J. Gen. Physiol.* **36**, 389–413 (1953).
[18] P. Perlmann, J. Couffer-Kaltenbach, and H. Perlmann, *J. Immunol.* **85**, 284–291 (1960).

two immune sera will give rise to a zone with a progressively diminished density and a progressively increased penetration as the concentration of this immune serum in the mixtures becomes lower (Fig. 10).

When the number of precipitation zones is small, the procedure may be simplified in the following way. The two sera are mixed (for example, in equal parts). Each of them is also diluted, to the same extent as in the mixture, with serum from a nonimmunized animal. These three mixtures

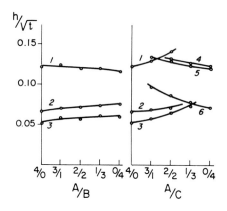

Fig. 10. Identification of the precipitation zones in the reactions of one antigen solution with three immune sera A, B, and C by mutual dilution of these immune sera two by two. *Abscissas:* Ratios of the two immune sera A and B (left-hand graph) or of immune sera A and C (right-hand graph). *Ordinates:* ratio of h (in centimeters) to the square root of t (in hours) for the various precipitation zones observed. The antigen solution was a pupal blood of cecropia moths. Immune sera A and B were two rabbit immune sera against adult blood; the three zones, in the reactions of the two immune sera A and B, were zones of the same three antigens 1, 2, and 3. Immune serum C was against larval (silkworm) blood; the three antigens with which this immune serum reacts, giving three zones 4, 5, and 6, are different from the three antigens involved in the reaction of immune serum A: each of the three zones in the reaction of each immune serum progressively fades out when that immune serum is diluted in the other one. Redrawn from Telfer and Williams.[17]

or dilutions are reacted in a comparable manner with the antigen solution. An antigen against which there are precipitating antibodies in both immune sera should give rise to a zone with smaller penetration (and as great or greater density) in the reaction with the mixture of immune sera than with either antiserum diluted with normal serum (Fig. 11).

(c) *Identification by "Profile" Analysis.* The penetration of a zone (h) is usually a linear function of the logarithm of the initial concentration of both reactants over a wide range of concentration (see Section 14.B.1.b.ii). It follows, therefore, that the difference in penetration at a

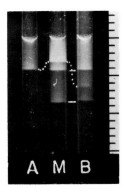

F𝚒𝚐. 11. An antigen solution was reacted, in tubes A and B, respectively, with two different immune sera A and B, each diluted 1:1 in a normal rabbit serum. In tube M, the same antigen solution was reacted with a 1:1 mixture of the two immune sera. Two zones are at the same level in tubes M and B; the antibodies which react in these two zones are lacking in immune serum A, so that their concentration is the same in tubes M and B. In tube M there is one zone whose penetration is much decreased, as compared to B and somewhat with respect to A (dotted). The concentration of the antibodies reacting in this zone is necessarily maximal in tube M, and therefore the penetration of the zone is minimal.

given time by the zone of an antigen in two different antigen solutions will be the same regardless of the antiserum employed. Stated formally (see Fig. 12): the penetration (h_{a1}) of antigen G in solution S_1 reacted with antiserum a, less the penetration (h_{a2}) of antigen G in solution S_2 reacted with antiserum a (i.e., $h_{a1} - h_{a2}$) equals the corresponding values ob-

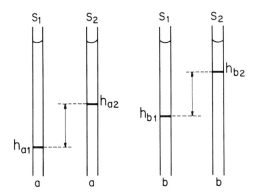

F𝚒𝚐. 12. Antigen solutions S_1 and S_2, containing different concentrations of antigen, reacted with antisera a and b, which in turn differ in antibody content. Penetrations h are labeled h_{a1}, h_{a2}, h_{b1} and h_{b2}, respectively. The linear relationships between penetration and the log of the antigen concentration or the log of the antibody concentration predict that $h_{a1} - h_{a2} = h_{b1} - h_{b2}$.

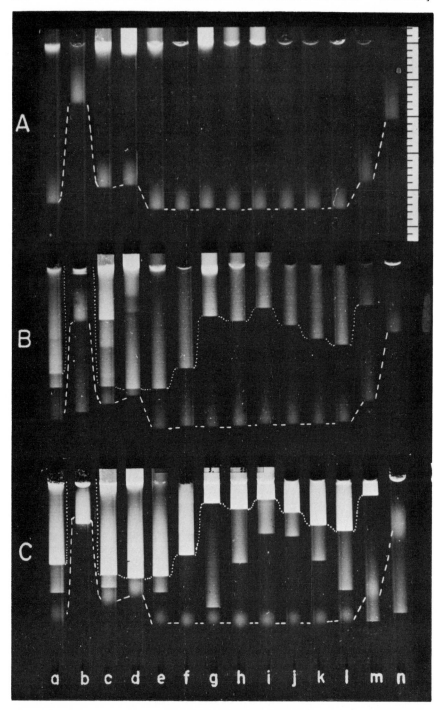

a b c d e f g h i j k l m n

tained with antiserum b (i.e., $h_{a1} - h_{a2} = h_{b1} - h_{b2}$). It also follows from this that $h_{a1} - h_{b1} = h_{a2} - h_{b2}$.

These relationships predict that a series of antigen solutions differing in concentration of a given antigen will produce a characteristic profile of h values with any antiserum which contains the appropriate antibody.

The application of this principle is illustrated in Fig. 13. In several rows of tubes a number of antigen solutions in the same sequence are reacted with several immune sera. All rows are photographed after the same length of time. A profile of the reactions of each antigen diffusing from the various solutions is visualized by connecting the leading edges of the zones of the same antigen by a line. This profile will be the same, or nearly so, in all rows of tubes in which an antigen reacts even though the actual penetrations of the zone are likely to be different, due to differences in antibody concentration in different immune sera.

Since the logarithmic laws apply only over a limited range of the antigen and antibody concentrations, and since certain variables such as the viscosity of the antisera may influence penetration, profiles may not superimpose perfectly. Nevertheless, this method is usually adequate to identify precipitation zones. The requirements mentioned above concerning the density of the antigen solution must be observed if the antigen layer is liquid, which is usually the most convenient.

One of the immune sera in the example of Fig. 13 precipitated only one antigen, so that the profile of this antigen was established simply and unambiguously. It is not necessary to start with reactions giving only one zone; it is sufficient that identity is tentatively suggested by the common appearance of a zone in the tubes of one row. The tentative profile is checked by superimposition on the profile of another row. Each time a zone is identified in a row of tubes, it becomes easier to identify the other zones so that, by going from the row showing the simplest patterns to those involving more complex patterns, the analysis of complicated reactions has proved possible in spite of fairly large numbers of zones involved. This identification becomes more certain as the number of the antigen solutions and antisera reacted is increased. Thus, this means of identification is particularly suitable for a thorough study of a large number of antigen solutions with a large number of immune sera. The determination of the number of reacting antigens cannot be separated from the identification of the precipitation zones, and the study may easily be made

---

Fig. 13. Tubes in rows A, B, and C, respectively, photographed after 7 days contain 3 different immune sera in the gel layer. Fourteen different antigen solutions, a through n, were placed in the upper layer of each set. The white dashed and dotted lines indicate the profiles of two distinct antigens.

quantitative by comparing the penetrations measured on the photographs to suitable calibration curves.[19]

Reactions may be simplified or identification confirmed by partial absorption of the immune serum as described above [Section 14.B.1.c.ii(b)]. It should be mentioned that cross-reactions of antigens in the same solutions with antisera may cause exceptions to the superimposability of precipitation profiles. In fact, the attempt to superimpose profiles of allotypic specificities of rabbit γ-globulins that showed systematic exceptions in turn led to the notion of mixed allotypes carrying two allotypic specificities on the same molecule.

(d) *Identification by Reactions of Adjacent Antigen Solutions.* Simple diffusion in one dimension in suitable cells, as described in Section 14.B.4 gives, with the same reagents, reaction patterns easily recognizable with those in tubes, thus supplying the possibility of identification of precipitation zones by the reaction of two adjacent antigen solutions with the same antiserum.

ACKNOWLEDGMENT

The author wishes to thank Dr. John Campbell for his help in the preparation of the English version of this section.

[19] J. Oudin, *J. Immunol.* **81**, 376–388 (1958).

2. DOUBLE DIFFUSION IN TUBES*

a. GENERAL PRINCIPLES

Initially designed for studies of antigens in short supply, but then found to offer special advantages, small columns were introduced by Preer[1, 2] for double diffusion (tubes of 3 mm o.d., 1.7 mm i.d.). Antigen and antibody in 0.02 ml portions are separated by a 5 mm neutral zone agar column into which the reactants diffuse from opposite directions; losses due to radial diffusion are avoided.† Band positions after diffusion are determined most readily under a binocular dissecting microscope at 6.5× power, using oblique illumination provided by placing the microscope mirror beyond the optical axis; a cross-hatched grid‡ in one eyepiece

---

* Section 14.B.2 was contributed by I. Finger.

† See Sections 14.A.1.b, 14.B.3.a and c, 14.B.4, 14.B.7, and 14.C.7.

‡ A useful device having 0.5 mm squares with accented line every 10 squares can be ordered from Graticule, Ltd., 57/60 Holborn Viaduct, London, E.C.1, as item E.10, by specifying the i.d. of the eyepiece.

[1] J. R. Preer, Jr., *in* "Developmental Cytology," (D. Rudnick, ed.), pp. 3–20. Ronald Press, New York, 1959.

[2] J. R. Preer, Jr., *J. Immunol.* **77**, 52 (1956).

allows measurement of the agar column, taken as 100%. The position of each band is measured from the antigen–gel interface and converted to percent of penetration. Typical examples are shown in Figs. 1 and 2, and Fig. 4 on page 335.

As with all double-diffusion methods, the position of the precipitate is determined by the diffusion coefficients of antigen and antibody, their initial concentrations, and other nonspecific factors, such as the length of the neutral zone and the nature of any diluent used. The one obvious requirement is that precipitates form within the agar column. This generally occurs within several doubling dilutions on either side of the equivalence ratio. For precipitates forming in the middle portion of the neutral zone there is a linear relationship between the location of a precipitate and the logarithm of a reactant concentration. There is a change in disc position of about 10% within the neutral zone with every doubling or halving of concentration of either antigen or antibody (see Fig. 1).

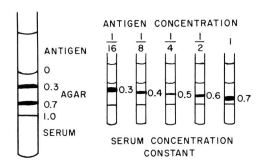

FIG. 1. The tube on the left is a Preer double-diffusion tube in which a partly purified antigen solution forms two bands at positions that are 30% and 70% of the total length of the agar column. The series of tubes drawn in the right shows the change in the lower band when serial dilutions of antigen are set against a constant antiserum concentration. From Preer.[1]

Generally the antigens used in double diffusion should be soluble; for some procedures such as mutual dilution analysis, it is essential. Particulate antigens such as certain viruses, however, have been studied with success in agar. With the profile method, also described below, there is no theoretical need to restrict comparisons to soluble antigens.

This efficient procedure serves in determining the number of Ag/Ab systems when polyvalent antisera react with crude antigens, such as entire serum or ragweed extract, or in following the course of purification of an antigen, or in studying cross-reacting antigens. If the same sera are employed for all comparisons and all nonspecific factors are kept constant, then two antigen samples may be analyzed to determine whether they are immunologically distinct. The distinguishing features are considered to represent qualitative, and possibly quantitative, differences in the determinants of the antigens. Should two antigens differ by any of the tests described below, they must be structurally different; however, two antigens identical by the same criteria may still differ in aspects which the method cannot resolve. An important immunological variable is the ability of a given animal to produce differentiating antibodies.

b. General Procedures

Preparation of Tubes

Double-diffusion tubes are prepared by cutting appropriate-sized tubing into 40-cm lengths, cleaning them with acid, rinsing with distilled water, and allowing the tubes to dry. The interior is coated with 0.1% agar; after drying the tubing is cut into 4-cm lengths. One end is sealed in a flame, using a microburner to retain sufficient of the agar subbing within the tube. The agar is highly purified (e.g., Oxoid I. D. No. 2 or the equivalent) and is dissolved in saline or buffer; Merthiolate 1:10,000 is added, and the hot solution is dispensed into small tubes sufficient for a day's tests to avoid repeated melting. Usually a concentration of 0.6% agar is used in 5 mm columns, but for special purposes the author has employed 2 mm columns of 0.3% agar. Variations in composition may include addition of 0.5 M glycine (for clarification of the agar) or Tween 20 in 0.01% (v/w).

To set up a Preer-type double-diffusion tube,[1, 2] a sealed, coated tube is placed upright and serum is layered by lowering a needle (e.g., 26 gauge, 2 inch) fitted on a syringe (0.25 ml tuberculin type) to the bottom of the tube and, with a twisting motion of the plunger, gently adding about 0.02 ml of serum. Then 5 mm of molten agar (ca. 60°) is added with a fresh syringe, making certain that the bevel of the needle faces the wall of the tube; 20-gauge blunt needles, commercially available, can be used also. The agar supply is kept at temperature suspended in hot water in a small thermos flask. The loading area and syringe can be held at 58–60° by a shielded infrared lamp. To prevent bubbles and to expel cooling agar from the needle shaft, the syringe plunger should be pushed forward and a single drop of solution expelled before the needle is inserted into the tube. The agar also should be added gradually in one motion to assure a level, unmixed serum–agar interface. For accurate comparisons of disk positions agar columns should be closely the same height for all tubes, as

5 ± 0.2 mm. Preer and Preer[3] described a tube loader and a mechanical device for advancing the syringe plunger. A scale mounted alongside the tube being filled is advantageous. After the agar has gelled, the antigen solution is introduced in the same fashion, avoiding air bubbles, and the tubes are sealed, as by Pyseal or paraffin or Criti-caps. The exact volumes of antigen (or serum) are not critical. Tubes are allowed to develop at room temperature, upright, but the temperature should be rather constant.

An alternative technique[3] makes use of tubes open at both ends. One end is lightly embedded in modeling clay, and a solution of agar and 0.01% (v/w) Tween 20 is inserted near the exposed end, leaving enough space for a serum layer. The tube is allowed to cool in a horizontal position. Serum is added and the end is sealed. After cooling, antigen is layered at the opposite end, and this end is sealed also. This method, although more difficult in its execution, avoids any admixture of antigen and serum prior to diffusion through the agar and gives more reprodubible results.

c. ANALYTICAL PROCEDURES

The most common application of "Preer-tube" analysis is the enumeration of the reactive systems according to the principle that one band represents a single antigen–antibody reaction. The test is probably the most sensitive for the detection of trace antigenic components of a mixture. Obviously, as multiple systems become more complex the likelihood of superposition of precipitates increases; and, of course no reaction with a single antiserum assures detection of all the antigens present.

Tubes should be examined for the presence of multiple bands within 6 hours if antigen and antibody are initially in high concentrations, or after 24 to 72 hours with weak systems. If intense disks appear within 6 hours, prolonged development may lead to artifactual splitting of initially single bands (compared with control tubes). Disk positions are measured most easily with a ruled reticule in one eyepiece of a binocular microscope (6.5× magnification); for very simple systems, a vernier caliper can be used. Photography and projection of negatives is possible but cumbersome. A tube will have at least three horizontal planes for measurement: a flat serum–agar meniscus, the middle of a disk, and the tangent to the curved agar–antigen meniscus. The measurements to be made are agar column height and disk position (agar–antigen meniscus to middle of disk).

Special procedures are required for analyses involving cross-reacting antigens. The *mutual dilution method* is a useful example. Identification

[3] J. R. Preer, Jr. and L. B. Preer, *J. Protozool.* **6,** 88 (1959).

of a band may present a problem when simple specific absorption of the antiserum is not feasible. The *profile method* may be valuable in such cases.

i. Mutual Dilution Method for Comparison of Antigens

In the mutual dilution method, two antigens to be compared are mixed in varying proportions and each mixture is allowed to diffuse against an antiserum prepared against one of the antigens.[4]

The first step in the mutual dilution method is to determine the approximate equivalence ratios for each of the antigens. This can be done by setting up one series of tubes with undiluted serum, against which a series of halving concentrations of antigen are reacted, and another series with the most concentrated preparation of antigen set against halving dilutions of serum. (To obtain sharp antibody–agar interfaces, the diluted antiserum must have the viscosity of serum, either by using normal serum as diluent or sucrose, etc.) The combination which represents the equivalence ratio is that tube in which the disk is dense and thinnest and whose position does not shift with time. Once the equivalence concentrations have been determined, mixtures of the two antigens, each at equivalence concentration, are made in varying volume ratios, e.g., 9:1, 3:1, 1:1, 1:3, and 1:9. Each mixture is reacted against the same serum. As controls, each antigen should be used undiluted and diluted 9:1 and 2:1 with saline or buffer. If the antigens are identical with respect to the antiserum, then all mixtures will form a single band, lower in the tube than with the single antigens. However, should the antigens be distinguishable by the antibodies present, two bands may form with the mixture in which the homologous antigen is the minority component. This occurs because the heterologous antigen will precipitate only a fraction of the antibodies and will allow the remainder to diffuse through the leading disk and form a trailing second disk. The occurrence of double bands with cross-reacting antigens in mutual dilution is strictly analogous to spur formation by double diffusion in plates or in cells. All are analogous to a liquid precipitin test for the presence of antibodies specific for homologous antigen after absorption with a cross-reacting antigen.

Figure 2 is an illustration of the results of a mutual dilution test using two cross-reacting *Paramecium* immobilization antigens. Two related, nonidentical antigens will form two disks only when the heterologous antigen is in excess of the homologous. The band formed with the homologous antigen only, the trailing disk, will be farther down the tube when

[4] J. R. Preer, Jr., *Genetics* **44,** 803 (1959).

compared with the appropriate control tube due to the removal (absorption) of cross-reacting antibodies by the leading disk. This is because as an antigen increases in concentration or antibody concentration decreases, a disk will appear farther toward the serum layer.

ii. Profile Method

Antigen solutions can also be compared in double-diffusion tubes by assigning each a "profile" derived from the relative positions of precipitates formed with several antisera. Since position reflects antibody concentration with a particular antigen, different sera may possess varying amounts of antibody to each antigen, bands will form at different levels with different sera.

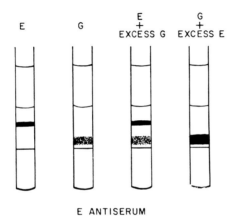

E ANTISERUM

Fig. 2. Reactions of cross-reacting purified antigens, G and E, in mutual dilution tests with an antiserum against E. The first two tubes are the control tubes with each antigen set up separately. In the third tube, the heterologous antigen is present in excess; in the last tube, the homologous antigen is in excess. From Preer.[1]

Serum concentrations should be adjusted in order that bands form well within the agar. Dilution of sera should be made with normal serum or with a viscous liquid, e.g., 1 M sucrose, that will allow liquid agar to be layered. The only other requirement is that an antigen solution be relatively homogeneous, or at least free from cross-reacting antigen or haptens since both of these can combine with antibody and affect band position. The profile of an antigen will be characteristic of the antigen because the *relative* position of the antigen–antibody precipitate with each serum will be unaffected by concentration; with a change in concentration of antigen the band in every tube will move an equal distance up or down.[5]

A cross-reacting antigen may share only some determinants with the homologous antigen and, therefore, only part of the antibody. Its precipitate with the same sera may form at different relative positions. Only when two antigens have the same number and kinds of determinants should their profiles be superimposable.

Precisely the same manipulations as outlined for the mutual dilution method are followed in setting up tubes for profiles. For maximum reproducibility, positions of disk should be measured after a constant interval of time and agar length should be uniform (the increment in shift in band position with concentration varies with agar height). The simplest way to record disk position is in terms of percent displacement from the agar-antigen meniscus. A sequence of band positions characterizes a profile. The data in Table I, taken from a study comparing five cross-reacting

TABLE I

PROFILES OF 5 CROSS-REACTING *Paramecium* ANTIGENS[a,b]

Serotype	Differences in band position				Number of preparations
	Sera				
	10–89	101–99	110–109	110–111	
1	28 ± 6	27 ± 2	33 ± 4	18 ± 5	5
2	34 ± 6	33 ± 9	11 ± 2	9 ± 6	5
3	20 ± 4	27 ± 5	23 ± 5	4 ± 7	4
4	55 ± 5	35 ± 5	14 ± 2	2 ± 2	3
5	—	38 ± 5	16 ± 6	2 ± 2	3

[a] From Finger and Heller[5] (modified).

[b] The profiles are expressed as differences in position (on a scale of 100) of the same antigen with two sera. For instance, a figure of 28 ± 6 in the column headed 10–89 means that the band formed with serum 10 was about 28% farther down the agar column than with serum 89. The standard deviation for each position is indicated in the conventional way. The larger the number, the greater is the discrepancy between the position of the band formed with the two sera used.[5]

antigens from *Paramecium*, indicate the method of recording a profile and the variability encountered.

iii. Other Methods

The principles of *hapten inhibition* are applied by mixing the serum with the suspected hapten prior to overlaying with antigen and noting whether

[5] I. Finger and C. Heller, *J. Mol. Biol.* **6**, 190 (1963).

there is a change in disk position in agreement with that expected from binding of antibody sites.

In the *displacement* method the precipitate develops in the agar in the usual fashion. Then the antigen layer is removed, the tube interior is rinsed twice with saline, and the antigen solution suspected of being related to the antigen initially used is added. An unrelated antigen should have no affect on the position of the band; an identical or cross-reacting antigen should cause a migration downward.

There are also variations in the manner of handling the reservoirs of antigen and serum. Preer double-diffusion tubes were devised as a modification of the tubes originally used by Oakley and Fulthorpe[6] in which serum was first incorporated into agar prior to being overlayered with plain agar. Polson[7] has retained the all-liquid serum and antigen reservoirs but has devised a multiple cell of three parallel plastic blocks that slide into place to form a continuous series of columns with three sectors: serum, agar, and antigen (see Section 14.C.2).

d. COMPARISON OF METHODS

Apart from the role played by artifacts, the major drawback of the mutual dilution method is that concentrated antigens and antibodies are required. Sufficient quantities of reactants must remain after "absorption" by the heterologous antigen to produce a precipitate visible as a trailing disk. With the profile method, highly concentrated antigen solutions are not required for maximum resolution of two closely related antigens. Great care must be exercised, however, in setting up tubes and in measuring the bands formed. The major disadvantage of this method is the reliance on variations in antibody response among individual animals when sera against cross-reacting antigens are not available. The profile method is probably the more sensitive of the two and most readily yields information about the number of classes of antigens. Often two antigens can be easily distinguished by using only two or three sera that provide an abbreviated but diagnostic profile.

For qualitative analysis of antigens, the greatest advantage offered by double diffusion in tubes is its sensitivity in comparison with either simple diffusion in tubes (see Section 14.C.1) or double diffusion on slides or plates (see Section 14.C.3). A serious difficulty with simple-diffusion tubes is the tendency for temperature striae to form, an artifact observed more rarely in double diffusion.

Double diffusion in plates is not as sensitive as tube methods, but it generally can yield more information with considerably less effort if care is taken to minimize artifacts.

[6] C. L. Oakley and A. J. Fulthorpe, *J. Pathol. Bacteriol.* **65**, 49 (1953).

[7] A. Polson, *Biochim. Biophys. Acta* **29**, 426 (1958).

3. DOUBLE DIFFUSION IN PLATES*

a. BASIC PRINCIPLES OF THE DOUBLE-DIFFUSION TEST

In double diffusion, antibody and antigen migrate toward each other through gel which originally contained neither of these reagents. As the reagents come in contact with each other, they combine to form a precipitate that is trapped in the gel matrix and immobilized. This test offers the unique advantage of not only enumerating the minimum number of antigen–antibody systems reacting in a given mixture, but also indicating the relationship among various antigens.

As in other precipitin tests, the double-diffusion test depends on the specific precipitation of antigen–antibody complexes at the proper ratios and on the solubility of the precipitate in excess of antigen or antibody. Only antigens that migrate through the gel and for which antibodies are present in sufficient concentration in the antiserum can form lines of precipitation. To determine the complexity of a mixture of antigens, therefore, it is important to utilize an antiserum containing antibodies to all the antigens involved. In practice, this is not an easy matter to control and frequently requires the use of several antisera. The position of the band of precipitate is determined by the relative diffusion rates of the antigen and antibody and their relative concentrations. The zones of precipitation "move" only when an excess of one reagent is present (unbalanced systems), appearing to migrate away from the reagent which is in excess. Formed precipitate dissolves on the excess side of the zone, and new precipitate is formed on the other side. Because of the multiple variables determining the position of precipitates and because of the formation of sharp bands of precipitate at equivalence, it is possible to demonstrate different antigen–antibody systems in a complex mixture as separate lines of precipitate. The simplest situation is illustrated diagrammatically in Fig. 1. Two antigens, a and b, in the right-hand well migrate through the gel at different rates and meet their respective antibodies, react and precipitate to form two distinct lines. Many systems can be demonstrated in this way, but there are practical limitations to the resolving capacity of this test. In a single reacting area, it is difficult to enumerate more than 10 to 15 bands with any degree of accuracy. By varying the relative concentration of the two reagents, by absorption of the antiserum and by fractionation of the antigenic materials, it is possible to detect most if not all antigens in the mixture for which antibodies are present in the antiserum.

* Section 14.B.3 was contributed by J. Munoz.

If the same antigen is diffusing from two different sources, the two diffusion patterns present a common front to the diffusing antibody. The resulting band of precipitate will have a shape which is the geometric resolution of the combined antigen front. This is usually in the form of an angle as illustrated in patterns 1 to 4 in Fig. 2. Pattern 5 shows double diffusion of two systems in a tube comparable to those shown on the plate in Fig. 1.[1,2,3] This method is described in Section 14.B.2.

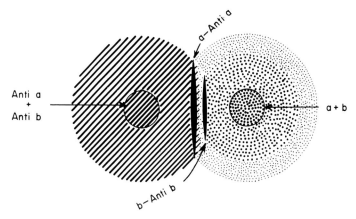

Fig. 1. Diagrammatic illustration of formation of two bands of precipitate in a double gel-diffusion type test. Dots represent antigens, and lines represent antibodies.

Other reviews which deal more extensively with principles should be consulted. See in particular those by Oudin,[1] Ouchterlony,[2,3] and Crowle.[4]

b. Materials and Procedures

i. Preparation of Gels

The most commonly used materials for gel diffusion are agar and agarose. Although these materials have certain disadvantages, no other is as practical. Gelatin, pectin, starch, silica gel, alginate, and cellulose acetate have been used (see Ouchterlony[2,3] and Crowle[4] for reviews). In this laboratory, 0.5% Ion agar (Oxoid) or 0.6% Noble agar (Difco) are satisfactory. Various methods of purifying cruder forms of agar have been published (see Section 14.F.1), but for most purposes, the two brands mentioned are satisfactory as purchased. Agar is dissolved in physiologi-

[1] J. Oudin, *Methods Med. Res.* **5**, 335 (1952).
[2] O. Ouchterlony, *Progr. Allergy* **5**, 1 (1958).
[3] O. Ouchterlony, *Progr. Allergy* **6**, 30 (1962).
[4] A. J. Crowle, "Immunodiffusion." Academic Press, New York, 1961.

cal salt solutions or in $\frac{1}{15}$ M phosphate-buffered saline at pH 7 to 7.2. Some workers prefer to dissolve the agar in distilled water, but this practice is not recommended because of possible nonspecific precipitation of some serum proteins. In this laboratory, saline solutions of agar are used. The suspension of agar is autoclaved at 15 pounds pressure for 5 minutes

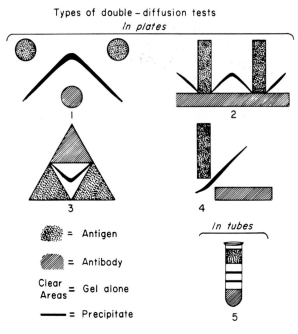

Types of double-diffusion tests
In plates

In tubes

= Antigen

= Antibody

Clear Areas = Gel alone

= Precipitate

FIG. 2. Examples of double-diffusion tests. 1. Ouchterlony double diffusion in plates. 2. Elek double diffusion in plates.[5] 3. Jennings double diffusion in plates.[6] 4. Elek-type double diffusion in plates. 5. Oakley and Fulthorpe double diffusion in tubes.[7]

and stored at 2° to 5° until needed. Before use, it is remelted and Merthiolate is added as preservative to a final concentration of 1:10,000. Routinely, 0.5 gm of Oxoid Ion agar is placed in 90 ml of saline, melted, cooled to about 50° to 60° and then 10 ml of 1:1000 merthiolate solution is added and mixed, and the plates are poured immediately.

Other preservatives that can be used are sodium azide in a concentration of 0.02% or greater, phenol at 0.1 to 0.5% concentration or a mixture of 100 units of penicillin and 500 μg of streptomycin per milliliter. Some workers have reported that certain preservatives interfere with the

[5] S. D. Elek, *Brit. J. Exptl. Pathol.* **30**, 484 (1949).

[6] R. K. Jennings and F. Malone, *J. Immunol.* **72**, 411 (1954).

[7] C. L. Oakley and A. J. Fulthorpe, *J. Pathol. Bacteriol.* **65**, 49 (1953).

agar diffusion test[8] and for this reason the investigator should make certain that the particular preservative employed has no adverse effects on the antigens being studied.

In general, buffered physiological saline is satisfactory, but if chicken antisera are employed, high (8%) salt concentration is usually necessary to produce good precipitation[9] (see Section 13.A.2.c).

ii. Preparation of Plates for Double-Diffusion Test

There are two principal methods of preparing plates for immunodiffusion: (1) A layer about 1 mm thick of 2% melted agar is poured into a petri dish and allowed to solidify so as to form a perfectly level surface. Another 1 to 2 mm thick layer of 0.5 to 0.6% agar is poured on top of this layer and allowed to solidify. Reagent wells are cut in the upper layer of agar. (2) Only one layer (1 to 2 mm thick) of 0.5 to 0.6% agar is poured and allowed to solidify, and reagent wells are cut. With glass petri plates the first technique gives more satisfactory results, but with plastic dishes the second technique is adequate, since the supporting surface is flat.

Some workers employ rectangular glass plates to support the layer of agar.[10] The plates are flooded with 0.5% melted agar, drained, and dried in an oven at 80° to 90°. This provides a surface to which the experimental layer will adhere. A layer of about 2 mm of 0.5 to 0.6% agar is poured on the plates, the agar is allowed to solidify and the reagent wells are cut. The same principle is applied to microscope slides (75 × 25 mm) in which case 2 to 2.5 ml of molten agar at 1% gives a diffusion layer of suitable thickness (see Section 14.B.3.b.v).

(a) *Procedures for Making the Wells.* For agar gel in petri dishes, a specially made Lucite template containing cylindrical openings is placed on top of the dish. The template is secured by means of a side screw, and the wells are cut by pressing a close-fitting metal cutter through each hole (Fig. 3). The agar plug is sucked out through a flattened end of a pulled glass tubing connected to a vacuum line. Some practice is needed to remove the agar plugs without damaging the sides of the wells, particularly when only one layer of gel is used in plastic dishes. Specially made molds that can be placed in the plate before the agar is poured are also convenient. An illustration of such molds is shown in Fig. 4. The mold should be coated with a film of silicon or other water repellent to prevent it from sticking to the gel when it is removed after the agar solidifies.*

[8] G. L. LeBouvier, *J. Exptl. Med.* **106**, 661 (1957).

[9] M. Goodman, H. R. Wolfe, and S. Norton, *J. Immunol.* **66**, 225 (1951).

[10] M. Kaminski, *J. Immunol.* **75**, 367 (1955).

* Some commercial sources for templates and cutters are: National Instrument Laboratories, Washington, D.C.; Gelman Instruments, Ann Arbor, Michigan; Colab Laboratories, Inc., Chicago Heights, Illinois.

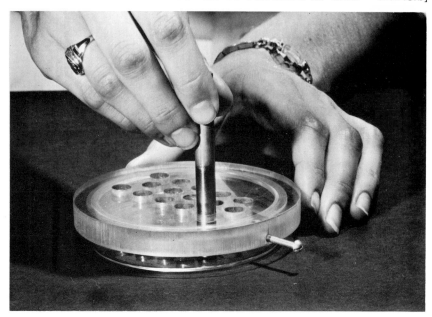

Fig. 3. Illustration of one type of template used in this laboratory to cut the wells in plates. Note screw on side to secure the template to the petri dish. The cylindrical cutter is shown in place for cutting the first well.

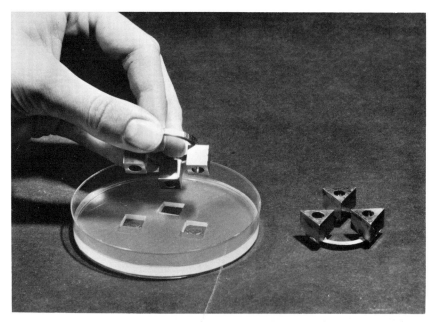

Fig. 4. Two types of mold used to form wells in gel. The melted gel is poured around the mold. After the gel has solidified, the template is carefully removed.

It is important to have the bottoms of the wells completely sealed with agar to prevent leakage of antigen or antibody between the gel and surface of the plate. This can be accomplished by filling the well with hot 0.5 to 0.6% melted agar and immediately removing the excess by means of suction. Alternatively, a artist's sable brush of appropriate size may be employed to apply the seal.

Metal or glass antibiotic assay cups can also be placed on the agar instead of wells cut in it. Care should be taken that a perfect seal exists between cups and agar, since irregular patterns will result if the antigen or antibody leaks underneath the cups.

(b) *Pattern of Wells.* Many different patterns of wells have been devised but, for the most part, the results are not different from the basic patterns

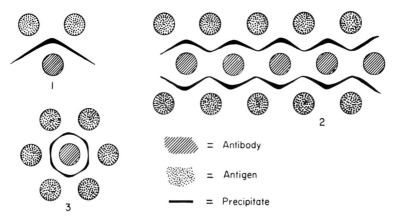

Fig. 5. Illustration of most commonly used patterns of wells for the double gel-diffusion test in plates.

originally described by Ouchterlony.[2, 3] Depending on the investigation, one pattern may be more suitable than another. The most commonly used patterns are shown in Fig. 5.

iii. Diffusion Conditions and Development of Precipitin Lines

Diffusion plates are usually incubated at temperatures ranging from 18° to 37° although, in the case of microdiffusion studies, cold room temperatures may be suitable since development is quite rapid. Diffusion of antigens and antibodies is accelerated by increasing the temperature. Whatever temperature is chosen, it should be kept relatively constant, since sharp changes in temperature cause artifacts (see Section 14.B.1). The double-diffusion test is not as sensitive to these artifacts as the tube single-diffusion test, but striae can be produced in double-diffusion test by sharp changes in temperature. If a daily record of precipitate lines is kept, the plates should be examined or photographed at the same temperature, care being taken that illumination does not warm the plates.

In order to prevent desiccation of agar, development should proceed in a closed chamber containing some source of moisture, such as a moistened sponge or towel. The length of development time varies directly with distance between wells and concentration of gel, and inversely with concentration of reagents (antigen and antibody) and temperature of incubation. With gels in standard petri dishes full development occurs within 4 to 5 days. When 0.2-ml wells are placed 5 mm apart and concentrations of reagents are high, 18 to 24 hours' incubation produces good development of precipitin lines. Microsystems develop rapidly, and overnight at ambient temperature may lead to overdevelopment if any reactants are in excess.

iv. Recording Results

The best method of recording agar diffusion tests is by photography, since the camera can record lines that are almost invisible to the eye. To observe or photograph the plates, dark-field illumination is most satisfactory. An easily constructed viewer is pictured in Fig. 6. Contrast Process Panchromatic film (Kodak) is employed; it is developed in Kodak's formula D-11 Panchromatic film developer. Other films and developing solution have given excellent results in other laboratories.[2-4] A Polaroid camera with PN55 film has also given good results in our hands. Dried agar film can be stained and then photographed. This procedure is described in detail in Section 14.E.1, and for the microtechniques it is recommended (see also Jackson[11]).

v. Micromethods

Diffusion in gels can be performed on microscope slides employing materials and methods similar to those described above.

The method of Wadsworth, as modified by Crowle,[4] is as follows: A clean microscope slide is dipped in hot 0.2% agar in distilled water and allowed to drain and dry in air. Two strips, each consisting of two layers of waterproof plastic insulating tape, are applied to the slide perpendicular to the long side 2 cm apart. About 0.3 ml of melted 1% agar (60°) is placed between the strips, and immediately a plastic template coated with a water-repellent grease is laid upon the agar. Air bubbles should not be

[11] R. Jackson, *J. Biol. Phot. Assoc.* **34**, 13 (1964).

trapped between the template and the agar. This template is slightly wider than 2 cm and has funnel-shaped holes which make good contact with the agar. It also forms a uniform layer of agar of the same thickness as the double layer of plastic tape (about 0.5 mm). When the agar solidifies, the holes in the template are filled with the proper reactants. Care must be taken not to trap the air between the gel and the reactant. The slides are incubated for 1 to 3 days at constant temperature in a petri

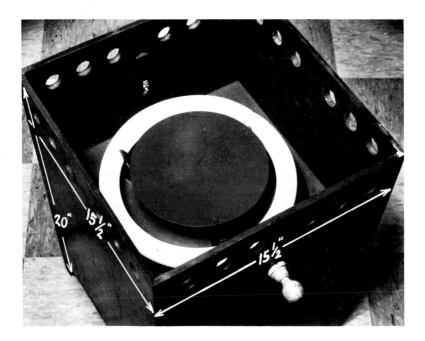

Fig. 6. Dark-field illuminator for viewing precipitates in gels. The source of light is a large circular fluorescent tube. The black shield in center of light projects above it so as to produce a uniformly dark background. A variety of lids (none shown) with a centrally located opening for viewing may be adapted to hold different sizes and shapes of plates. The dimensions of the box are indicated in inches. The size can be reduced with some loss of clarity.

dish containing a piece of moistened filter paper and then photographed. The slides can be washed by soaking in 2% NaCl to remove unreacted protein, then briefly in water to remove the salt, covered with a moistened filter paper and left to dry at room temperature. The filter paper can then be removed and the dried gel film stained with Amido Black or any other suitable protein stain (see Section 14.E.1). Other modifications of the Wadsworth technique have been employed.[12, 13]

A second method[14] that has been used successfully is as follows: Clean microscope slides (75 × 25 mm) are overlayered with 2 to 2.5 ml of a 2% solution of agar in 0.9% saline containing 1:10,000 Merthiolate. The agar is allowed to spread uniformly over the slide and solidify. Wells are cut with the help of a template, similar to but smaller than the one shown in Fig. 3, by punching through the agar with a cut-off and sharpened hypodermic needle.* Wells 1.7 mm diameter whose edges are 3.6 mm apart are satisfactory. After the wells are punched, the agar plugs remaining in them are removed by means of a capillary pipette connected to a vacuum. Care must be taken not to damage the walls. Wells arranged in a suitable pattern are charged with antigen and antibody and incubated in a humid chamber for a few hours to 3 days at the temperature desired.

The reactions can then be recorded as above. The interpretation of precipitation patterns obtained in microdiffusion tests is identical to that given for macrodiffusion.

c. INTERPRETATION OF PRECIPITATION PATTERNS

The double-diffusion test is uniquely suited for comparing different antigen preparations either for numbers of corresponding antigens present in each or for the degree of correspondence among single antigens which are structurally similar.

i. Reaction Patterns

The four basic patterns that can be obtained with an antiserum and preparations of single antigens are illustrated in Fig. 7. These can be interpreted as follows:

Pattern I, called "pattern of identity" or "pattern of coalescence," indicates that both antigens have a set of identical determinant groups with respect to the antiserum employed. Although the antigens may differ in other determinant groups, an antiserum may lack antibodies to those antigenic groups.

Pattern II, called "pattern of nonidentity" or "absence of coalescence pattern," indicates that the antiserum used does not contain antibodies to any determinant groups common to both antigens, and thus the two lines formed are completely independent of each other and cross without interaction or significant interference.

---

[12] S. E. Holm, *Intern. Arch. Allergy Appl. Immunol.* **26**, 34 (1965).

[13] U. Krause and V. Raunio, *Acta Pathol. Microbiol. Scand.* **71**, 328 (1967).

[14] J. Hirschfeld, *Sci. Tools* **10**, 45 (1963).

* Some commercial sources for templates and cutters are: National Instrument Laboratories, Washington, D.C.; Gelman Instruments, Ann Arbor, Michigan; Colab Laboratories, Inc., Chicago Heights, Illinois.

Pattern III, called the pattern of "partial identity" or "partial coalescence," indicates that one antigen (left) reacts more fully with the antibodies employed, while the other antigen (right) reacts with fewer of these antibodies, thus allowing the formation of a "spur" which projects beyond the point of partial coalescence. The spur is generally considered to be due entirely to determinants found in one antigen (left) but not the other (right). The "deficient" antigen does not impede the diffusion of those antibodies responsible for the spur.

Pattern IV indicates that the two antigens have at least one type of determinant group in common and, in addition, each has at least one type, and probably more types, of antigenic groupings not shared by the other. In other words, the antiserum used has antibodies to the common as well

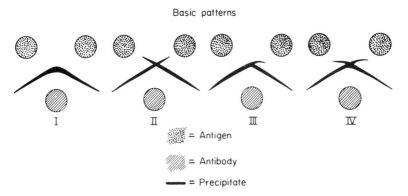

Basic patterns

I   II   III   IV

= Antigen

= Antibody

= Precipitate

FIG. 7. Basic precipitate patterns obtained in double gel diffusion. I. Complete coalescence. Reaction of identity. II. Absence of coalescence. No cross-reaction. III. Partial coalescence of one antigen. Cross-reaction. IV. Partial coalescence of two antigens.

as to the specific determinants of both antigens. Thus the reaction obtained is that of partial coalescence on both sides and formation of double spurs. These spurs should be less dense than the main portion of the line of precipitate, since they are due to a reaction with only a fraction of the antibody present in the serum. This pattern could easily be confused with pattern II (absence of coalescence), but when seen it is likely to involve two cross-reacting antigens different from the antigen used in the preparation of the antiserum. This type of pattern is sometimes seen with enzymatically produced fragments of antigens and also between various classes of immunoglobulins.

Depending on concentration of antibodies and antigens involved, many modifications of these four basic patterns can be obtained. The best and least ambiguous results are always obtained when both antigens are at equivalence with the antiserum. As a rule it takes less of the cross-reacting antigen to achieve equivalence than of the homologous antigen. In artificially made systems and in unusual circumstances this rule might not be applicable.

ii. Guiding Principles

Certain rules should be helpful when interpreting gel-diffusion tests.

1. The intensity of the precipitate line is controlled mainly by the amount of antibody.

2. At constant antigen concentration the precipitate band will form closer to the antibody well as the concentration of antibody is reduced and farther as it is increased. Similarly, at constant antibody concentration the band will form closer to the antigen well as the concentration of antigen is reduced.

3. Since antibody activity to different determinants are on separate immunoglobulin molecules, they can act independently of each other if the antigenic determinants occur in different molecular species. Each antibody molecule will recognize its corresponding determinant and will contribute only to the line of precipitation with antigens possessing that determinant. If the determinants are all in one molecule, only one line will be formed.

4. When two antigens of different complexity but with some common antigenic determinants with respect to an antiserum are placed in the same well of a double-diffusion plate and made to react with antiserum against the more complex antigens, the lines of precipitate formed vary depending on the relative concentration of the two antigens. If the more complex antigen is in a higher concentration and diffuses faster than the simpler antigen, it reacts with all the antibodies available, and only one line of precipitate is formed. On the other hand, if the simpler antigen migrates ahead of the more complex antigen, it reacts with the antibodies for which it has determinant groups and leaves untouched those antibodies still capable of reacting with the more complex antigen. Thus, two lighter lines of precipitate are formed instead of the one denser line formed when the complex antigen diffuses at a faster rate.

5. Single antigens can, under certain conditions, be degraded or broken down to smaller fragments with specificities which are either found in the intact molecule or which are completely new or at least previously unexposed.[15,16,16a]

[15] T. Ishizaka, D. H. Campbell, and K. Ishizaka, *Proc. Soc. Exptl. Biol. Med.* **103**, 5 (1960).

[16] C. Lapresle, *Ann. Inst. Pasteur* **89**, 654 (1955).

[16a] T. Webb and C. Lapresle, *J. Exptl. Med.* **114**, 43 (1961).

6. Artifacts can be produced by rapid changes in temperature, defects in the reservoirs, or denaturation of antigen during migration. Formation of multiple lines or zones from a single system has been observed in greatly unbalanced systems, but it is not certain in all cases that the phenomenon was not due to temperature artifacts.

7. More than one band of precipitate produced by a presumed single antigen–antibody, observed by some workers, finds no acceptable general explanation. The most frequently observed example is that of immunoglobulin G reported in immunoelectrophoetic patterns by Williams and Grabar[17] and since by many authors. Certain observations suggested that different sets of antibodies directed against distinct portions of the antigen molecule might be responsible for the double lines.[18, 19] Mannik and Kunkel showed, however, that the two bands with normal IgG were distinguished by their cross-reactivity with type I (κ) and type II (λ) myeloma proteins.[20] It is evident, therefore, that antigenic heterogenicity within a class of antigen can be detected by double diffusion depending on the antiserum used. Probably, this is a special case of guiding principle 4 above.

Recently, Paul and Benacerraf[21] have clearly shown that two lines of immune precipitate can be formed by hapten–protein conjugates reacting with specific antihapten sera. One complement *independent* line forms close to the antibody well and another complement *dependent* close to the antigen well. The complement component involved is apparently C′l. The same workers also observed formation of false partial identity (spurs) lines in both reactions depending on the solubility of antigen–antibody precipitates in antigen or antibody excess. Most workers have failed to demonstrate true double bands with antigens known to be pure, even when deliberately attaching two antigenically distinct haptens to the same carrier.[22]

The fact that double bands by apparently single systems have been observed does not necessarily contradict the rule that one antigen–antibody system always gives only one band of precipitation, because the possibility still exists that the bands observed may have actually been due to two systems. For example, a pure antigen can break down or denature during migration through the gel to produce antigenic derivatives

[17] C. A. Williams, Jr. and P. Grabar, *J. Immunol.* **74**, 404 (1955).

[18] G. M. Edelman, J. Heremans, M. T. Heremans, and H. G. Kunkel, *J. Exptl. Med.* **112**, 203 (1960).

[19] J. J. Heremans, "Les Globulins Seriques du Systeme Gamma," Chapter VII. Masson, Paris, 1960.

[20] M. Mannik and H. G. Kunkel, *J. Exptl. Med.* **117**, 213 (1963).

[21] W. E. Paul and B. Benacerraf, *J. Immunol.* **95**, 1067 (1966).

[22] M. Richter, B. Rose, and A. H. Sehon, *Can. J. Biochem. Physiol.* **36**, 1105 (1958).

with completely different serological specificities[15, 16]; or an antigen may have different sets of antigenic determinants, one giving rise to the production of antibodies that precipitate only in presence of complement while another set stimulating production of antibodies which precipitate with the antigen in the absence of complement. This latter possibility might explain Paul and Benacerraf's results.[21] If this is shown to be the case, the observation of multiple bands with apparently single systems would emphasize the high degree of resolving power that the gel diffusion test actually has. In practice, the investigators should always be aware of the possibility that more than one band of precipitation can be observed with what appears to be only a single antigen–antibody system.

Nonspecific rhythmic bands of precipitation similar to the Liesegang bands observed when solutions of certain chemical substances diffuse into each other has not been of serious consequence in the hands of most investigators; and should they be observed, one might consider the regularity of previous examination of the plate, particularly if this practice involved periodic removal from low or ambient temperature to a warm illumination stage.

iii. Sensitivity of Double-Diffusion Tests

The sensitivity of the double immunodiffusion test depends to a large extent on the distance between wells and the relative concentration of reactants. The closer the wells, the smaller the amount of reactants needed. Sensitivity also depends on the concentration, thickness, and viscosity of the gel employed. With wells 0.5 cm apart, as little as 0.1 μg of rabbit antibody N per well can be detected when 0.01 μg of antigen (egg albumin) N per well is used (0.05 ml of reagent per well). If the antigen concentration is increased to 0.1 μg per well, 0.1 μg of antibody N cannot be detected but 1 μg can. Therefore, if the antigen is too concentrated, minute amounts of antibody are not detected. Similarly, at a level of 10 μg of antibody N per well, 0.01 μg of antigen could be detected 18 hours later but not 96 hours later. In systems highly soluble in excess antibody (e.g., horse antiprotein antibody), the effect of antibody excess would be more pronounced. Various workers have found that minute concentrations of antibody can be detected if the wells are large. Sometimes refilling the wells to provide a continuous diffusion of antibody or antigen permits detection of low concentrations. In most cases, however, this procedure is not useful and can produce undesirable artifacts.[1]

iv. Limitations

Identification of bands is simple when a source of pure antigen is available, but difficult when it is not. The gel-diffusion test can sometimes resolve about 10 to 15 antigen–antibody systems with some reliability, but not a greater number. Dense broad lines can completely obscure weaker lines. It is also possible that two or more lines may migrate at exactly the same rate and fail to resolve. Greatly unbalanced systems, even under controlled conditions, may produce double bands due to a single antigen species. Most of these difficulties can usually be overcome by fractionation of the antigenic mixture into less complex mixtures.

The gel-diffusion test is further limited to antigenic substances to which antibodies are present in the particular antiserum used. Various workers erroneously have assumed purity because a single precipitin band was obtained. One band does not indicate chemical or immunological purity. Antigens which stimulate antibody production in some species of animals may not in others, and even different individuals of the same species react differently to the same antigens.

Only antigens that diffuse freely through the gel can be expected to form good lines of precipitation. These antigens should also be relatively stable under the conditions of gel diffusion. If an antigen denatures or precipitates during diffusion, false precipitates can result. If specificity of an antigen changes during denaturation, extra bands may appear if antibodies to the "new" antigen are present in the antiserum used.

Certain antigens may break down during chemical or physical manipulations with the formation of fragments with two separate or cross-reacting specificities. Analyses of extracts of certain tissues and microorganisms which are known to contain proteolytic enzymes must be interpreted with this in mind.

d. Applications

The gel-diffusion test in plates is uniquely suited for the enumeration of antigens in a given mixture and for the determination of antigenic relationships among various antigens and has been used extensively for these purposes in systematic biology[22a, 23, 23a, 24] and in immunogenitics to establish relationships among proteins in sera of different individuals of the same species.[24a, 25]

The methods are used to follow fractionation of antigenic substances, to establish presence of common antigens in different mixtures, and to assess relative homogeneity. If one reagent, antigen or antibody, is kept constant, the gel-diffusion test can give the relative concentration of the other reagent in different samples.

[22a] C. A. Williams, Jr., in "Evolutionary and Genetic Biology of Primates" (J. Buettner-Janusch, ed.), Vol. 2, pp. 25–74. Academic Press, New York, 1964.
[23] M. Kaminski and J. Nouvel, Bull. Soc. Chim. Biol. **37**, 758 (1952).
[23a] M. Kaminski, Bull. Soc. Chim. Biol. Suppl. 1, 85 (1957).
[24] M. Goodman, Human Biol. **34**, 104 (1962).
[24a] J. Oudin, Compt. Rend. Acad. Sci. **242**, 2489 (1956).
[25] S. Dray and G. O. Young, J. Immunol. **81**, 142 (1958).

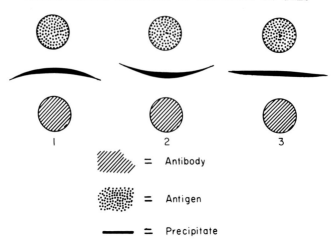

FIG. 8. Illustration of effect of molecular weight of antigen on curvature of precipitate band. 1. Antigen with smaller molecular weight than antibody. 2. Antigen with greater molecular weight than antibody. 3. Antigen with approximately the same molecular weight as antibody.

By the use of special staining procedures, it is also possible to determine the general nature or biochemical activity of antigens in complex mixtures (see Section 14.E.1).

An interesting application involved estimation of diffusion coefficients and molecular weights of antigens. Antigens with molecular weights close to that of γ-globulin produce straight lines of precipitate at equivalence, while antigens with much lower molecular weights and higher diffusion coefficients than γ-globulin form lines of precipitate that bend toward the antibody well. Antigens with higher molecular weights and low diffusion rates form lines that bend toward the antigen well, as illustrated in Fig. 8.[26, 27]

[26] L. Korngold and G. van Leeuwen, (1957). *J. Immunol.* **78**, 172 (1957).
[27] A. C. Allison and J. H. Humphrey, *Immunology* **3**, 95 (1960).

4. SIMPLE AND DOUBLE DIFFUSION IN CELLS*

Cells with parallel walls have been used for antigen–antibody reaction in gels by simple diffusion[1, 2] in the same manner as cylindrical tubes (see Section 14.C.1). Their advantage over tubes at the time they were devel-

* Section 14.B.4 was contributed by Jacques Oudin.

[1] J. Oudin, *Bul. Soc. Chim. Biol.* **29**, 140–149 (1947).
[2] J. Oudin, *Ann. Inst. Pasteur* **75**, 30–51 (1948).

oped was that they facilitated photometric analysis of the density of precipitation zones.[2] Such density curves can now be obtained with tubes with the aid of special equipment, and the quantitative information is described in Section 14.C.1.

Cells can also be used for comparison in the same gel of reactions of two antigen solutions with the same immune serum, or of two immune sera with the same antigen solution. Several types of cells have been suggested for this purpose. The main ones are described below. The general techniques and precautions associated with their use are the same as described in Section 14.C.1.

a. CELLS WITH PARTITIONS

Cells of the type shown in Fig. 1[3] and of a slightly different version described earlier, with a larger number of compartments,[4] are made of

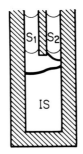

FIG. 1. Cell with two upper compartments (drawn after Ransom *et al.*[3]). IS is gel layer containing the immune serum. S_1, S_2 indicate two antigen solutions (or bacterial suspensions) whose reactions with the immune serum are compared. The leading edges of two precipitation zones are represented: one due to an antigen present in S_2 but not in S_1, the other due to an antigen present in both S_1 and S_2.

Lucite. As described for simple diffusion in tubes (Section 14.C.1) they are internally coated with dried 1% agar prior to introducing the reactants.

The cells are filled with immune serum–agar mixture (containing Merthiolate as preservative), just to the lower end of the center dividing strip. Once this mixture has solidified, each of the two antigen solutions (or bacterial suspensions) to be compared is placed in one of the two compartments. Figure 1 gives an example of a precipitation zone of an

[3] J. P. Ransom, S. F. Quan, M. D. Hogan, and G. Omi, *Proc. Soc. Exptl. Biol. Med.* **88**, 173–176 (1955).
[4] M. J. Surgalla, M. S. Bergdoll, and G. M. Dack, *J. Immunol.* **69**, 357–365 (1952).

antigen diffusing from only one compartment, and that of a zone of another antigen diffusing from both compartments.

b. CELLS WITHOUT PARTITIONS

Cells for double diffusion have been described, which employed forms to be removed after one gel had set, making a reservoir for the gel con-

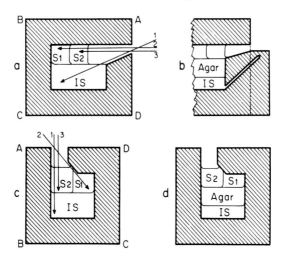

FIG. 2. Noncompartmented cells for simple and double diffusion reactions. The rubber or plastic inner piece is represented by hatched areas. (a) Simple diffusion. The position of the pipet for delivering the layer of immune serum with agar (IS) is represented by arrow 1; for delivering the layer of the first antigen solution (S_1) by the arrow 2 after layer IS has gelled and the cell is standing on its side BC (see text); for delivering layer S_2, by arrow 3. (b) Slightly modified cell, used for double diffusion. The first layer IS is introduced through the channel in the inner piece, a part of which remains outside the glass walls (whose limit is represented by a broken line). A layer of pure agar is poured onto layer IS. Then S_1 and S_2 are poured as in diagram a. (c) An alternative use of a cell similar to that in diagram a for simple diffusion. The layer of immune serum IS is poured according to arrow 1 and allowed to gel. Then, the cell standing on its side CD, layer S_1 is introduced (arrow 2). Finally the cell is put in its original position (standing on its side BC) and the S_2 layer is delivered according to arrow 3. (d) Double diffusion in a cell carried out in a manner similar to that described for diagram c.

taining the complementary reactants.[5] The cells described here (Fig. 2) have neither compartments nor form and can be used either for simple or double diffusion. Even when two or more antigen solutions are reacted with one immune serum in such cells, diffusion in one dimension is realized.

[5] C. L. Oakley, *Discussions Faraday Soc.* **18**, 358–361 (1954).

i. Preparation of the Cells

Initially these cells were made of cemented glass or plexiglass.[6] It is very easy, however, to make them in the laboratory, cutting the desired shape and size from a rubber or plastic sheet.[7] These templates are inserted between two agar-coated glass slides which are held together with clamps. To ensure the tightness of the cells, it is convenient to have the border of the inner part of the cell at least 2 cm wide and to apply a thin layer of grease around the periphery. In the author's laboratory, the inner piece is generally 1 mm thick, sometimes less (0.5 or 0.6 mm). The glass walls are carefully cleaned (sulfochromic mixture or detergents) and rinsed. They are smeared on the inner surfaces with one drop of melted agar solution, and rapidly dried.

The use of clamps may be avoided by the following procedure, if the inner piece is made of plastic. The three parts of the cell (two glass slides coated with agar and the plastic inner piece) are held in a press at a temperature of 110° for 4 to 6 hours. The plastic sheet then adheres to the glass.[8]

ii. Procedure

Each of the antigen solutions and immune sera (or antibody solutions) is mixed with melted agar at approximately 48°, the final agar concentration being 0.6 to 1 % according to the grade of agar. These mixtures should be introduced in the cells as soon as possible after they are prepared, since the turbidity which sometimes develops in these hot mixtures increases with time. The reagent layers are distributed as indicated in Fig. 2, using a drawn, warmed Pasteur pipet, whose delivery is controlled by a mouth tube. Alternatively, a syringe and needle may be used. It is convenient to distribute the agar mixture under an infrared bulb which may be switched off in order to allow the layers to solidify.

As an example, the reaction of an immune serum with two or more antigen solutions will be considered. First the immune serum, mixed with agar, is poured and allowed to gel. Then the cell is allowed to stand on its end so that this level becomes vertical (for this step the gel must be sufficiently firm). Then the first antigen–agar solution is poured. Once this layer has solidified, a second antigen–agar solution is poured above it and allowed to gel; a third and possibly more layers may be successively poured. It is advisable that each antigen layer be sufficiently wide (e.g.,

---

[6] J. Oudin, *Ann. Inst. Pasteur* **89**, 531–555 (1955).

[7] A. Bussard, *Proc. 7th Intern. Congr. Microbiol., Stockholm*, 1958, pp. 152–153. Almquist & Wiksell, Uppsala, 1958.

[8] P. Dupouey, personal communication (1960).

15 mm or more unless one intends to observe the reaction for only a short time). Care must be taken that the part of the cell designed for one reagent is contaminated as little as possible by another reagent.

If double diffusion is to be used, a 5 to 10 mm layer of pure agar is poured on top of the first layer containing antiserum–agar. The antigen layers are subsequently poured as before. If two or more immune sera are to be reacted with the same antigen solution, the layer of antigen solution is poured first. In this case, it is better to use double diffusion, which usually gives reactions with better characteristics.

These versatile cells lend themselves to many other possibilities, which cannot be described here. Whatever the precise use of the cells, they must be hermetically sealed, for example with melted beeswax, sealing wax, or the same mixture as that used for gel tubes (Section 14.B.1). Artifacts seem to be related to evaporation due to imperfect sealing of the cell. Also a very small amount of reagent from one of the layers may seep into the interface between two adjacent layers.

Cells are photographed in a manner similar to that described for simple diffusion tubes (Section 14.C.1). Cells might also be used for contact prints,[2] but the results are less satisfactory.

c. ANALYSIS OF REACTIONS

   i. One Immune Serum with Different Antigen Solutions

Reactions of two adjacent antigen solutions with an immune serum are illustrated by Figs. 3, 4, and 5. There are three main types of precipitation zones.

Type a. An antigen present in sufficient concentrations in both solutions S_1 and S_2 gives rise to a single precipitation zone, shown schematically in Fig. 3a. As soon as the precipitation zone is visible, it is continuous from one side of the cell to the other because of the contiguity of layers S_1 and S_2, from which the antigen diffuses. However, the penetration of this zone (i.e., the distance from the interface to the leading edge) will differ for S_1 and S_2 if the concentration of the reacting antigen is not the same. The penetrations are the same as they would be in tubes and, therefore, obey the laws described in Section 14.C.1 except in front of the interface between S_1 and S_2, where they have an intermediate value.

The precipitation zones appear very rapidly with this procedure, which is generally true for simple diffusion techniques, thus allowing rapid identification of common antigens. If one is dealing with double diffusion, the appearance of the precipitation zones will not be immediate, the length of time required for a precipitation zone to appear increasing as the width of the intervening neutral layer is increased. Theoretically, the length of time needed for the reagents to meet each other is proportional to the square of the initial distance between diffusing reactants.[9] Another difference between double diffusion and simple diffusion is that the density of the zone, instead of rapidly becoming constant as in simple diffusion, increases for a relatively long period of time even when the antigen is in excess. In double diffusion also, however, the zones are continuous from the moment they appear in front of the antigen reservoirs.

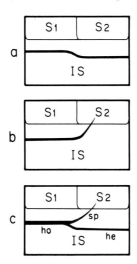

FIG. 3. Schematic representation of three cases in which an immune serum (IS) is reacted with two antigen solutions (S_1 and S_2) in a simple diffusion cell. (a) An antigen in excess in both S_1 and S_2 solutions relative to the precipitating antibodies in IS, but more concentrated in S_2, would give rise to a precipitation zone with a leading edge that is represented by the heavy line. (b) The heavy line represents the leading edge of the precipitation zone of an antigen, lacking in S_2, but in sufficient excess in S_1. (c) Reactions of a homologous antigen (in S_1) and a cross-reacting antigen (in S_2) with an immune serum IS. The antibodies reacting at *he* are those which are precipitable by the heterologous antigen (in S_2); at *ho*, all the antibodies which precipitate the homologous antigen.

Of course, the fact that an antigen in S_1 and an antigen in S_2 are not distinguished by the immune serum (i.e., giving a continuous zone with this technique) does not necessarily mean that they are immunochemically identical. With other immune sera they may appear quite distinct.

Type b. Figure 3b shows a schematic example of the zone of an antigen present in one reservoir but not in the other. Some of the antigen diffuses from the S_1 reservoir into the S_2 antigen layer, explaining the

[9] J. Oudin, *Methods Med. Res.* **5**, 335–378 (1952).

deflection of the zone into the S_2 layer, where it fades out in antibody excess. If two antigens were present, one in solution S_1 and the other in solution S_2, their zones would obviously cross each other.

In Fig. 4, precipitation zones of type a and type b are shown in a simple diffusion cell (Fig. 4A) and in a double diffusion cell (Fig. 4B).

Type c. Cross-reactions. Certain cross-reactions give rise to precipitation zones having characteristics intermediate between those described under types a and b. A schematic example of such a cross-reaction is

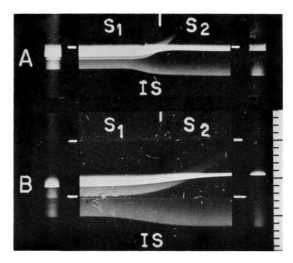

Fig. 4. Reaction, in a cell and in two tubes, of two antigen solutions S_1 and S_2 with an immune serum IS. The interfaces between the various agar layers are indicated by white dashes in the margins. (A) Simple diffusion. Two precipitation zones of type a, and one zone of type b (see legend of Fig. 3) can be seen. Photograph taken after 4 hours. (B) Double diffusion. In A and B, corresponding zones are easily recognized in the two tubes and in the cell. Photograph taken after 2 days. Scale at right is graduated in millimeters.

given in Fig. 3c, and an actual example in Fig. 5. In these examples, the immune serum is homologous with the antigen in solution S_1 (hen ovalbumin) and heterologous with the antigen in solution S_2 (duck ovalbumin). Part of the antibodies are precipitable by either antigen; it may be assumed that, if these were the only antibodies in the serum, they would give a precipitation zone of the above type a. However, another part of the antibodies is precipitable only by the homologous antigen. If only these antibodies were present in the immune serum, they would give rise to a precipitation zone of type b, occurring only in front of the gel layer containing the homologous antigen. Of course, even though these two distinct kinds of antibodies take part in the reaction, a single precipitation zone is observed in front of the homologous antigen, regardless of the proportions of the two kinds of antibodies, since both kinds are combining with the same antigen molecules.

Comparison of the density of precipitate in the different parts of the precipitation zone can give an idea of the extent of the cross-reaction. In simple diffusion, the density is more directly related to the comparative concentration of the two kinds of antibodies. In the drawing of Fig. 3c, the three arms of the precipitation zone are designated: *he*, those

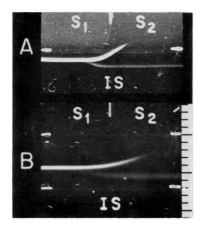

FIG. 5. Cross-reaction of two antigens, diffusing from layers S_1 and S_2, respectively, with an immune serum IS to the antigen in S_1. The white dashes indicate the interfaces between the various layers. (A) Simple diffusion. The appearance of the reaction is like the diagram in Fig. 3c. Photograph taken after 4 hours. (B) Double diffusion. Photograph taken after 24 hours.

antibodies which precipitate with the heterologous antigen without distinguishing it from the homologous; *sp*, those which precipitate specifically with the homologous antigen (and not the heterologous one); *ho*, the whole of the antibodies which precipitate with the homologous antigen, i.e., the sum of the preceding two. The greater the density in *he* as compared to *sp* the closer or the stronger is the cross-reaction; at the limit one finds the case represented in Fig. 3a. The smaller the density of *he* as compared to *sp* and *ho*, the weaker is the cross-reaction; at the limit one finds the case represented in Fig. 3b.

This simple kind of cross-reaction is the easiest to recognize. If the immune serum were homologous for both cross-reacting antigens in S_1 and in S_2, the appearance of the cross-reactions would be less characteristic, especially if these cross-reactions were weak.

ii. Single Antigen Solution with Different Immune Sera

An example of such a reaction in double diffusion is given in Fig. 6. An antigen against which precipitating antibodies are present in a sufficient concentration in two adjacent layers of immune sera gives rise to a precipitation zone which is continuous in these two layers or in front of them, a situation somewhat comparable to case a of Fig. 3. An indication of the relative concentrations of the antibodies against this antigen is given by the relative density and the position of the two parts of the zone. The zone is denser and nearer the antigen layer on the side of the greater antibody concentration. An antigen against which antibodies are present in

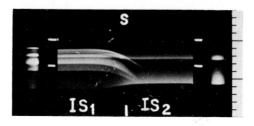

FIG. 6. Reactions of an antigen solution S with two immune sera IS₁ and IS₂ by double diffusion in a cell and in two tubes. Photograph taken after 25 hours. Dashes in margin indicate interfaces. Serum IS₂ is deficient in several antibodies to antigens in solution S. (See text.)

only one immune serum (e.g., IS₁ in Fig. 6) will give rise to a zone similar to that in case b of Fig. 3, the penetration increasing and the zone fading out in the layer of IS₂ deprived of antibody.

5. DOUBLE DIFFUSION IN CELLULOSE
ACETATE MEMBRANE (CAM)*

a. INTRODUCTION

CAM is homogeneous, microporous, wettable, chemically inert, and relatively pure. It permits the free migration of large molecules without absorption, thus fulfilling the requirements for a satisfactory supporting medium for diffusion. It was found to be a simple and convenient alternative and substitute for the commonly used gels and has been adapted to

* Section 14.B.5 was contributed by J. Kohn.

immunoelectrophoresis analysis and other immunochemical techniques, based on diffusion in stabilized media.[1-4]

i. Advantages

CAM is immediately available for use without preliminary preparations, and there is no need for any supporting materials. No wells or troughs are necessary, hence no cutting devices are needed. As the continuity of the supporting medium is not interrupted, there is no distortion or masking of the precipitation lines. CAM is easily cut, and the marking is very legible. Economy of reactants results from high sensitivity conferred by the high ratio of sample volume to cross section of supporting medium. This is further enhanced by Nigrosin staining. The presence of as little as 0.2 μg of γ-globulin can be easily demonstrated with a commercially available antiserum. Using the "microspot" technique (Section 14.B.5.d.iii), even smaller quantities can be detected. Whole blood may be used as the reactant; the RBC's and the hemoglobin are removed during the washing procedure. Storage problems are negligible. CAM can be rendered completely transparent, both for projection and enlarging purposes. Elution of nonprecipitated reactants is rapid and complete, and there is hardly any background staining left.

ii. Disadvantages

The formation of precipitation lines cannot be observed without staining. The volumes of samples to be applied are limited. Some care and skill in handling is required. Some reactants may leave traces on the application sites.

b. CAM CHARACTERISTICS

CAM for immunodiffusion techniques is the same as that used for CAM electrophoresis (see Chap. 6.C.2, Vol. II). The thickness, the average pore size, the water absorption ratio, and the degree of acetylation vary according to the commercial source; but these factors do not materially affect the suitability of CAM as a supporting medium for immunodiffusion. The procedure described here was carried out on Sartorius and Oxoid CAM, but other brands should be equally suitable.

[1] R. Consden, and J. Kohn, *Nature* **183**, 1512 (1959).

[2] J. Kohn, *in* "Chromatographic and Electrophoretic Techniques" (I. Smith, ed.), Vol. 2, pp. 120–137. Heinemann, London, 1968.

[3] J. Kohn, *in* "Protides of the Biological Fluids" (H. Peeters, ed.), pp. 120–121. Elsevier, Amsterdam, 1961.

[4] J. Kohn, *Nature* **217**, 5135 (1968).

c. Procedure for Double Diffusion[4]

i. Diffusion Chamber

For two-dimensional double diffusion, round or square holes (about 3 cm in diameter) are cut out from filter paper pads, 4 to 6 mm thick (for example a few layers of Whatman No. 3 MM). This forms a support which is placed on a piece of filter paper in a suitable flat container (e.g.,

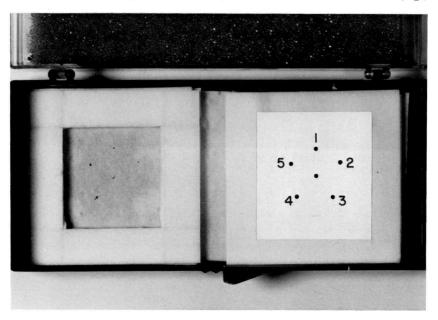

Fig. 1. Diffusion chamber with square filter paper pads. One CAM square in position with application sites marked. Note lid lined with plastic foam.

plastic box about 2 to 3 cm high) with a tight fitting lid (see Fig. 1). The lid should be lined with foam which when wetted will maintain a high humidity in the chamber and also absorb condensation. The pad is soaked with an appropriate electrolyte solution, the excess fluid being drained off; it should not be too wet.

ii. Preparation of CAM

The application sites and the appropriate legends are marked on suitable size and shape CAM, e.g., 4 × 4 cm squares or disks; equal distances from a central point are obtained by means of a pair of dividers. The distance between the application sites will vary, usually about 5 to 10 mm.

The CAM is then impregnated with a suitable electrolyte solution, blotted (as for electrophoresis, see Vol. II, Chap. 6.C.2), and placed on the pad in the diffusion chamber in such a way that the diffusion area spans the gap and the periphery is in contact with the support, overlapping it by about 5 to 10 mm.

iii. Application of Reactants

The samples containing antigen and antibody are applied to the surface of the CAM as discrete drops by means of a micropipet, capillary, or suitable automatic dispensing pipet, taking care to avoid "blow out" bubbles. A very convenient device for the delivery of small samples is a blood-aspirating tube, fitted at one end with a perforated rubber stopper so that a drawn-out capillary can be inserted. The addition of suitable marker dyes (e.g., bromophenol blue) to the reactants is recommended. The stained sample shows up against a white background and also indicates whether any spilling or irregular spreading has occurred. The volumes that can be applied are relatively small compared with those commonly used in gel methods. The optimal relative volumes and the distances between the application sites vary with the antigen–antibody system and are best determined by preliminary experiments: 0.5 to 2 μl would be the usual volume for the peripheral applications and about twice as much for the central one. An alternative and possibly more precise method of application consists of using small filter paper disks (e.g., Whatman No. 1) or squares, impregnated with the sample fluid. The impregnated disks are easily placed in exactly the desired position and at the exact distance chosen. More fluid can be added after the first application has partly soaked in, until the desired volume has been applied. Using this technique larger volumes can be applied because of the additional absorptive capacity provided.

iv. Diffusion

Diffusion under oil as previously recommended[1,2] is a very reliable method but it has minor drawbacks. Great care must be taken to avoid drying out of the CAM during application of the samples. A somewhat tedious procedure of oil removal is involved.

The simplest and most practical procedure is carrying out the diffusion in the specially designed diffusion chamber, as described in Section c.i. A system of immunodiffusion on cellulose acetate, using compression between a suitable support and a template, has been introduced and is commercially available.*

* NIL-Saravis ALL-Plastic Immunodiffusion Kit. Millipore Filter Corporation, Bedford, Massachusetts.

The diffusion time depends on the nature and concentration of the antigen and antibody, the distance of application sites, and the temperature. With 1 cm distance, diffusion for 16 to 24 hours at room temperature is usually adequate. After diffusion the CAM is removed and placed in an eluting fluid, such as 0.2% Haemo-Sol [Meinecke and Co. Inc., U.S.A.; Alfred Cox (Surgical), Ltd., U.K.], buffer or saline for about 10 to 20 minutes, preferably with agitation.

v. Analysis

After elution the CAM is stained, washed, dried, and (if required) cleared as recommended for CAM electrophoresis (See Vol. II, Chap.

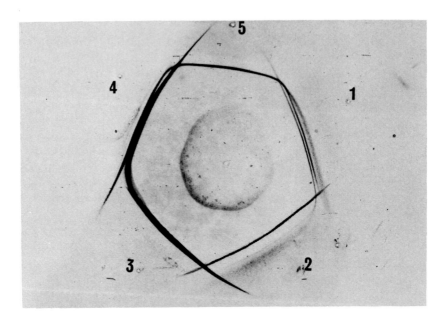

FIG. 2. Two-dimensional double diffusion on CAM. Twenty hours' diffusion. Bacterial antigens on periphery; human serum in center.

6.C.2). For weak precipitates 0.002% Nigrosin stain in 2% acetic acid is a most useful stain.

The stained CAM is best inspected against a strong source of light. Photographic enlargement of stained and cleared CAM greatly facilitates the analysis of complex (Fig. 2), often crowded precipitation pattern. The most common errors are careless and irregular application of sample.

d. USEFUL MODIFICATIONS AND ADAPTATIONS

i. Titrations

By applying increasing dilutions of one of the reactants placed around the other reactants in the center, the last line of precipitation to be still seen constitutes a crude "titer." This technique was found to be useful for the estimation of C-reactive protein.

ii. Quantitative Determination of Serum Immunoglobins by Simple Single Radial Immunodiffusion on Cellulose Acetate[5]

(a) *Preparation of Antiserum-Impregnated Strip.* CAM of 2.5 × 18 cm held taut by clips in a moist chamber is sprayed with 0.8 ml of diluted antiserum and then spread evenly by means of a glass rod. Anti IgG, IgA, and IgM are diluted 1:5, 1:6, and 1:12 with saline, respectively. The strip is then left for 30 minutes in a moist chamber to ensure homogeneous distribution and impregnation.

(b) *Application of Sample.* One microliter of test and standard sample is applied on the CAM accurately with a microsyringe. Test sera are diluted in 5% Dextran in saline, the concentration of immunoglobulin not exceeding 0.6 mg/ml. The recommended dilutions are: 1:40 for IgG (∼0.3 mg/ml), 1:10 for IgA (∼0.2 mg/ml), and 1:10 for IgM (∼0.1 mg/ml). One-microliter samples of standard serum at different dilutions are applied to the impregnated CAM strip in order to plot the calibration curve having at least three reference points.

After the samples have soaked in, the CAM is placed gently under oil (e.g., Ondina oil 17), and left for 48 hours at 37° until diffusion is completed. Following this, the CAM is removed from the oil and the excess oil wiped off mechanically (e.g., between lid and wall of the container). In order to elute the nonprecipitated proteins as well as to remove traces of oil, the CAM is transferred for 10 to 30 minutes into a 0.2% aqueous solution of Haemosol or a similar type of detergent. Gentle shaking accelerates the process. When the CAM has been eluted, it is rinsed in running tap water and placed in a staining solution, e.g., Ponceau S, Amido Black, or Nigrosin; the staining and washing procedure is as for electrophoresis.

(c) *Reading and Recording of Results.* Squares of the diameters of the precipitation rings are plotted against standard antigen concentrations. A straight line is obtained from which values for test sera are read off. About 0.06 μg of immunoglobulin can be detected with this method.

[5] C. Vergani, R. Stabilini, and A. Agostoni, *Immunochemistry* **4**, 233 (1967).

The other advantages of simple diffusion on CAM are that (1) precipitation rings are sharply outlined, (2) the problem of uniformity of thickness of the carrier medium is eliminated, and (3) smaller amounts of sera and particularly of antisera are required. It shares a disadvantage with two-dimensional CAM double diffusion, however, in that the technique is more exacting than when an agar gel is used.

iii. "Microspot" Technique[6]

This is an immunodiffusion method and, like the one above, is based on the impregnation of the CAM with one of the reactants and the subsequent application of discrete microspots of the other reactants. A strip of CAM is marked into squares, numbered, and impregnated with antiserum appropriately diluted in a suitable fluid, e.g., saline-phosphate buffer. Usually the antiserum is diluted 1:10 and 1:20, but the optimal dilutions are best determined for each system. The impregnated CAM is blotted and placed on a suitable support. Small drops of the antigenic substances and suitable controls are then placed in the center of the marked squares. The CAM is placed under oil to permit the development of antigen–antibody precipitate and is then processed as described above. Nigrosin should be used for staining. Precipitates appear as spots or concentric circles against a white background. The microspot test has been found very convenient for the grouping of β-hemolytic streptococci[7] and was also applied with success to the detection of autoimmune antibodies.[8] By applying serial dilutions and recording the end point or the diameter of the rings compared with that obtained with a known standard, quantitative estimations can be obtained.

[6] J. G. Feinberg, *Nature* **194**, 307 (1962).
[7] M. Goldin and A. Glenn, *J. Bacteriol.* **87**, 227 (1964).
[8] J. G. Feinberg and A. W. Wheeler, *J. Clin. Pathol.* **16**, 282 (1963).

C. Quantitative Determinations by Precipitation Analysis in Gels

1. DETERMINATION OF DIFFUSION COEFFICIENT OF ANTIGENS BY SIMPLE DIFFUSION IN TUBES*

a. Introduction

In single diffusion in tubes, determination of the diffusion coefficient of the antigen responsible for a given precipitate band is useful in identifying the antigen, in aiding in relating bands in different tubes to each other, and as one of the steps in obtaining the concentration of a protein

* Section 14.C.1 was contributed by Elmer L. Becker.

antigen in absolute weight units (Section 14.C.7). As will become evident from a description of the method, it is only for these special purposes, particularly the last, that the technique of simple diffusion in tubes is to be recommended. The determination of diffusion coefficients using either double diffusion in tubes (Section 14.B.2), or double diffusion in plates (Section 14.B.3) is at least as accurate, and the measurements and calculations are much simpler. For general purposes, because of this greater simplicity, either of the latter two methods is preferable except in those few instances where there is uncertainty whether the antibody is a 7 S or 19 S. This is due to the fact that, unlike the double diffusion methods, the calculated value of the diffusion coefficient of the antigen determined by the technique of single diffusion is almost independent of the value chosen for the diffusion coefficient of the antibody.[1, 1a]

b. MATHEMATICAL BACKGROUND

Three methods[1, 2, 3] are available for determining the diffusion coefficient of antigens by single diffusion in tubes. Only the last will be described here. This utilizes Eq. (1).[1, 4]

$$\log \frac{Ag}{Ab} + \log \left(\frac{1 - \operatorname{erf} y}{1 + \operatorname{erf} z} \right) = -0.434 \left(1 - \frac{D_1}{D_2} \right) y^2 + \log R_0 \qquad (1)$$

where Ag = the antigen concentration in the upper layer, Ab = the antibody concentration in the lower layer.

$$z = k/2(D_1)^{1/2} \qquad (2)$$

where k is the slope obtained by plotting the distance, x, that the leading edge of the precipitate band moves in time, t, against $t^{1/2}$, and D_1 is the diffusion coefficient of the antigen.

$$y = (k/2)(D_2)^{1/2} \qquad (3)$$

where D_2 is the diffusion coefficient of the antibody and erf is the error function,

$$\frac{2}{\sqrt{\pi}} \int_0^w l^{-u^2} \, dw$$

where $w = (k/2)(D)^{1/2}$. R_0 is the "immobilization ratio," i.e., the ratio of antigen to antibody at which there is no movement of the band ($k = 0$).

[1] E. L. Becker, *Arch. Biochem. Biophys.* **93**, 617–30 (1961).
[1a] E. L. Becker, unpublished calculations (1961).
[2] E. L. Becker, J. Munoz, C. Lapresle, and L. Lebeau, *J. Immunol.* **67**, 501–11 (1951).
[3] E. L. Becker and J. C. Neff, *J. Immunol.* **83**, 571–81 (1959).
[4] J. A. Spiers and R. Augustin, *Trans. Faraday Soc.* **54**, 287–95 (1958).

Although this equation holds over a very wide range of antigen and antibody concentrations, at sufficiently high antibody concentrations the calculated values for the diffusion coefficient will be too low. However, under conditions of greatest use (see Section 14.C.7) this is not a problem. The equation assumes undisturbed diffusion of antigen in the upper antigen layer. This assumption is met in practice by putting not only the antibody but the antigen in agar.

c. PROCEDURE

In practice, tubes for simple diffusion are prepared and filled as described in Section 14.B.1., the only modification being that the antigen as well as the antibody is incorporated in agar of a final concentration of 0.3%. We have used tubes of 7 mm o.d. as well as tubes 4 mm o.d.; tubes of smaller diameter should also work.

Duplicate tubes at each of four or five concentrations of antigen and a fixed concentration of antiserum are generally sufficient. Usually, doubling dilutions of antigen are employed; the antiserum concentration is chosen to give the least dense band which is easily readable. The times at which the tubes are filled are noted, and immediately after filling the tubes are placed in a water bath or some other device which will allow the temperature to be kept constant to within at least one-half a degree. Any temperature suffices which can be conveniently maintained; we use 25°.

The distance, x, the leading edge of the band has moved from the meniscus at the time of measurement, t, is determined daily for 4 to 5 days. Measurements may be taken more or less frequently than this depending on the rate of movement of the band. We use a traveling microscope capable of reading to 0.01 mm for making the measurements; however, calipers or straight edge capable of reading to ± 0.1 mm suffices for any but the most exacting measurements. The distance in centimeters that the band moved is plotted against the square root of the time in seconds. The slope of the straight line obtained is k.

d. CALCULATIONS

By means of Eqs. (2) and (3) y, y^2, and z are calculated for each k, provisional values for D_2 and D_1 being used. The usual provisional value chosen for D_2, the diffusion coefficient of the antibody, is 3.9×10^{-7}. If nothing is known about the magnitude of the coefficient of the antigen, 3.9×10^{-7} is a convenient choice of the provisional value of D_1. By means of Table I, numerical values for log $(1 - \text{erf } y)$ and log $(1 + \text{erf } z)$ are calculated.

Log Ag/Ab for each measured k is also calculated. In this computation the units of concentration are not important; they may be in terms, for

TABLE I[a]

$Y = 0.00 - 0.85$

Y	Y^2	$-\log(1 - \operatorname{erf} y)$	$\log(1 + \operatorname{erf} y)$	Y	Y^2	$-\log(1 - \operatorname{erf} y)$	$\log(1 + \operatorname{erf} y)$
0.00	0.00	0.0000	0.0000	0.43	0.1849	0.26511	0.16343
0.01	0.0001	0.00493	0.00488	0.44	0.1936	0.27264	0.16619
0.02	0.0004	0.00991	0.00971	0.45	0.2025	0.28024	0.16894
0.03	0.0009	0.01495	0.01444	0.46	0.2116	0.28790	0.17164
0.04	0.0016	0.02005	0.01916	0.47	0.2209	0.29563	0.17426
0.05	0.0025	0.02520	0.02383	0.48	0.2304	0.30343	0.17690
0.06	0.0036	0.03041	0.02841	0.49	0.2401	0.31129	0.17947
0.07	0.0049	0.03567	0.03298	0.50	0.2500	0.31917	0.18199
0.08	0.0064	0.04100	0.03747	0.51	J.2601	0.32720	0.18446
0.09	0.0081	0.04638	0.04191	0.52	0.2704	0.33526	0.18693
0.10	0.0100	0.05181	0.04630	0.53	0.2809	0.34338	0.18935
0.11	0.0121	0.05731	0.05061	0.54	0.2916	0.35158	0.19170
0.12	0.0144	0.06286	0.05492	0.55	0.3025	0.35984	0.19404
0.13	0.0169	0.06848	0.05915	0.56	0.3136	0.36817	0.19634
0.14	0.0196	0.07415	0.06330	0.57	0.3249	0.37656	0.19860
0.15	0.0225	0.07988	0.06744	0.58	0.3364	0.38502	0.20082
0.16	0.0256	0.08566	0.07151	0.59	0.3481	0.39355	0.20301
0.17	0.0289	0.09151	0.07555	0.60	0.3600	0.40215	0.20518
0.18	0.0324	0.09742	0.07951	0.61	0.3721	0.41081	0.20728
0.19	0.0361	0.10339	0.08343	0.62	0.3844	0.41954	0.20935
0.20	0.0400	0.10942	0.08732	0.63	0.3969	0.42835	0.21139
0.21	0.0441	0.11549	0.09114	0.64	0.4096	0.43722	0.21341
0.22	0.0484	0.12165	0.09493	0.65	0.4225	0.44615	0.21537
0.23	0.0529	0.12786	0.09864	0.66	0.4356	0.45516	0.21733
0.24	0.0576	0.13413	0.10233	0.67	0.4489	0.46424	0.21922
0.25	0.0625	0.14046	0.10595	0.68	0.4624	0.47338	0.22110
0.26	0.0676	0.14685	0.10954	0.69	0.4761	0.48259	0.22292
0.27	0.0729	0.15330	0.11307	0.70	0.4900	0.49187	0.22474
0.28	0.0784	0.15982	0.11657	0.71	0.5041	0.50123	0.22652
0.29	0.0841	0.16639	0.12001	0.72	0.5184	0.51065	0.22825
0.30	0.0900	0.17304	0.12339	0.73	0.5329	0.52014	0.22996
0.31	0.0961	0.17974	0.12675	0.74	0.5476	0.52971	0.23165
0.32	0.1024	0.18651	0.13004	0.75	0.5625	0.53934	0.23330
0.33	0.1089	0.19333	0.13332	0.76	0.5776	0.54904	0.23490
0.34	0.1156	0.20022	0.13653	0.77	0.5929	0.55881	0.23649
0.35	0.1225	0.20717	0.13969	0.78	0.6084	0.56865	0.23805
0.36	0.1296	0.21419	0.14280	0.79	0.6241	0.57856	0.23957
0.37	0.1369	0.22128	0.14588	0.80	0.6400	0.58855	0.24107
0.38	0.1444	0.22842	0.14891	0.81	0.6561	0.59860	0.24254
0.39	0.1521	0.23563	0.15189	0.82	0.6724	0.60873	0.24398
0.40	0.1600	0.24290	0.15485	0.83	0.6889	0.61892	0.24539
0.41	0.1681	0.25024	0.15776	0.84	0.7056	0.62919	0.24677
0.42	0.1764	0.25764	0.16062	0.85	0.7225	0.63954	0.24814

$Y = 0.86 - 1.77$

Y	Y^2	$-\log(1 - \operatorname{erf} y)$	$\log(1 + \operatorname{erf} y)$	Y	Y^2	$-\log(1 - \operatorname{erf} y)$	$\log(1 + \operatorname{erf} y)$
0.86	0.7396	0.64995	0.24947	1.32	1.7424	1.20806	0.28738
0.87	0.7569	0.66043	0.25076	1.33	1.7689	1.22196	0.28780
0.88	0.7744	0.67099	0.25205	1.34	1.7956	1.23593	0.28823
0.89	0.7921	0.68160	0.25329	1.35	1.8225	1.25097	0.28865
0.90	0.8100	0.69231	0.25452	1.36	1.8496	1.26409	0.28905
0.91	0.8281	0.70307	0.25573	1.37	1.8769	1.27829	0.28943
0.92	0.8464	0.71393	0.25691	1.38	1.9044	1.29257	0.28981
0.93	0.8649	0.72483	0.25806	1.39	1.9321	1.30692	0.29019
0.94	0.8836	0.73582	0.25919	1.40	1.9600	1.32135	0.29055
0.95	0.9025	0.74688	0.26029	1.41	1.9881	1.33585	0.29090
0.96	0.9216	0.75801	0.26136	1.42	2.0164	1.35043	0.29124

TABLE I (Continued)

Y = 0.86 -1.77

Y	Y²	-log (1 - erf y)	log (1 + erf y)	Y	Y²	-log (1 - erf y)	log (1 + erf y)
0.97	0.9409	0.76922	0.26243	1.43	2.0449	1.36509	0.29157
0.98	0.9604	0.78049	0.26345	1.44	2.0736	1.37983	0.29188
0.99	0.9801	0.79185	0.26446	1.45	2.1025	1.39464	0.29219
1.00	1.0000	0.80327	0.26545	1.46	2.1316	1.40954	0.29250
1.01	1.0201	0.81477	0.26642	1.47	2.1609	1.42450	0.29279
1.02	1.0404	0.82635	0.26736	1.48	2.1904	1.43954	0.29308
1.03	1.0609	0.83797	0.26830	1.49	2.2201	1.45467	0.29334
1.04	1.0816	0.84970	0.26921	1.50	2.2500	1.46986	0.29361
1.05	1.1025	0.86151	0.27007	1.51	2.2801	1.48515	0.29387
1.06	1.1236	0.87335	0.27093	1.52	2.3104	1.50051	0.29411
1.07	1.1449	0.88529	0.27180	1.53	2.3409	1.51593	0.29436
1.08	1.1664	0.89733	0.27261	1.54	2.3716	1.53145	0.29460
1.09	1.1881	0.90939	0.27342	1.55	2.4025	1.54703	0.29482
1.10	1.2100	0.92154	0.27420	1.56	2.4336	1.56269	0.29504
1.11	1.2321	0.93379	0.27497	1.57	2.4649	1.57845	0.29526
1.12	1.2544	0.94612	0.27573	1.58	2.4964	1.59426	0.29546
1.13	1.2769	0.95849	0.27646	1.59	2.5281	1.61016	0.29568
1.14	1.2996	0.97094	0.27717	1.60	2.5600	1.62613	0.29585
1.15	1.3225	0.98347	0.27786	1.61	2.5921	1.64220	0.29605
1.16	1.3456	0.99611	0.27855	1.62	2.6244	1.65833	0.29623
1.17	1.3689	1.00877	0.27921	1.63	2.6569	1.67455	0.29642
1.18	1.3924	1.02153	0.27985	1.64	2.6898	1.69184	0.29658
1.19	1.4161	1.03437	0.28049	1.65	2.7225	1.70721	0.29675
1.20	1.4400	1.04728	0.28110	1.66	2.7556	1.72365	0.29691
1.21	1.4641	1.06026	0.28172	1.67	2.7889	1.74017	0.29706
1.22	1.4884	1.07331	0.28228	1.68	2.8224	1.75679	0.29721
1.23	1.5129	1.08645	0.28287	1.69	2.8561	1.77348	0.29737
1.24	1.5376	1.09966	0.28341	1.70	2.8900	1.79022	0.29750
1.25	1.5625	1.11295	0.28396	1.71	2.9241	1.80707	0.29763
1.26	1.5876	1.12631	0.28448	1.72	2.9584	1.82500	0.29776
1.27	1.6129	1.13975	0.28499	1.73	2.9929	1.84097	0.29789
1.28	1.6384	1.15325	0.28549	1.74	3.0276	1.85808	0.29800
1.29	1.6641	1.16685	0.28598	1.75	3.0625	1.87507	0.29813
1.30	1.6900	1.18051	0.28646	1.76	3.0976	1.89245	0.29824
1.31	1.7161	1.19425	0.28693	1.77	3.1329	1.90978	0.29835

Y = 1.78 - 2.69

Y	Y²	-log (1 - erf y)	log (1 + erf y)	Y	Y²	-log (1 - erf y)	log (1 + erf y)
1.78	3.1684	1.92716	0.29846	2.24	5.0176	2.81344	0.30070
1.79	3.2041	1.94462	0.29855	2.25	5.0625	2.83484	0.30071
1.80	3.2400	1.96218	0.29866	2.26	5.1076	2.85608	0.30073
1.81	3.2761	1.98080	0.29874	2.27	5.1529	2.87742	0.30075
1.82	3.3124	1.99753	0.29883	2.28	5.1984	2.89884	0.30076
1.83	3.3489	2.01533	0.29892	2.29	5.2441	2.92031	0.30077
1.84	3.3856	2.03320	0.29901	2.30	5.2900	2.94188	0.30079
1.85	3.4225	2.05110	0.29909	2.31	5.3361	2.96353	0.30080
1.86	3.4596	2.06918	0.29918	2.32	5.3824	2.98527	0.30081
1.87	3.4969	2.08728	0.29925	2.33	5.4289	3.00709	0.30082
1.88	3.5344	2.10547	0.29933	2.34	5.4756	3.02899	0.30083
1.89	3.5721	2.12374	0.29940	2.35	5.5225	3.05097	0.30084
1.90	3.6100	2.14209	0.29946	2.36	5.5696	3.07303	0.30085
1.91	3.6481	2.16052	0.29953	2.37	5.6169	3.09517	0.30086
1.92	3.6864	2.17902	0.29959	2.38	5.6644	3.11740	0.30087
1.93	3.7249	2.19761	0.29966	2.39	5.7121	3.13970	0.30088
1.94	3.7636	2.21628	0.29970	2.40	5.7600	3.16209	0.30089
1.95	3.8025	2.23502	0.29977	2.41	5.8081	3.18456	0.30089
1.96	3.8416	2.25386	0.29981	2.42	5.8564	3.20710	0.30090
1.97	3.8809	2.27276	0.29988	2.43	5.9049	3.22974	0.30090
1.98	3.9204	2.29175	0.29992	2.44	5.9536	3.25246	0.30090

TABLE I (*Continued*)

Y = 1.78-2.69

Y	Y^2	- log (1 - erf y)	log (1 + erf y)	Y	Y^2	-log (1 - erf y)	log (1 + erf y)
1.99	3.9601	2.31082	0.29996	2.45	5.0025	3.27525	0.30092
2.00	4.000	2.33096	0.30001	2.46	6.0516	3.29813	0.30092
2.01	4.0401	2.34919	0.30005	2.47	6.1009	3.32109	0.30092
2.02	4.0804	2.36850	0.30010	2.48	6.1504	3.34413	0.30092
2.03	4.1209	2.38788	0.30014	2.49	6.2001	3.36725	0.30094
2.04	4.1616	2.40736	0.30018	2.50	6.2500	3.39046	0.30094
2.05	4.2025	2.42691	0.30023	2.51	6.3001	3.41374	0.30094
2.06	4.2436	2.44654	0.30025	2.52	6.3504	3.43711	0.30094
2.07	4.2849	2.46624	0.30029	2.53	6.4009	3.46056	0.30096
2,08	4.3264	2.48604	0.30031	2.54	6.4516	3.48410	0.30096
2.09	4.3681	2.50592	0.30036	2.55	6.5025	3.50770	0.30096
2.10	4.4100	2.52586	0.30038	2.56	6.5536	3.53142	0.30096
2.11	4.4521	2.54589	0.30042	2.57	6.6049	3.55519	0.30096
2.12	4.4944	2.56601	0.30044	2.58	6.6564	3.57905	0.30096
2.13	4.5369	2.58620	0.30046	2.59	6.7081	3.60300	0.30098
2.14	4.5796	2.60648	0.30049	2.60	6.7600	3.62703	0.30098
2.15	4.6225	2.62683	0.30051	2.61	6.8121	3.65113	0.30098
2.16	4.6656	2.64726	0.30053	2.62	6.8644	3.67533	0.30098
2.17	4.7089	2.66778	0.30057	2.63	6.9169	3.69960	0.30099
2.18	4.7524	2.68837	0.30058	2.64	6.9696	3.72395	0.30099
2.19	4.7961	2.70905	0.30060	2.65	7.0225	3.74839	0.30099
2.20	4.8400	2.73081	0.30062	2.66	7.0756	3.77291	0.30099
2.21	4.8841	2.75065	0.30064	2.67	7.1289	3.79751	0.30099
2.22	4.9284	2.77157	0.30066	2.68	7.1824	3.82220	0.30099
2.23	4.9729	2.79258	0.30068	2.69	7.2361	3.84698	0.30101

Y = 2.70 - 3.00

Y	Y^2	-log (1 - erf y)	log (1 + erf y)
2.70	7.2900	3.87183	0.30101
2.71	7.3441	3.89674	0.30101
2.72	7.3984	3.92176	0.30101
2.73	7.4529	3.94684	0.30101
2.74	7.5076	3.97204	0.30101
2.75	7.5625	3.99732	0.30101
2.76	7.6176	4.02265	0.30103
2.77	7.6729	4.04808	0.30103
2.78	7.7284	4.07359	0.30103
2.79	7.7841	4.09919	0.30103
2.80	7.8400	4.12486	0.30103
2.81	7.8961	4.15062	0.30103
2.82	7.9524	4.17646	0.30103
2.83	8.0089	4.20239	0.30103
2.84	8.0656	4.22840	0.30103
2.85	8.1225	4.25449	0.30103
2.86	8.1796	4.28066	0.30103
2.87	8.2369	4.30692	0.30103
2.88	8.2944	4.33326	0.30103
2.89	8.3521	4.35968	0.30103
2.90	8.4100	4.38618	0.30103
2.91	8.4681	4.41277	0.30103
2.92	8.5264	4.43944	0.30103
2.93	8.5849	4.46619	0.30103
2.94	8.6436	4.49304	0.30103
2.95	8.7025	4.51995	0.30103
2.96	8.7616	4.54696	0.30103
2.97	8.8209	4.57404	0.30103
2.98	8.8804	4.60121	0.30103
2.99	8.9401	4.62845	0.30103
3.00	9.0000	4.65578	0.30103

[a] Prepared by Mrs. A. T. Randall, National Institutes of Health, Bethesda, Maryland.

example, of nitrogen per milliliter or of percent of stock antigen solution and undiluted antiserum.

Log Ag/Ab + log $(1 - \text{erf } y)/(1 + \text{erf } z)$ is then plotted against y^2, and the slope, s, of the resulting straight line is determined. D_1, the diffusion coefficient of the antigen, is calculated from Eq. (4).

$$D_1 = D_2/(2.303s + 1) \tag{4}$$

If D_1 so determined, is greater than two times or less than one-half the provisional D_1, the calculated D_1 should be used as a provisional D_1 and the computation be repeated.

It is necessary to correct D_1 for the viscosity of the antiserum and buffer, and the temperature at which the diffusion is carried out if this is other than 20°. This is done by means of the usual formula (Section 14.A.2). In general, however, we have found that if the concentration of antiserum is less than, or not much above, 10%, diffusion coefficients obtained by the above procedure at 25° agree with those obtained at 20° and corrected to the viscosity of water.

2. DETERMINATION OF DIFFUSION COEFFICIENTS BY A METHOD OF DOUBLE DIFFUSION IN GELS*

a. THEORETICAL

Quantitative gel precipitin technique (QGP)[1] is a modification of double-diffusion tube technique of Oakley and Fulthorpe.[2]

The theoretical part of this section is based on the original equations derived by Mitchison and Spicer[3] in their work on the estimation of streptomycin concentration in the body fluids from the extent of the antibiotics' inhibition of bacterial growth in agar gel into which the streptomycin was allowed to diffuse. By using the Gaussian error function in its expanded form, they have shown that the concentrations of the antibiotic could be calculated from one of two equations. These were:

$$\log C_0 = \log (2C \sqrt{\pi}) + \log \frac{x}{2 \sqrt{Dt}} + \frac{x^2}{4Dt} \tag{1}$$

and

$$\log C_0 = \log 2C + \frac{x}{\sqrt{\pi Dt}} \tag{2}$$

---

* Sections 14.C.2.a–e were contributed by Alfred Polson.

[1] A. Polson, *Sci. Tools* **5**, 17, (1958).
[2] C. L. Oakley and A. J. Fulthorpe, *J. Pathol. Bacteriol.* **65**, 49–60 (1953).
[3] D. A. Mitchison and C. C. Spicer, *J. Gen. Microbiol.* **3**, 184 (1949).

In these equations C_0 is the original concentration of antibiotic, C is the concentration of bacterial inhibition, D is the diffusion coefficient of the antibiotic, t is the diffusion time in seconds, and x is the depth of inhibition. When x is large, Eq. (1), containing the second power of x, is applicable; when x is small, Eq. (2) holds as a first approximation. This indicates that for short distances $\log C_0$ is a linear function of x. These equations are also applicable to the double diffusion technique of Oakley and Fulthorpe.[2]

The concentration of each of the reactants (antibody and antigen) at the position of the precipitin band is given by an equation similar to Eqs. (1) or (2). It follows, therefore, that

$$\log \frac{C_{0g}}{C_{0b}} = \log \frac{C_g}{C_b} + \log \frac{x_g}{x_b} + \log \sqrt{\frac{D_b}{D_g}} + \frac{x_g^2}{4D_g t} - \frac{x_b^2}{4D_b t} \qquad (3)$$

when x is large, and

$$\log \frac{C_{0g}}{C_{0b}} = \log \frac{C_g}{C_b} + \frac{x_g}{\sqrt{\pi D_g t}} - \frac{x_b}{\sqrt{\pi D_b t}} \qquad (4)$$

when x is small. In these equations the subscripts g and b refer to antigen and antibody, respectively. (For example, x_g is the distance from the antigen meniscus to the center of the band of precipitate.)

It was found empirically, during investigations of a number of systems ranging from low molecular weight antigens such as myoglobin, to giant protein molecules such as the hemocyanins and their antibodies, that the distance from the antigen meniscus where a precipitin band was formed was a linear function of the log antigen concentration when-gel column lengths of 1 and 1.5 cm were used. It therefore indicates that Eq. (4) was valid. Equation (3) can therefore be disregarded.

At the position of optimal proportions C_g/C_b is constant and if C_{0b} is kept constant, Eq. (4) may be written in the form

$$K \log C_{0g} = \log y + \frac{x_g}{\sqrt{\pi D_g t}} - \frac{x_b}{\sqrt{\pi D_b t}}$$

or

$$K \log C_{0g} = \log y + x_g \left(\frac{1}{\sqrt{\pi D_g t}} + \frac{1}{\sqrt{\pi D_b t}} \right) - \frac{x_g + x_b}{\sqrt{\pi D_b t}}$$

where K and y are constants. This equation may be reduced to its simplest form

$$x_g = k \log C_{0g} + Z \qquad (5)$$

where k and Z are constants.

If the antigen and antibody are present in optimal proportions

$$\frac{C_{0g}}{C_{0b}} = \frac{C_g}{C_b}$$

it follows that

$$\frac{x_g}{\sqrt{\pi D_g t}} = \frac{x_b}{\sqrt{\pi D_b t}}$$

or

$$\frac{x_g^2}{x_b^2} = \frac{D_g}{D_b} \tag{6}$$

From Eq. (6) it is clear that if the relative position of the precipitin band at optimal proportions of the reactants is known, the relative diffusion coefficients may be calculated.

b. Apparatus and Method

If accurate measurements are to be made of the positions of precipitin bands relative to the original levels of antigen and antibody in double gel diffusion, it is essential that the menisci should be flat, as concavity may introduce serious errors. Plane menisci are formed most readily in the apparatus especially designed for QGP reactions. The apparatus shown in Fig. 1 consists of 3 rectangular Perspex (Lucite) bars 20 × 2 × 1.5 cm and a section 20 × 2 × 0.5 cm through which 10 cylindrical holes 0.5 cm in diameter are drilled at regular intervals along their lengths. The cylinders form cuplike cavities, 1 cm deep, in one of the bars. To ensure maximum clarity the surfaces of the holes are well polished. Prior to assembly the surfaces of the sections are well greased with vacuum grease. The sections are pressed tightly together and held in this position with strong rubber bands. By moving the assembled sections relatively to one another excess grease is pressed out into the cylinders and may be removed with a cotton wool swab. The sections are moved until the cylindrical cavities are in exact apposition.

Antibody at the appropriate dilution is introduced in the cuplike bottom holes, and the excess is removed after sliding the section above it to the cutoff position. Traces of antibody are removed by thorough washing of the cavities with saline and drying with a cotton wool swab.

Gelling substance at the lowest possible concentration dissolved in the appropriate solvent is cooled to a temperature near its gelling point and introduced into the holes in the next section.* The following section is

---

* Agarose has several advantages over agar as a medium in which to produce precipitin bands. The main advantages are the absence of charged groups which may influence the diffusion of basic antigens, such as lysozyme, and its superior gel strength, which allows QGP experiments to be conducted in gels of much lower concentrations than

moved across. The excess gel is removed with a Pasteur pipet and suction. The top cavities are then filled with the antigen diluted serially. To ensure accurate results it is advisable to have the dilution interval as small as possible. The top cavities are closed by moving the lid to the closed position, and the cavities brought to exact apposition by moving the section containing the gel across. The rubber bands are then replaced with "cellotape" and the apparatus is left at room temperature and examined

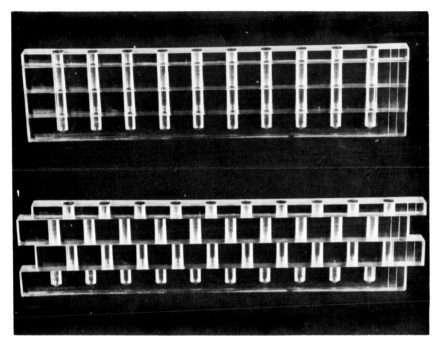

Fig. 1. Apparatus for quantitative gel precipitin reactions. *Top:* Apparatus when the cylindrical cavities are in apposition. *Bottom:* Apparatus immediately prior to start of the gel diffusion experiment. Antibody is contained in bottom cavities of the apparatus, the agarose gel in the next, and the dilutions of the antigen in the top.

daily for the appearance of precipitin bands. When these appear, their widths and positions relative to the antigen menisci are recorded with the aid of a microcomparator (a suitable apparatus is made by Precision Grinding, London). The data obtained are plotted against the logarithm of the dilution series.

would be possible if agar were used. Agarose prepared from the seaweed *Gelidium pestoïdes* may be used successfully in concentrations as low as 0.15 % on account of its superior gel strength over agarose derived from other sources.

c. ILLUSTRATION OF METHOD

Figure 2 is a contact photograph of the system human γ-globulin and antihuman γ-globulin prepared in the rabbit. The positions of the precipitin bands and their widths as recorded over a period of several days may be seen in Fig. 3. The dilution for optimal ratio between antigen and antibody may be read off on the abscissa at the point of intersection between the two limbs of the V. By interpolation of this position into the straight line, the exact position of x_g of Eq. (6) may be determined. x_b is

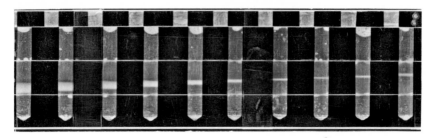

FIG. 2. Gel precipitin reaction of human γ-globulin at twofold dilutions against its antibody at constant concentration after 5 days at 25°.

obtained from $X - x_g$, where X is the length of the gel column (1.5 cm in the present case).

d. REFERENCE DIFFUSION COEFFICIENT

Equation (6) enables the calculation of the diffusion coefficient of the antigen relative to that of the antibody. If the value of D_b is known, D_g may be calculated. In general, antibodies are of the 7 S type, and it is to be expected that these antibodies would have the same diffusion constant at infinite dilution. This is probably true, but QGP experiments are always performed at finite serum dilutions (e.g., 1:5 to 1:20 dilution of the serum). The value for the diffusion coefficient of γ-globulin at infinite dilution is 4.81×10^{-7} cm²/sec at 20°.[4] This figure cannot be used as total protein of the diluted serum would have a depressing effect on the diffusion coefficient of the antibody. This difficulty was overcome by determining the diffusion coefficient of antibody with reference to that of human serum albumin at different dilutions of the antialbumin serum. The diffusion coefficient of human albumin is fairly well established and it is generally accepted that the value is 5.95×10^{-7} cm²/sec at 20°.[5]

[4] J. F. Largier, *Arch. Biochem. Biophys.* **77**, 350 (1958).
[5] R. L. Baldwin, L. J. Gosting, J. W. Williams, and R. A. Alberty, *Discussions Faraday Soc.* **20**, 13, (1955).

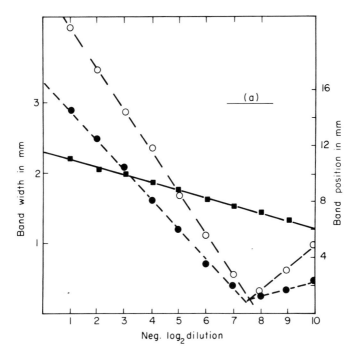

Fig. 3. Determination of diffusion constant of human γ-globulin by quantitative gel precipitin reaction. The rectangular points indicate the central precipitin band positions after 3 days, the solid circles the precipitin band widths after 3 days' diffusion, and the open circles the same after 5 days. Line (a) indicates the gel column length (15 mm) in the region of minimum line width.

Using this figure for albumin, a value of 4.6×10^{-7} cm²/sec was determined for the diffusion of antialbumin antibody when the antiserum was diluted fivefold in saline and 4.7 when diluted twentyfold.

e. Diffusion Coefficients of Components in a
   Mixture of Antigens

It was found feasible to determine the diffusion coefficients of the separate components in a mixture of antigens. Using a mixture of albumin and γ-globulin and diffusing the mixture against a mixture of their antisera, diffusion coefficients that differ very little from values obtained by the conventional optical techniques were obtained. The QGP technique is applicable even in such cases when the diffusion coefficient of two antigens are identical but differ in antigenicity.

In Table I are the results of diffusion coefficients as determined by QGP and by other methods.

TABLE I
DIFFUSION COEFFICIENTS DETERMINED BY QGP AND BY OTHER METHODS[a]

Substance	Diffusion coefficient by QGP	Diffusion coefficient by other methods
Serum albumin	—	5.95[b] Baldwin et al.[5]
Ovalbumin	7.9	7.76 Polson[6]
Serum γ-globulin	4.7	4.81 Largier[4]
Jasus lalandii hemocyanin	3.6	3.4 Polson[7]
Myoglobin (whale)	11.3	10.9 Crumpton and Polson[8]
Burnupena cincta hemocyanin	1.2	1.2 Polson and Deeks[9]
Type II poliovirus	1.2	— Polson et al.[10]

[a] Reference diffusion coefficient of antibody 4.6×10^{-7} cm²/sec. Serum diluted tenfold in saline and antigens serially twofold in same solvent.

[b] Reference diffusion constant.

f. A DENSITOMETRIC METHOD FOR DETERMINING THE POSITION OF OPTIMUM PROPORTIONS IN THE DOUBLE-DIFFUSION APPARATUS*

A worthwhile improvement in the method of measuring the position of lines of precipitation in the double-diffusion apparatus has been developed. The technique, which utilizes a densitometer (Analytrol, Beckman) makes it possible to plot the position of precipitin bands accurately and may also detect the presence of bands that are not readily observed directly. To demonstrate the method, an experiment to determine the diffusion coefficient of *Jasus lalandii* hemocyanin will be described.

An all-glass apparatus was used with serial dilutions of hemocyanin in the top wells and a constant concentration of antibody in the bottom wells. A 0.33% (w/v) solution of agarose in normal saline was introduced into the center section and allowed to gel. The experiment was started by sliding the upper and lower wells so that they were in apposition with the gel columns.

It has been noticed that the relatively heavy solutes employed tend to set up convection currents if the apparatus is kept in the same position for more than approximately 24 hours. This results in anomalous diffusion. The problem is easily overcome by turning the apparatus over twice each day.

[6] A. Polson, *Kolloid-Z.* **87**, 149 (1939).

[7] A. Polson, *Biochim. Biophys. Acta* **21**, 185 (1956).

[8] M. Crumpton and A. Polson, *J. Mol. Biol.* **11**, 722 (1965).

[9] A. Polson and D. Deeks, *Biochim. Biophys. Acta* **39**, 208 (1960).

[10] A. Polson, J. W. F. Hampton, and D. Deeks, *Biochim. Biophys. Acta* **44**, 18 (1960).

* Section 14.C.2.f was contributed by A. Polson and B. Russell.

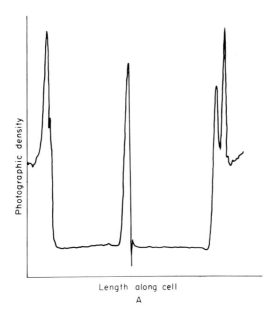

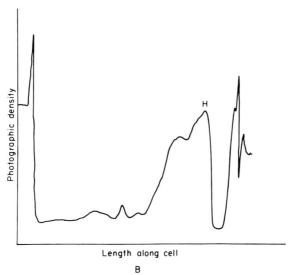

FIG. 4. (A) Densitometer trace of the precipitin band (center peak) of the main antigen in a cell where the antibody–antigen ratio is very close to optimal. Antigen well
(top of column) is peak on far left. Antibody is to the right.

(B) Densitometer tracing of a cell showing several separate precipitin bands; the
main antigen (band H) is in extreme excess.

As soon as precipitin bands first become visible, usually after 24 hours, their position is recorded photographically. This may be achieved by laying the apparatus on a high contrast negative and making a contact exposure. The method of illumination is important; parallel light should be used. If a point source of light is used, especially if it is not directly above the apparatus, parallax effects cause the image of the precipitin bands to be wider than in reality, and this reduces the accuracy of the experiment. Alternatively, the bands may be photographed against a black background using diffused side lighting. At least 3 exposures should be made over a period of 3–7 days, depending on the diffusion coefficient of the material under investigation.

The exact position of the precipitin bands in relation to the length of the agarose column is then determined by measuring the photographic density of the negative. Two densitometric tracings are shown in Fig. 4.

The distance of the peaks representing the precipitin bands may now be measured from the top of the agarose column which is shown by the sharp left-hand peak. This distance, plotted against the respective cell number, results in a straight line. Different straight-line curves, obtained for different diffusion times, are found to cross at a point which gives the exact position of optimum proportion.

This figure together with the total length of the cell, found by measuring the distance between the peaks at the start and finish of the densitometer trace, and the known diffusion coefficient of the antibody are used to calculate the diffusion coefficient of the antigen. In the case of *J. lalandii* hemocyanin, 3.3×10^{-7} cm^2/sec was found. This diffusion coefficient was calculated for the main antigen present.

The method may, therefore, be used to determine the diffusion coefficient of macromolecules when a suitable immune serum is available, and the presence of contaminating material may also be detected and its diffusion coefficient measured. If the antigen molecules can be shown to be approximately spherical, the molecular weight may be calculated.

3. MEASUREMENTS OF DIFFUSION COEFFICIENTS IN AGAR PLATES*

a. MEASUREMENTS OF DIFFUSION OF LABELED ANTIGEN OR ANTIBODY

Since the supporting medium stabilizes the system against convection and does not significantly impede random movement of most protein molecules when it is pure and dilute, diffusion in agar gels follows quite

* Sections 14.C.3–4 were contributed by A. C. Allison.

closely that expected from theory. Allison and Humphrey[1] showed that the rates of diffusion of radioactively labeled proteins from a small well through agar gels can be estimated by measuring the radioactivity present in small uniform cylindrical samples punched out of the agar at various times and at various distances from the well.

If diffusion takes place from an infinitely thin pencil source through a uniform layer, the concentration C at any point in the agar, distant r from the center of the source is given by

$$C = \frac{M}{4\pi hDt} \cdot e^{-r^2/4Dt} \tag{1}$$

where M is the quantity of material present in the source, h is the depth of the layer, t is the time allowed for diffusion, and D is the diffusion coefficient of the material used. Taking logarithms in expression (1) and differentiating with respect to r^2 we obtain

$$\frac{d}{d(r^2)} (\log_e C) = \text{slope at time } t = -\frac{1}{4Dt} \tag{2}$$

The slopes S_1 and S_2 at time t of two materials of diffusion coefficients D_1 and D_2 are related by the expression

$$\frac{S_1}{S_2} = \frac{D_2}{D_1} \tag{3}$$

In practice, provided that the value of t is large, plots of the logarithm of the concentration of material against the square of the distance from the center of the well give satisfactory straight lines, from the slopes of which D_1 and D_2 can be calculated. This eliminates uncertainties arising from the fact that the source is of finite size and makes it unnecessary to measure accurately the amount of material introduced at the start of the experiment.

Convenient experiments can be carried out with 4–5 mm layers of 1.2% (w/v) highly purified agar or preferably 0.7% agarose in saline buffered at pH 7.0 in carefully leveled, flat-bottomed petri dishes. With lower concentrations of agar or agarose gel, strengths are insufficient to allow handling of the punch samples. After 24 hours at room temperature, wells 3.5 mm in diameter are cut and carefully filled to the brim with material to be studied. The dishes are kept in a moist atmosphere at room temperature; after about 19 and 40 hours, four or five punch samples 1 mm in diameter are taken at various distances from the centers of the wells.

[1] A. C. Allison and J. H. Humphrey, *Immunology* **3**, 95 (1960).

An example of the use of this technique is the comparison by Humphrey of the diffusion coefficients of labeled human serum albumin and of complexes of human serum albumin with nonprecipitating antibody.[2] It was not practical to separate small amounts of nonprecipitating antibody from other proteins in sufficient quantity to permit conventional measurement of diffusion coefficients.

b. ESTIMATION OF DIFFUSION COEFFICIENTS FROM OUCHTERLONY PLATES

i. Theory

Theoretical analyses of double diffusion in agar were given by Ouchterlony[3] and Korngold and van Leeuwen.[4] The latter drew a conclusion of practical interest, namely that the zone of precipitation is concave toward the antibody well when the diffusion coefficient of antigen is greater than that of antibody, and vice versa. Later workers[5, 6] analyzed some of the complications that should be taken into consideration, including the facts that diffusion does not take place from a point source, that a finite amount of precipitate must be built up before it can be detected, and that the precipitate may not remain in the same place. A serious complication is the "sink effect"—removal from solution of both antigen and antibody where the precipitate is formed, so that movement of molecules in the neighborhood is nonrandom. This can be shown to occur with labeled molecules and can be treated theoretically by Bessel functions—which are, however, outside the mathematical experience of many immunologists (see Section 14.A.2).

It was partly to overcome this difficulty and partly to provide a simple technique requiring only elementary mathematics that Allison and Humphrey developed the L-plate system of estimating diffusion coefficients.[1] Elek and Ouchterlony had previously observed that if antigen and antibody are inserted at right angles to one another, precipitates are sometimes formed along a plane which, when viewed from above, appears as a straight line. This is likely to occur only if precipitation continues to take place along the plane at which the molecules first meet at optimal proportions, so that the "sink effect" is largely avoided. Furthermore, it can be shown that the ratio of diffusion coefficients of antigen (D_g) and antibody (D_b) is given by $\tan \theta = (D_g/D_b)^{1/2}$, where θ is the angle between the precipitation line and the antigen trough (Fig. 1).

[2] J. H. Humphrey, *Immunology* **7**, 462 (1964).
[3] O. Ouchterlony, *Arkiv Kemi* **1**, 43 (1949).
[4] L. Korngold and G. van Leeuwen, *J. Immunol.* **78**, 172 (1957).
[5] J. Engelberg, *J. Immunol.* **82**, 467 (1959).
[6] F. Aladjem, R. W. Jaross, R. L. Paldino, and J. A. Lackner, *J. Immunol.* **83**, 221 (1959).

ii. Procedure

In practice, a template is made by fixing to a support two stainless steel bars 30 × 1 × 5 mm deep at right angles to one another, separated by 1 mm. A flat glass plate of convenient size has a thin layer of agar dried onto it. The template is placed in position and a layer of agar 4 mm deep is poured. When the agar has cooled the template is removed and one of the 30 × 1 mm troughs is filled with antigen, the other with antibody. Usually concentrations found to be equivalent by the method of optimum proportions give good, straight precipitates, but it may be necessary to dilute antigen or antibody. If one is present in excess, the

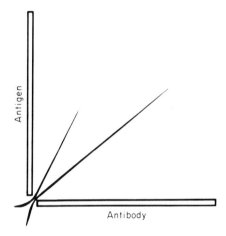

FIG. 1. Estimation of diffusion coefficients of antigens by the L-plate technique. The antigens in this experiment are human serum transferrin ($\theta = 51°$) and human serum β-lipoprotein ($\theta = 28°$); the precipitation lines are copied from a photograph.

precipitation line will be curved and diffuse toward the trough containing the other. When a long, straight precipitate has been formed (usually after 48 hours or more), the angle of the precipitation line with the antigen trough is measured with a protractor, preferably on an enlarged image. This value should be reproducible to within one degree. In the calculation, the diffusion coefficient of antibody can be taken as 3.8×10^{-7} cm^2 sec^{-1}, whence $D_g = 3.8 \times 10^{-7}$ (tan θ) cm^2 sec^{-1}. If the antibody is IgM (as can be shown by suitable control experiments such as demonstration of mercaptoethanol sensitivity), a diffusion coefficient of 1.8×10^{-7} cm^2 sec^{-1} can be used. Two or more antigens can be examined in the same system, although it may be necessary to adjust proportions of antibody to antigen so as to give equivalence precipitates of each separately.

4. DETERMINATION OF THE EFFECTIVE SIZE OF ANTIGENS AND ANTIBODIES

a. GEL FILTRATION

i. Gelatin and Agar "Plug" Methods

As the concentration of solid material in a gel increases, the effective pore size becomes smaller. The movement of large molecules through the gel is progressively retarded until the pore size approaches the Stokes radius of the molecule, when the movement of the molecules through the gel is prevented altogether. This cutoff can be relatively sharp, and provides information about molecular size. Allison and Humphrey[1] used a system in which antigens were allowed to diffuse through cylinders of

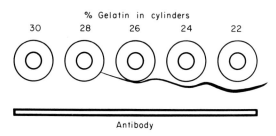

FIG. 2. Determination of molecular size by gel filtration. Each cylinder is composed of gelatin gel at a different concentration. Antigen (human serum albumin 1 mg/ml) was placed in the cylinders, and rabbit antiserum in the trough. Antigen diffused through 26% gelatin with some retardation, but not through 28%. From Allison and Humphrey.[1]

agar or gelatin of different concentration (Fig. 2). A series of holes of equal size (7.5 mm in diameter) and 5 mm apart are cut in a plate of 1.5% (w/v) buffered agar or 0.7% agarose and filled with agar gels of concentration 3 to 8% or of gelatin 5 to 40%. The gelatin is poured in at 60°; later, holes 3 mm in diameter are cut in the agar or gelatin plugs, a narrow trough for antiserum is cut about 7.5 mm from the row of holes, and the plate is set aside in a moist chamber for 24 hours for the gels to mature. Equal concentrations of antigen solution are then added to the holes, and antiserum to the trough. The concentration of agar or gelatin preventing precipitate formation is readily determined, and the system can be calibrated empirically. This is necessary for each sample of agar or gelatin used. Some cutoff points are given in Tables I and II.

A theoretical analysis of diffusion through agar gels and a technique for measuring transport across a thin agar membrane are given by

TABLE I
PERCENTAGES (W/V) OF AGAR LIMITING PENETRATION OF ANTIGENS[a,b]

Protein	Estimated molecular weight	Agar concentration
Caminella hemocyanin	6,600,000	3
Human serum β-lipoprotein	2,770,000	5
Sheep thyroglobulin	660,000	7
Jasus hemocyanin	450,000	7

[a] From Allison and Humphrey.[1]
[b] The values for hemocyanins are taken from Polson.[7]

TABLE II
PERCENTAGES (W/V) OF GELATIN LIMITING PENETRATION OF ANTIGENS[a]

Protein	Estimated molecular weight	Gelatin concentration
Human serum β-lipoprotein	2,770,000	5
Sheep thyroglobulin	660,000	7
Human and rat serum γ-globulin	177,000	18
Human serum transferrin	88,000	26
Human serum albumin	70,000	28
Hen's ovalbumin	44,000	32
Mouse urinary protein	17,000	40

[a] From Allison and Humphrey.[1]

Ackers and Steere.[8] Even at low agar concentrations slight restriction of diffusion of protein molecules was observed, possibly owing to ion exchange effects with charged groups in agar. It is well known that basic proteins such as lysozyme interact with sulfate groups of agar. For these reasons the use of agarose gels, in which the concentration of total solid is decreased and sulfate is largely eliminated, is desirable in all quantitative work.

ii. Sephadex Columns

An alternative gel-filtration technique which is useful for determining the size of unknown antigens is the use of Sephadex G-200 columns; this is discussed in Volume II. The antigen is passed though the column with suitable markers (e.g., labeled IgM, IgG, and hemoglobin), and the posi-

[7] A. Polson, *Biochim. Biophys. Acta* **19**, 53 (1956).
[8] G. K. Ackers and R. L. Steere, *Biochim. Biophys. Acta* **59**, 139 (1962).

tion in the effluent is determined by placing the fractions (concentrated, if necessary) in peripheral wells in an Ouchterlony plate and reacting with antibody. The maximum concentration of antigen is shown by the position of the precipitate (see Fig. 4). Such empirical determinations in the presence of markers are adequate for most practical purposes. For the theoretically minded, Ackers[9] has shown that, from experimental measurements of equilibrium solute partitioning and of corresponding column effluent volumes with Sephadex G-200 gels, the effective gel pore radius can be calculated. A column thus calibrated can be used for the determination of Stokes radii or diffusion coefficients of other macromolecules, and an upper limit for the hydrated molecular weight can be obtained.

iii. Thin-Layer Sephadex Chromatography and Immunodiffusion

The development of Superfine Sephadex dextran gels has allowed the use of thin-layer separation of macromolecules for molecular weight determinations. A convenient adaptation of this method for chromatography of proteins and nucleic acids, and for immunodiffusion, has been described by Williamson and Allison,[10] who give references to earlier work with the thin-layer system.

(a) *Preparation of Plates.* Discarded photographic 1/2 plates (16.6 × 12.1 cm) are freed from the emulsion coating, carefully cleaned and scribed with a diamond transversely 3 cm from one end. Alternatively, standard 20 × 10 cm plates are satisfactory. Gel suspensions are prepared by thoroughly mixing 4 gm of Sephadex G-200 Superfine (Pharmacia) with 100 ml of 0.5 M sodium chloride buffered with 0.05 M sodium phosphate, pH 7.0. The gel suspension is stored in a covered beaker for at least 72 hours to allow adequate swelling of the dextran particles. The gel is then applied to the unscribed side of the glass plates in a 0.25-mm layer with any standard spreader, such as that described by Stahl.[11] The quantities given are sufficient for 12 plates.

(b) *Chromatographic System.* Lucite food boxes (22.5 × 13.5 × 8 cm), with tightly fitting lids, are used as containers (C) for the plates (P) as shown in Fig. 3. A Whatman No. 3 MM filter paper wick (W) leads the solvent from a 13 × 3 × 3 cm Lucite trough (T) onto the gel 1 cm from the upper edge. Liquid is drawn from the bottom of the plate by a filter paper pad (F) which is moistened to ensure good contact with the gel. The trough is placed so that the plate is at an angle θ of about 10 degrees from the horizontal. Solvent is allowed to flow overnight before applica-

[9] G. K. Ackers, *Biochemistry* **3**, 723 (1964).
[10] J. Williamson and A. C. Allison, *Lancet* **II**, 123 (1967).
[11] E. Stahl, *Chemiker-Ztg.* **82**, 323 (1958).

tion of samples. To stop eluant flow for sample application, the box is tilted by placing a cork of suitable size under one end so that the plate is horizontal. A single drop (approximately 1 μl) of test sample from a capillary pipet (drawn from 3 to 4 mm quill tubing and attached to a rubber tube with mouthpiece) is applied to the origin, i.e., the scribed line visible through the gel from the uncoated underside of the plate. The pipet tip should not touch the gel, and samples should not be applied closer than 1.5 cm to the side of the plate. Precisely known volumes of sample, if required, can be delivered from a micrometer pipet. Each row of samples has a suitable colored marker, e.g., hemoglobin, ferritin, or a mixture of both. The cork is then removed and the tilt of the box is adjusted by support at either end so as to allow 1.4 to 1.6 cm movement of the hemoglobin marker per hour. Samples are run 4 to 5 hours.

(c) *Staining*. Plates are dried for 15 to 30 minutes in an oven at 50° to 60°. They are immersed for 5 to 10 minutes in a filtered saturated solution

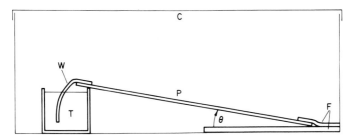

Fɪɢ. 3. Apparatus for thin-layer chromatography of proteins. See text for details.

of Amido Black 10B in methanol–water–glacial acetic acid (50:40:10, v/v) and destained in the dye solvent for 5 to 10 minutes in each of two successive wash baths. The position and relative staining intensity of proteins, including reference markers, can be determined accurately by transmission densitometric scanning. The apex of the density peak (Fig. 2) is used to estimate to the nearest millimeter the migration of a sample spot from the origin.

The following stain has proved most satisfactory for nucleic acids (DNA and RNA): Dried plates are immersed for 10 minutes in each of the following solutions in turn: (i) 0.5% Toluidine Blue in 50% aqueous methanol; (ii) and (iii) 2 wash baths of 25% aqueous methanol; (iv) 5% ammonium molybdate in 25% aqueous methanol; (v) 1 wash bath of 25% aqueous methanol. Densitometry is carried out as before. Other procedures are given in Section 14.E.1.

(d) *Autoradiography*. Dried stained plates are kept in contact with Ilflex X-ray film for an appropriate time, usually 2 to 7 days. Proteins labeled with ^{14}C, ^{125}I, or ^{131}I can be used, and densitometric readings show the positions of samples and relative concentration of radioactivity.

(e) *Immunochromatography.* Immediately after chromatography a strip of Whatman 3 MM paper 16 cm long and 5 mm wide, marked in pencil in numbered centimeter divisions, is applied to the wet gel on the plate, beginning at the top edge and extending along the line of run of the sample. The strip is left in place until visibly damp (2 minutes). After careful removal the whole strip, or an appropriate section of it, is placed on the surface of a thin layer of agar or agarose on a glass slide. For most purposes 1.5 ml of 0.5% agarose gel made up in phosphate-buffered saline on an ordinary microscope slide is satisfactory. A similar strip of filter paper 2 mm wide soaked in an appropriate dilution of antibody is placed on the gel parallel to the first strip and about 3 mm from it. Slides are left in a moist chamber until precipitation occurs; usually overnight is enough. The pattern should resemble those of immunoelectrophoretic analyses. The apices of precipitation arcs correspond to the positions of maximum antigen concentrations.

(f) *Determination of Molecular Weights.* Migration distances of proteins are expressed as fractions of the migration distances of human hemoglobin (R_{Hb} values). When R_{Hb} values are plotted against the logarithms of molecular weights of proteins in the range 15,000 to 200,000, a linear relationship is found (Fig. 4); proteins which are highly asymmetric or associated with much carbohydrate may give anomalous results.[12] Below molecular weight 15,000 and above 200,000 there is deviation from linearity. In the appropriate range, molecular weights can be calculated from the equation describing the linear part of the curve:

$$\log_{10} \mathrm{MW} = 1.53\, R_{\mathrm{Hb}} + 3.0$$

This gives a molecular weight for the hemoglobin marker (33,900) corresponding closely to the predicted half-unit value. Determinations of molecular weights of nucleic acids in this range also show satisfactory correspondence with those calculated from sedimentation coefficients in the range 1 S to 16 S. Soluble and ribosomal RNA, for example, are widely separated.

(g) *Sensitivity and Reproducibility.* In samples of 1-μl amounts of protein down to 0.5 to 1 μg can be detected and estimated by staining of plates. The sensitivity is such that traces of bovine plasma albumin dimer are detectable in samples of crystalline protein. Densitometry of stained spots permits estimation of amounts of nucleic acids down to about 1 μg. The sensitivity of detection of radioactive samples obviously

[12] P. Andrews, *Biochem. J.* **96**, 595 (1965).

depends on the level of labeling, but at levels of iodination commonly used, sensitivity is at least twentyfold greater than that possible by staining. Detection of antigens by precipitation is also more sensitive than direct staining by a factor of at least five.

The R_{Hb} values of the proteins used to construct the reference curve (Fig. 4) were means of 5 to 11 determinations, the standard deviations of

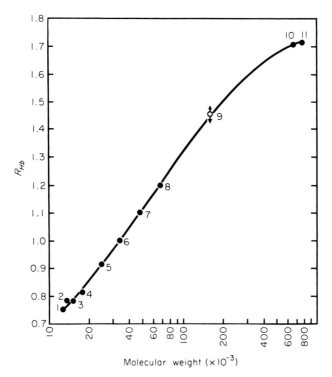

Fig. 4. Log₁₀ molecular weight as a function of R_{Hb} values of purified proteins run on thin-layer Sephadex G-200 Superfine gel. Point 1, cytochrome c; 2 and 3, pancreatic ribonuclease (A, B, respectively); 4, myoglobin; 5, chymotrypsin; 6, hemoglobin; 7, streptokinase; 8, bovine plasma albumin; 9, bovine γ-globulin; 10, thyroglobulin; 11, ferritin. From Williamson and Allison.[10]

which averaged approximately ±5% of the mean value for proteins lying on the linear part of the curve and up to ±10% for the largest proteins tested.

(h) *Characterization of Antibodies.* Samples containing antibodies can likewise be separated in the thin-layer Sephadex system, and their mobilities can be detected by suitable techniques. Thus, filter paper strips can be tested on slides for precipitation with antigen, the reverse of the procedure described for immunochromatography. Alternatively, strips can be tested against specific antisera defining the main immunoglobulin classes. The system described gives wide separation of IgG and IgM, with IgA extending from the position of IgG into the intermediate zone. Moreover, samples of antibody eluted from appropriate sections of the filter paper strips can be tested for hemagglutination or its inhibition, complement fixation, etc. Satisfactory separations can also be obtained of immunoglobulin subunits produced by enzymes, or by reduction and alkylation.

(*i*) *General Comment.* The usefulness of the immunochromatographic method for detection, separation, and characterization of small amounts of protozoal or viral antigens and of immunoglobulin fractions has already been established. Further applications, for example in the analysis of proteins in urine and other body fluids can be envisaged. For some purposes it is useful to determine the positions of antigens by enzyme assays. Marked filter paper strips can be stained by standard histochemical procedures or by applying them to substrate in agar. An example would be the lysis of fibrin included in an agar layer by streptokinase. Similarly, ribonuclease can be detected using a convenient plate method.[13] Such assays can detect enzyme protein in submicrogram amounts.

The apparatus is simple and inexpensive. For many types of analytical work with protein fractions, the thin-layer Sephadex system, used alone or in combination with electrophoresis, seems likely to replace the more tedious and elaborate column system. For most preparative purposes column fractionation retains its obvious advantages, but for certain types of preparation, when many samples or small amounts of highly active materials are available, the thin-layer system with elution from paper strips is satisfactory.

b. SEDIMENTATION COEFFICIENTS

Sucrose-density gradient centrifugation provides a convenient system for determining sedimentation coefficients of antigens. The technique is discussed in Volume II; the variation which we have used has been shown by Charlwood[14] to give satisfactory measurements of sedimentation coefficients of proteins, even when fixed-angle rotors are used instead of the swinging-bucket type; the former are useful for preparative work and allow many samples to be run simultaneously. Discontinuous gradients were set up with concentrations of sucrose ranging from 100 gm/liter at the top of the tube to 200–500 gm/liter at the bottom; these were allowed to diffuse for 24 hours before the sample was inserted with small

[13] J. Martin-Esteve, P. Puig-Munet, and F. Calvet, *Rev. Espan. Fisiol.* **12,** 243 (1956).
[14] P. A. Charlwood, *Anal. Biochem.* **5,** 226 (1963).

amounts of suitable markers (usually IgM labeled with ^{125}I and IgG labeled with ^{131}I, using pulse-height analysis in scintillation counters for measurements of radioactivity of fractions). The ultracentrifuges were run overnight ($\sim$16 hours) at speeds of 23,000 to 40,000 rpm according to the needs of the particular experiment. Temperatures of 16° to 10°

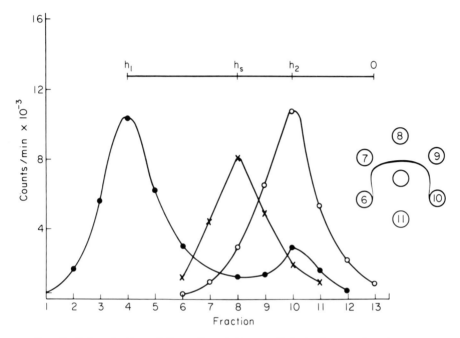

FIG. 5. Determination of the sedimentation coefficient of an antigen by sucrose density gradient centrifugation. Centrifuged (rotor 40) for 16 hours at 25,000 rpm in 100 to 300 gm/liter sucrose in phosphate buffer (pH 7.0, $I = 0.01$). The marker corresponding to h_1 was [125]I $-$ IgM (19.6 S), the marker corresponding to h_2 was [131]I $-$ IgG (6.8 S), and the sample with peak at h_s was beef liver catalase, the concentration of which was determined spectrophotometrically at 406 mμ. On the right, fractions have been set up in an Ouchterlony plate with rabbit anticatalase serum in the center well. From the position of the precipitate, it is clear that the maximum concentration of catalase is in fraction 8.

were used; since internal markers were present, accurate temperature controls were unnecessary. Fractions were counted for radioactivity and then placed in peripheral wells of Ouchterlony plates, with antibody in the center well; the sucrose was not dialyzed out since it did not interfere with precipitation in the systems used. Antigen peaks were taken as coinciding with the fractions in which the precipitate was farthest from the antigen well (Fig. 5). The sedimentation rates, S_1 and S_2, refer to the faster and slower markers, the peaks of which have traveled fixed distances h_1 and h_2 measured radially from the origin; under these conditions distances traveled are directly proportional to sedimentation coefficients (see Charlwood).[14] The sedimentation rate of the unknown sample (S_s), which has moved a distance h_s from the origin, is obtained from

$$S_s = S_2 + \left(\frac{h_s - h_2}{h_1 - h_2}\right)(S_1 - S_2)$$

hence in practice only differences between positions of peaks need be measured. Sedimentation coefficients of known antigens determined immunologically in this way have been in satisfactory agreement with accepted values ($\pm 25\%$). From sedimentation coefficients thus measured, and diffusion coefficients measured as described above, useful information about the molecular parameters of antigens can be obtained even in mixed and impure systems.

5. ANTIGEN AND ANTIBODY CONCENTRATION IN RELATIVE UNITS ON DIFFUSION PLATES*

a. PRINCIPLES OF METHOD

The method described here is a quantitative adaptation of Ouchterlony's original double-diffusion technique. It is based on the well known observation that, when an antigen and antibody diffuse toward one another in a gel to give a band of precipitate, there is no movement of the band at the equivalence point. In antigen excess, however, the band will move toward the antibody source and the higher the concentration of antigen used, the faster the band will migrate. Thus by measuring the position of the leading edge of the band after a standard incubation period and under carefully standardized conditions, it was found possible to estimate the antigen concentration with an accuracy of $\pm 5\%$ (95% confidence limits).[1, 2] A dilute antiserum which gives as few extraneous bands as possible is chosen as the standard and is calibrated against a standard antigen solution. A straight line calibration curve is usually obtained when the distance of the leading edge of the precipitate from the antigen source is plotted against the logarithm of the antigen concentration (Fig. 2).

Methods based on other principles include those of Gell,[3] in which the band pattern given by two dilutions of the unknown is matched against

* Sections 14.C.5.a–b were contributed by D. A. Darcy.

[1] D. A. Darcy, *Immunology* **3**, 325 (1960).
[2] D. A. Darcy, *Nature* **206**, 826 (1965).
[3] P. G. H. Gell, *J. Clin. Pathol.* **10**, 67 (1957).

that of a standard dilution series on the same plate, that of Feinberg,[4] which employs an antibody gradient in the agar so that the end-point dilution is indicated by a precipitate band which just encircles its antigen well, and that of van Oss and Heck[5] in which the equivalence point is determined. This and other more rapid but less precise methods are described below in Subsection c. More recently the diameter of the ring of precipitate produced by antigen diffusing into antibody agar has been widely used for estimating immunoglobulins (see Section 14.C.6).

b. Procedure for Estimating Antigens

i. Preparation of Antiserum

The method depends on having available a strong precipitating antiserum (or else a large quantity of a weak one). The purer the antiserum is (i.e., the fewer extraneous bands obtained with it) the better, so that immunization should be carried out with the purest available sample of the antigen which is to be estimated. A simple method used in this laboratory is to give a rabbit 2 ml of a strong solution (1 to 3%) of the antigen emulsified with 2 ml of complete Freund's adjuvant subcutaneously on the back on three occasions spaced 1 month apart. Bleeding is done 2 weeks after the last injection. Tubercle bacilli are omitted after the first injection. Other methods of immunization are described in Volume I, Chapter 2.

ii. Testing the Antiserum

Tests are carried out in a petri dish filled to a depth of 3 mm with 1 or 1.5% agar in 0.9% NaCl containing 0.01% Merthiolate. Holes are cut in the agar as the pattern shown in Fig. 1. The holes should be as near as possible to 1 cm in diameter, and the outer holes should be 1 cm from the center hole at the nearest point.

The center hole is used for the antiserum, and in it is placed 0.2 ml of a dilution of the antiserum in Merthiolated saline. A useful series of antiserum dilutions is 1:2, 1:4, 1:8 and 1:16. The same volume of four different dilutions of a solution of the antigen are placed in the outer wells, the same series being used for each plate. The plates are then incubated in a moist chamber for 3 days at 37° or at room temperature for 4 to 5 days. At the end of this time precipitate bands should be present, the ones formed by identical antigens being linked together by arcs. The antigen solution should be as crude as those later to be titrated. The ideal antiserum is one which gives a single measurable band at a 1:8 or higher

[4] J. G. Feinberg, *Intern. Arch. Allergy* **11**, 129 (1957).
[5] C. J. van Oss and Y. S. L. Heck, *Z. Immunitaetsforsch.* **122**, 44 (1961).

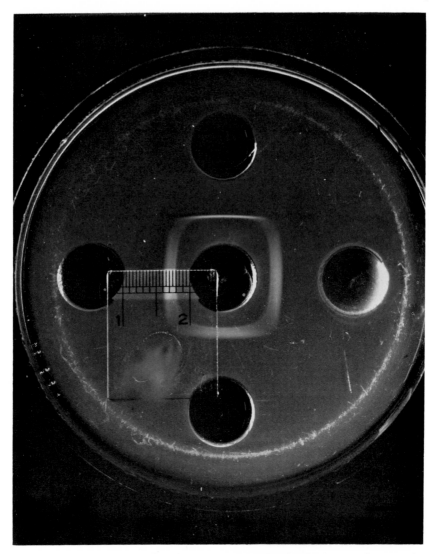

FIG. 1. The standard agar diffusion plate at the end of incubation showing the ruler method of measuring the position of the precipitate edge.

dilution. The band need not be dense, but its leading edge (the one nearest the antiserum well) should be sufficiently well defined under $2|\times|$ to $|10|\times$ magnification that its position can be measured. Suitable antisera may be pooled. Pooled antiserum is retested by diluting in narrower intervals. The highest dilution which gives a measurable band is chosen as the standard antibody solution. A purified preparation of the antigen is used to demonstrate that a precipitate band is formed by the antigen under consideration, not by a contaminant in a crude antigen preparation. If a purified preparation of the antigen is not available, the other methods of identification, such as immunoelectrophoresis (Section 14.D), specific staining (Section 14.E.1), determination of diffusion coefficient (Section 14.C.3), may be used to identify the correct band.

iii. Preparation of the Standard Agar Plate

For precision work it is necessary to use special flat petri dishes, and it is desirable that they should remain level when in stacks of four. If the gels are not incubated in a level position, considerable errors will result. Suitable dishes of 2.5 inch or 6.3 cm bottom diameter were obtained from Shandon Scientific Company, Ltd. A precision 5-hole cutter of the type designed by Feinberg[4] is used in this laboratory to make the gel pattern shown in Fig. 1. It cuts holes exactly 1 cm in diameter, with the outer holes 1 cm from the center hole at the nearest points; this cutter also was supplied by Shandon. A simpler, though less accurate tool would be a single cork borer and a guide block drilled with 5 holes of appropriate size.

The only essential requirement for the agar gel is that it should not vary in quality during the lifetime of the standard antiserum. In practice it is advisable to choose a purified agar (e.g., Oxoid I.D. agar or Difco Noble) and to start with a batch of at least 500 gm. A 1 or 1.5% solution is made up in buffered saline containing an antiseptic. It is important that the agar be fully dissolved. In this laboratory 15 gm of I.D. agar is added to a liter of buffered saline in a conical flask and heated in a bath of boiling water (3-liter beaker) with motor stirring for 1 to 2.5 hours.

A leveling table, or a level surface on which to let the plates gel and on which they are subsequently incubated, is required. The petri dishes are assembled on the leveled surface, and a predetermined amount of agar is dispensed into each so that the layer is 3 mm deep. The agar should be near boiling point to facilitate dispensing and even spreading. The covers of the plates are put on at once, and the plates are not moved until the agar has set. They are stored in a moist chamber, where they keep for months, or they may be used immediately. Any liquid in the holes is removed with a Pasteur pipet before they are filled with reactants.

The holes are then filled by pipetting 0.2 ml of the diluted antiserum on the center hole and 0.2 ml of the various antigen solutions on the outer holes. A convenient pipet is the Folin type recalibrated for blow-out delivery and fitted with a small rubber bulb. The plates are then incubated at 37° for 3 days (precise to within 30 minutes) and then read. A suitable incubating chamber is a desiccator jar of 10-inch diameter in which the desiccant is replaced with water. If the platform of the desiccator is not strictly flat, it should be replaced by a disc of plate glass which is then carefully leveled for each incubation. The plates are inserted in stacks of four preferably, but if heavy condensation occurs it may be necessary to put dummy plates at top and bottom of the stack to overcome it. When an air incubator is used it will be found that faster migration of bands will occur if the whole jar is wrapped with metal foil. Faster migration of the bands is desirable because it acts differentially; the bands of higher antigen concentrations move faster than the lower, hence better separation is achieved. If a water bath is used, the plates can be sealed with grease and put directly into the water on a level surface.

iv. Reading the Plates

A good viewing device is one consisting of illumination coming obliquely from below and a black background against which to see the precipitates. In fact, an adequate viewer consists of a beaker placed upsidedown on a piece of black paper with a partly shaded electric lamp shining upward through the side and bottom of the beaker. The petri dish is seated on the beaker bottom.

For accurate measurements, a magnifying lens (about 2 X) must be added. Measurement of the precipitate band can be carried out with a segment of clear plastic ruler, containing a centimeter ruled in half-millimeters, to which a small plastic handle is attached. The ruled centimeter is laid on the gel surface and lined up so that its limits coincide with the centimeter distance between the center hole and one of the outer holes along the line between their centers (Fig. 1). The distance from the edge of the outer hole to the sharp leading edge of the precipitate (the edge nearest the antiserum well) is estimated to the nearest 0.1 mm. If the distance between the 2 holes is slightly more or less than 1 cm, then the ruler is centered so that its 5-mm mark is approximately at the center of the distance between the two holes. This method of measurement is subject to some parallax error but is nevertheless capable of a good degree of precision and may be used routinely so that the overall error for the titration is only about ±5% (95% confidence limits).[6] A more accurate method of measurement is to use a microscope with a low-power objective (about 1 X) which throws the image on an ocular micrometer scale (a centimeter ruled in 0.1-mm divisions) fitted into the eyepiece. When such an instrument is used for measuring, the petri dish must be maneuvered until the centimeter scale is exactly centered between the center hole and the outer one. It is important to focus on the top edges of

[6] D. A. Darcy, *Nature* **191,** 1163 (1961).

the holes, as this is the only satisfactory point. Finally, it must be pointed out that different observers may consistently give different readings for the same line. This can occur even with the measuring microscope when faint lines are being measured. It is essential, therefore, that the person who made the calibration measurements measure the unknown titrations, unless the two persons are known to agree in their observations.

v. Calibration of the Standard Antiserum

The standard antibody solution (see Section ii) must be calibrated against known concentrations of the antigen or against dilutions of the antigen, selected as the standard, which contains a known (or assigned) number of arbitrary units. This antigen standard need not be pure; indeed it is preferable to choose the sort of solution (e.g., serum, concentrated urine, or tissue extract) that will later be titrated by the method. The highest concentration of the antigen that should be normally used is one that gives a reading about 9.0 mm against the standard antiserum under the standard incubation conditions. Higher readings, in addition to being less precise, may not be on the straight-line calibration curve (Fig. 2). The lowest concentration that will give a point on the logarithmic portion of the curve is approximately that concentration which gives just-measurable movement of the precipitate band (or its leading edge) toward the antiserum hole; this is tested at room temperature. The highest and lowest antigen concentrations having been selected, two intermediate values are selected and the calibration measurements are begun. The sharpest and narrowest line occurs at the equivalence point, but since there is no movement of the band, the present method operates in the antigen excess region.

When incubating the plates in a desiccator jar, it is convenient to incubate 16 plates (in 4 stacks) at once. Each plate contains the 4 antigen dilutions in its outer holes and the standard antiserum in the center one. It is necessary to see that each antigen dilution gets its fair share of outer (near the wall of the jar) and inner positions. This can be done by appropriate rotation of the plates in the stack. It is advisable to assemble the stacks in given positions in the jar, and the jar in a given position in the incubator; in this way information can be obtained about the characteristics of the incubator.

The above experiment should be repeated at least once to obtain 32 readings for each antigen dilution. A third or even fourth run is desirable, especially if the mean differences between the first two runs were appreciable. The readings for each dilution are finally assembled, the means are found, and the distances are plotted against the logarithm of the concentrations. The result, in most cases, will be a straight line. If it is not,

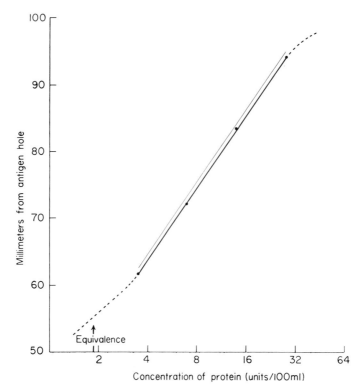

Fig. 2. Titration curve for an α_1-glycoprotein of rat serum, showing the distance traveled by the precipitate with increasing concentrations of the protein. The faint lines show the 95% confidence limits for the mean of 4 observations.

the reason may be that the highest antigen concentration was too high, or the lowest too low. This can be rectified by measuring less extreme concentrations. Alternatively, logarithms can be abandoned and a curved line obtained that will be less accurate but satisfactory enough for most purposes.

vi. Titration of Unknown Solutions

The same conditions are used as in the calibration experiments. Four 0.2-ml samples of each unknown are distributed to four representative positions in the incubator (e.g., one in each stack, one in each plate position within the stack, and two inner and two outer hole positions) according to a prearranged plan. Along with the unknowns should be a standard solution of the antigen, preferably one that gives a high reading, to serve as a check on the batch. If the titer obtained for the standard antigen solution indicates that the whole batch reads too high or too low, possibly because of temperature, then the appropriate percentage correction may be applied. Where the standard antiserum gives more than one band of precipitate it may be necessary to include the standard antigen in every plate so that it gives a "reaction of identity" with the appropriate band on either side of it. If fewer than 16 solutions per batch are to be incubated, then dummy plates (containing agar) can be substituted, or some other distribution of the unknowns can be arranged.

It is useful to have a standard form on which the readings are recorded and on which the 4 readings for each unknown can easily be assembled by means of the key. The form should also have space for the calculation of the means, for the calibration reading, the dilution factor, etc. This system enables the plates to be read blind so as to avoid subjectivity in the readings.

vii. Estimation of Antibody

The antibody titer of new antisera may be estimated in a manner similar to the above method for titration of antigens. A standard antiserum and a standard antigen solution are required, and the details of technique are as before. A single dilution of the antigen is used throughout—one that gave a reading approximately in the middle of the titration curve for antigens. The standard antiserum is diluted in a series that covers the expected range of strength of the new antisera, e.g., 1:5 to 1:20. Plates are set up with the standard antiserum dilutions in the center hole and the antigen solution in the outer holes, and a calibration curve is constructed with 32 or more readings for each point. A straight line is obtained when distance is plotted against logarithm of the standard antiserum concentration. The unknown antiserum is run similarly, a dilution is chosen that can be expected to give a result lying on the curve, and four plates are incubated with this. The result is a titer in terms of the standard antiserum.

This arrangement is not as efficient as that of putting the unknown antiserum dilution in the outer holes and the standard antigen in the center and measuring from the center hole outward. This method should be excellent for most purposes, but it gives readings different from the first one.

More direct methods, based on the equivalence point, are described below in Subsection c.

viii. Micromethod

This method has the advantage not only that it uses less of the reactants (about one-eighth), but that it requires only overnight incubation, needs no quantitative pipets, and can be carried out on microscope slides instead of petri dishes. Its error of estimation (95% confidence limits) in this laboratory was ±8%.[2]

The method is essentially a half-scale version of the macromethod employing the same pattern of holes as in Fig. 1, but these are now 5 mm in diameter and the outer ones are 5 mm from the center hole at the nearest points. If petri dishes are employed, they are filled to 1.5 mm with agar and a hole-pattern is cut in the center of the plate or in the 4 quadrants of the plate if a 9-cm plastic one is used. For microscope slides, a plastic tray of the kind designed for immunoelectrophoresis (e.g., Shandon Scientific Company or Gelman Instrument Co.) may be used. Gels of about 1.5 mm to 2.0 mm depth on the slides should be used. Gels of 1.0 to 2.5 mm thickness give the same readings, but it is essential that all holes in a given 5-hole pattern should be of the same depth. The agar is allowed to gel on a level surface and covered to prevent excessive evaporation. As with the petri dishes it is stored in a moist chamber before use. Two 5-hole patterns may be cut per slide.

The holes are filled to give a flat meniscus (or approximately so) using fine Pasteur pipets. No adjustment is made to the meniscus after about 10 seconds, since imbibition occurs fairly rapidly. The gels are incubated at 37° on a level platform in a well saturated moist chamber. After 18 hours (or other convenient standard interval) the position of the precipitates is measured as above. Other details are as in the macromethod. As before the 4 observations for each unknown are distributed over 4 different hole patterns.

ix. Sources and Calculation of Error

The accuracy of the method depends on standardization. Everything (agar gels, incubation temperature, the standard antiserum, etc.) must be kept as constant as possible from the time the antiserum is calibrated. A major source of error is failure to level the plates: aberrant readings are often traceable to a tilted plate. Interference from nonspecific substances in the antigen solutions has not been observed so far, thus a purified preparation of a protein should not give a different reading from the same concentration of the protein in a mixture such as serum,[1] but the investigator would be wise to check this possibility when applying the method to solutions of his antigen radically different in composition from that used to construct the calibration curve. Denaturation or other qualitative change of the antigen molecule may be expected to give false readings.

To determine the error of titration, the standard deviations are first calculated for the readings of the standard antigen dilutions and these are plotted on the calibration curve above and below the mean values (Fig. 2). When these new points are joined up they give two lines which represent the 95% confidence limits for using the mean of 4 readings for each unknown. This is the usual number of observations employed in the method. The 95% confidence limits for any single reading are two standard deviations, σ, from the means. Since in practice the estimate of the unknown is usually made from the mean of N readings, the 95% confidence limit, for practical purposes, will be represented by $2\sigma/\sqrt{N}$. Thus, to double the confidence in the routine (4-observation) method, 16 observations per unknown would be required. It may be noted that, if one of the calibration points lies a little way off the logarithmic straight line, the error for the new point can be assumed for practical purposes to be the same percentage of the new mean as it was for the observed mean.

c. SEMIQUANTITATIVE METHODS FOR EQUIVALENCE DETERMINATION*

The two micromethods described in this section are convenient overnight assays for either antigen or antibody. Both require standard solutions of known antigen concentration and antibody content.

i. Excess Deflection Method[7]

A gel punch† or a plastic template or guide is employed to produce the pattern of wells shown in Fig. 3. Three rows of wells are arranged so that any three wells determine an equilateral triangle. If a homemade template for microslides is employed, holes should be drilled to accommodate a 13-gauge hypodermic needle. When the point of the needle is ground off and the blunt tube is sharpened at its inner surface, it cuts a hole 2 mm in diameter. The needle punch may be connected to a vacuum trap so that the plugs are aspirated as they are cut.

The middle row of wells is filled alternately with standard antigen (A) and antiserum (S) at equivalent combining concentrations. The outer rows are filled with antigen–antibody mixtures, prepared in advance by adding antigen in quantities obtained by doubling dilutions.

If the objective is to titrate unknown antisera, for example a trial bleeding from an animal being immunized, then that serum is mixed with known amounts of antigen. Milligram amounts per milliliter of antiserum

* Section 14.C.5.c was contributed by Curtis A. Williams.

[7] M. M. H. Sewell, *Sci. Tools* **14**, 11 (1967).
† Gelman Instrument Co., Ann Arbor, Michigan.

are shown in Fig. 3, but these total quantities are not required. Wells in the outer rows may be filled immediately after the mixtures are made. If antigen concentrations are to be estimated, then serial dilutions are mixed with the standard antiserum.

The slides are placed in a humid chamber and are allowed to develop at room temperature. The reactions may be speeded by development at 37°, but then preservatives such as Merthiolate (0.01%), must be used in the agar.

Lines of precipitate will form between the alternating standard antigen (A) and antiserum (S) in the middle row. These lines will be deflected by an excess of either antigen or antibody in a well of the outer row. For

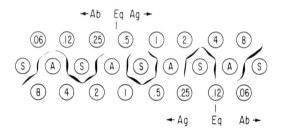

Fig. 3. Titration of two antisera by excess deflection method. S indicates standard antiserum, A indicates standard antigen. The outer rows of wells contain equal volume mixtures of antigen and antiserum made with antigen in concentrations (mg/ml) indicated. Deflection of standard precipitate around an A well indicates excess antibody; deflection around an S well indicates excess antigen in the mixture. No deflection indicates equivalence. Adapted from Sewell.[7]

example, in the well containing the mixture of 0.25 mg antigen per milliliter of antiserum (third from left on top row), there is an excess of antibody since the contents are seen to react with the standard antigen A. In the next well with a mixture at 0.5 mg of antigen per milliliter of antiserum, the antigen is in excess and reacts with the standard antiserum. With some precipitating systems it should be possible to employ smaller intervals in antigen concentration to define narrower limits of equivalence. The series represented in the bottom row seems to present an unambiguous equivalence reaction at 0.12 mg per milliliter of antiserum. But this is a relatively weak antiserum, and even if there were excess antibody it may not be sufficient to deflect the strong standard reaction between A and S.

This test is convenient since it does not require that precise amounts of reactants be pipetted to the wells in the agar. The precision, if desired, is introduced in the test tubes where the antigen and antisera are mixed.

ii. Band Width and Position Methods

Figure 4 illustrates the principle that a double diffusion precipitate at equivalence is sharp, narrow, and stationary. The pattern was cut free-hand with a 13-gauge needle punch on 5-mm centers using graph paper as a guide. In 2-mm thick agar, the holes accommodate 5 μl of fluid, which may be added precisely with micropipets. Alternatively holes may be filled to just brimming on the assumption that all holes are the same size. The only requirement is that all holes receive the same amount of fluid once the desired antigen dilutions are prepared.

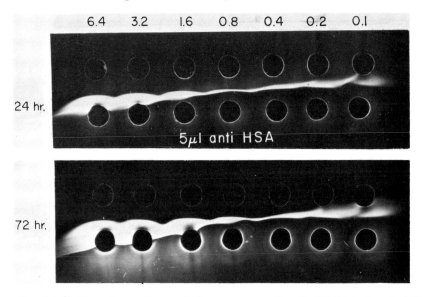

Fig. 4. Titration of an antiserum to human serum albumin (HSA) by band width and mobility method. Equal volumes (5 μl) of HSA solutions in concentrations (mg/ml) noted are added to wells of upper row. Equivalence is indicated by the narrow, stationary precipitate between 0.8 and 0.4 mg HSA/ml.

The numbers over the antigen wells (upper row) refer to the concentration (mg/ml) of human serum albumin (HSA). Since antiserum is added in equal volume to the wells of the lower row, the concentration values would also be equivalence notations. At 24 hours the estimate of equivalence in Fig. 4 would be slightly less than 0.8 mg HSA per milliliter of antiserum. By 72 hours, however, the equivalence reaction is seen to occur about half way between the 0.8 and 0.4 well; clearly 0.8 is in antigen excess and 0.4 is in antibody excess. Actually, true equivalence point of this system was determined at 0.55 mg/ml by quantitative precipitation.

(The periodic striae seen in antigen excess precipitate after 72 hours' diffusion are temperature artifacts induced by daily observation at a higher temperature than that at which the slides were stored for diffusion; see Section 14.B.1.c.)

Figure 5 illustrates a method making use of the principle that the position of the precipitate at equivalence is determined by the relative diffusion rates of the antigen and antibody. The position could be determined on an empirical basis for any soluble antigen. Human IgG is employed here to demonstrate the method. Since the human IgG antigen and rabbit IgG antibody can be assumed to diffuse at the same rate in agar, the equivalence precipitate, in addition to being immobile and sharp, should occur equidistant between the two wells.

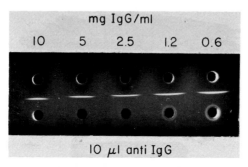

Fig. 5. Titration of an antiserum to human IgG by band position method. Equal volumes (10 μl) of IgG solutions at concentrations (mg/ml) noted are added to the wells of the upper row. For IgG, equivalence is indicated when precipitate is equidistant between the antigen and antiserum wells. The equivalence position for other antigens would depend on their diffusion rates relative to that of the antibody.

Measurement being more critical in this technique than in the previous one, a machined pattern punch or template is desirable. The pattern in Fig. 5 was cut by a Gelman punch giving holes 3 mm in diameter on 13-mm long centers and 10-mm short centers. Since only the position of the early precipitate is being considered, the development can be accelerated by incubation at 37°. In this case results are obtained in a few hours and no preservative need be employed in the agar.

It is seen that the reaction with 10 μl of antigen solution at 2.5 mg IgG per milliliter give a precipitate nearly equidistant from the antiserum and antigen wells. The slide was developed for 6 hours at 37°.

Any of these rapid micromethods can be carried out with a central-well pattern described above in Section 14.C.5.b, and suitable machined pattern punches are available commercially. In this laboratory linear patterns are preferred since direct visual comparison of reactions is more readily made and measurements are made simply by placing the slide on milli-meter-ruled paper. For accurate measurements, the Bausch and Lomb Measuring Magnifier can be used; of the various scales available the most useful is the metric scale measuring 0.1-mm interval up to 20 mm.

If narrower limits of equivalence are desired, it may be possible to use antigen dilutions with smaller intervals, but great care is required. The *excess deflection* method described above (i) may be more sensitive.

6. ANTIGEN TITRATION BY SIMPLE RADIAL IMMUNODIFFUSION IN PLATES*

a. PRINCIPLE OF THE METHOD

Simple radial immunodiffusion is the procedure whereby an antigen is deposited at a single point (practically in a small cylindrical well) of a thin layer of gel containing a uniform concentration of antibody. As the antigen diffuses into the antibody field, a disk-shaped immune precipitate is formed (Fig. 1). It has been known for a long time that a quantitative

* Section 14.C.6 was contributed by Joseph F. Heremans.

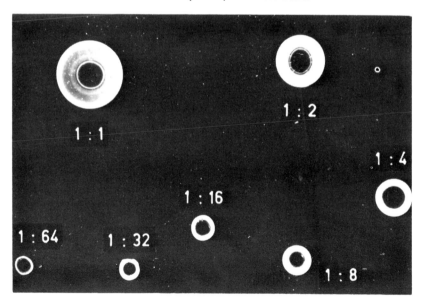

Fig. 1. Unstained immunodiffusion plate. The agar contained rabbit antiserum against human serum albumin. The antigen wells were filled with serial dilutions of a 1% albumin solution, as indicated on the photograph. The plate was photographed on a dark background, using indirect light. This picture was taken on day 5 of the experiment, when diffusion had ceased. From Mancini et al.[8]

relationship exists between the amount of antigen applied to the well and the size of the resulting precipitate.[1] Semiquantitative methods based on the end-point dilution principle have been proposed to exploit this principle,[2-4] and a more reliable technique, in which the diameter of the ring is measured after a short time of diffusion, has been described.[5, 6] The latter two methods are in fact simplified versions of a slightly more elaborate technique which was developed in 1963 at the author's laboratory by Mancini et al.,[7, 8] and which, with minor modifications, has also been used by other writers.[9]

The Mancini method, which is described below in some detail, is based on two empirically discovered principles: (1) The area of a given precipitate, after a period of growth due to diffusion of the antigen from the well, will eventually reach a maximum size, after which no further development will be noted (Fig. 2). (2) This terminal size (S) of the precipitate (or the square of its diameter, which is of course equivalent), is linearly proportional to the amount of antigen (Q_{Ag}) applied to the well, and to the reciprocal of the antibody concentration (C_{Ab}) in the gel, over a very wide range (Fig. 2):

$$S = a + b \frac{Q_{Ag}}{C_{Ab}} \tag{1}$$

It is essential to note that this simple concentration–size relationship holds true only after termination of the diffusion, a process usually taking a few days. Before that time, measurements have to be referred to a complex calibration curve, and the accuracy of the results will only rarely be better than 10 to 20%. If time is not important it is clearly advantageous to wait until the curve has straightened out, since by then the standard error will have become as low as 2% of the mean[8] and three reference dilutions of the antigen will be satisfactory for a standard curve.

The first explanation suggesting itself for the straight relationship between antigen concentration and area of the precipitate, would be that the ring stops growing when all the available antigen from the well has combined with antibody from the gel; that the terminal area therefore

[1] Ö. Ouchterlony, Acta Pathol. Microbiol. Scand. 26, 507–515 (1949).

[2] J. G. Feinberg, Intern. Arch. Allergy 11, 129–152 (1957).

[3] B. J. Hayward, and R. Augustin, Intern. Arch. Allergy 11, 192–205 (1957).

[4] A. J. Crowle, J. Lab. Clin. Med. 55, 593–604 (1960).

[5] T. B. Tomasi and S. D. Zigelbaum, J. Clin. Invest. 42, 1552–1560 (1963).

[6] J. L. Fahey and E. M. McKelvey, J. Immunol. 94, 84–90 (1965).

[7] G. Mancini, J. P. Vaerman, A. O. Carbonara, and J. F. Heremans, in "Protides of the Biological Fluids" (H. Peeters, ed.), pp. 370–373. Elsevier, Amsterdam, 1964.

[8] G. Mancini, A. O. Carbonara, and J. F. Heremans, Immunochemistry 2, 235–254 (1965).

[9] P. Rümke and P. J. Thung, Acta Endocrinol. 47, 156–164 (1964).

represents a volume of gel containing just sufficient antibody to consume the amount of antigen available; and that this amount of antibody (i.e., this area) is simply related to the amount of antigen through the equivalence ratio, which is a constant of each antigen–antibody system. However, recent work by Mancini at the author's laboratory has shown that this theory is an oversimplification. When antigen is allowed to

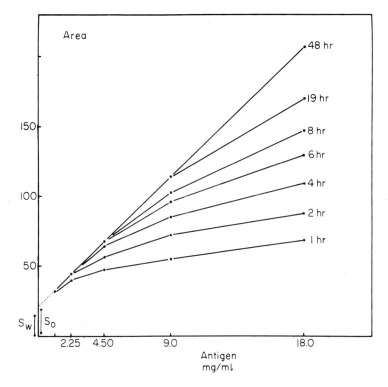

Fig. 2. Relation between area of precipitate and amount of antigen after different times of diffusion. The relative areas of the precipitates are given as milligrams of paper weight. S_w = area corresponding to the antigen well. S_0 = intercept of the final straight line with the vertical axis, indicating the fictitious area corresponding to zero antigen concentration. The antigen was human serum albumin, and the antibody was obtained from a rabbit. From Mancini et al.[8]

diffuse into a gel containing purified antibody, to the exclusion of other proteins, and when the protein distribution in and around the growing precipitate is assessed at various time intervals by staining the gel with Amido Black and recording the absorbancy curve along the radius of the precipitate disk (Fig. 3), it is found that: (a) The protein concentration inside the ring is far from uniform at termination of the diffusion, as would be anticipated by the theory; (b) instead, protein accumulates

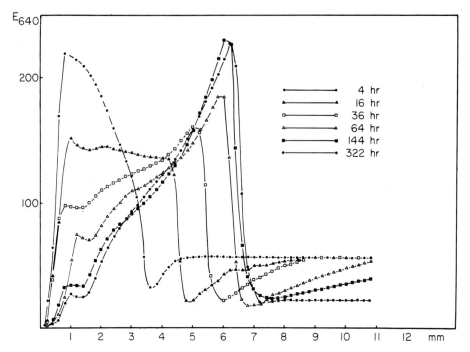

FIG. 3. Changes in distribution of protein during development of the precipitate in single radial immunodiffusion. The gel contained purified rabbit antibody against human serum albumin. The wells received identical amounts of antigen. After different incubation times, individual precipitates were stained with Amido Black and the absorption curve at 640 mμ was recorded by means of a traveling microscope, along a line passing from the center of the well (at left) to some distance beyond the rim of the precipitate (right).

along the rim of the precipitate, while moving out of the center of the system; (c) and antibody from the surrounding gel is constantly diffusing toward and being included into the precipitate. This creates a halo of protein-poor gel around the rim of the latter. It has been found that very large precipitates are capable of clearing all the antibody present in a whole plate.

b. RECOMMENDED TECHNIQUE*

i. *Preparation of the Agar*

To 100 ml of barbiturate buffer of pH 8.6 and ionic strength 0.1 (made by dissolving 9 gm of sodium diethylbarbiturate, 65 ml of 0.1 N HCl, and

* According to Mancini et al.[8]

0.5 gm of sodium azide in distilled water and adjusting the volume to 1 liter) is added 3 gm of Special Agar-Noble (Difco). The suspension is stirred on a boiling waterbath until dissolved, and distilled water is added to replace losses due to evaporation. This stock agar solution is distributed over a number of well-stoppered test tubes, these may be stored for several weeks at 4°.

ii. Preparation of the Agar–Antiserum Mixture

The required amount of solidified 3% agar gel is melted on a boiling water bath and cooled to 60°. A suitable dilution of the antiserum (in barbiturate buffer) is warmed to 55° and mixed at equal volumes with the molten agar. The mixture is thoroughly stirred (avoiding bubbling) by means of a pipet preheated to 60° in the water bath. The antiserum–agar mixture is then poured, without delay, into the mold described below, the same heated pipet being used.

To find the appropriate antiserum concentrations one has to set up a few plates with different dilutions of antiserum, the antigen wells being filled with serial dilutions extending over the range contemplated for practical applications. The antigen must be in significant excess whatever the most useful antibody concentration chosen.

iii. Preparation of the Immunodiffusion Plate

At the author's laboratory use is made of the mold illustrated in Fig. 4. It consists of a U-shaped brass frame, 1 mm thick, whose sides measure 8 mm in width, their lengths corresponding to the dimensions of a 10 × 7 cm photographic glass plate. This frame is used to separate two such glass plates, one of which (the top plate) has its side facing the frame siliconized. The other plate (the base one) should *not* be siliconized. The three pieces of the mold are held tightly together by means of a few clamps.

The mold is held in a slanting position, and the tip of the heated pipet containing the antiserum–agar mixture is applied to the lower corner of the 1-mm wide slit between the glass slides. Filling the mold in this way prevents the inclusion of air ꞈbbles. After solidification (10 to 15 minutes), the clamps are removed and the siliconized top plate is carefully slid off from the gel, after which the brass frame is in turn removed. The bottom plate is left to support the gel. It is recommended to use the plate without delay.*

* Ready made plates containing antisera against various plasma proteins including the three major human immunoglobulins (IgG, IgA, and IgM) are available commercially from Hyland laboratories, Los Angeles, California (Immuno-plates) or Behringwerke AG., Marburg, W. Germany.

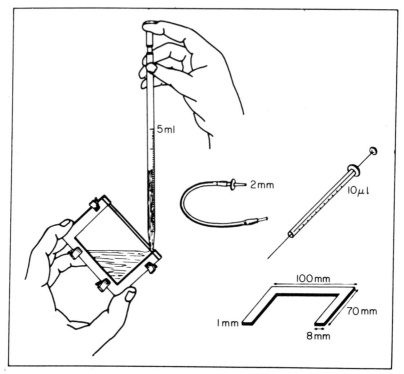

FIG. 4. Preparation of an immunodiffusion plate. See text. From Mancini et al.[8]

iv. Application of the Antigen Samples

Circular wells are punched out of the gel at chosen intervals. For this purpose the use of a template is recommended.[6] At the author's laboratory a needle of 2-mm bore is used, but the choice of this caliber is of course arbitrary. The small cylinders of gel cut out by the needle are removed by suction. Each well receives a measured amount out antigen solution (e.g., 2 μl). If accuracy is not essential, it is sufficient to fill each hole to the brim by blowing out the antigen solution from a finely drawn-out Pasteur pipet with its tip bent in the flame. For truly quantitative work the use of a microsyringe* is recommended.

When all wells are filled, the plate is kept for 10 to 30 minutes in a strictly horizontal position, in a moist box, in order to allow the gel to imbibe the antigen solutions. The plate is then transferred to the incubation box, where it is kept immersed under paraffin oil (containing a few crystals of thymol to prevent the growth of anaerobic microorganisms). To speed up diffusion it is preferable to store the incubation box at 37°.

* Microliter syringe +701-N, Hamilton Co., Whittier, California.

v. Recording the Results

After removal of the oil by a short rinse in petroleum ether, the plate is ready to be recorded.

For rough semiquantitative work (e.g., screening tests), it may be sufficient to read the plate after 1 night of incubation, but, as already stated, highly accurate results are obtained if the measurements are postponed until the rings no longer grow in size. The required incubation time will depend upon the final size to be attained, as well as upon the diffusion coefficient of the antigen. Usually 4 days are sufficient with serum albumin, 7 days with IgG, and 10 or more days with antigens such as IgM.

Some workers limit themselves to measuring the diameter of each ring (by holding a comparator scale against the plate under oblique illumination), and plotting the diameters on a semilogarithmic scale (or by plotting the square of the diameter on an ordinary scale). As this method is likely to give erroneous results in cases where the precipitin rings depart from the ideal circular shape, we prefer the more cumbersome but decidedly more accurate method of measuring the area encompassed by the precipitin rings. For this purpose we project the magnified silhouettes of the rings on a sheet of bristol-type cardboard paper, using a photographic enlarger, and pencil out the contours of the paper. The paper disks are then cut out, and their weights are used as the final data to be plotted on ordinary graph paper. The values thus obtained correspond to the sum of the area of the wells plus the area of the precipitates. It is not necessary to make a correction for the wells, since even if this is done the standard curve may not be expected to pass through the origin (Fig. 1).

Weak precipitates can be brought out by staining. This is by all means advantageous if the plates are to be stored for reference or future study. For this purpose the plates are washed with normal saline, in petri dishes, for 2 or 3 days, with several daily changes of the washing fluid. The preparations are then soaked for a few hours in distilled water (renewed 3 times), in order to remove the salt. After drying at room temperature or at 37°, the plates are immersed for 30 minutes in an aqueous solution containing 1 gm of Amido Black, 4.1 gm of sodium acetate, and 30 ml of acetic acid per liter. The background color is removed by three successive baths in a aqueous solution containing 50 ml of acetic acid and 5 ml of glycerin per liter.

c. LIMITATIONS AND PROBLEMS

i. Technical Notes

(a) *Lower Limit of Sensitivity.* If the antigen concentration is below that required for precipitate to form in the gel, the sensitivity of the method can be multiplied by diluting the antiserum [cf. Eq. (1)]. There is, however, a limit to this procedure, since the intensity of the precipitate ring will decrease in proportion with the dilution of the antiserum. It has been found useful in such cases to dilute the antiserum, not with plain saline, but with serum from a nonimmunized animal. As the antigen–antibody complexes will coprecipitate some of the protein from this source, precipitin rings may thus acquire an intensity sufficient to make them visible after staining. A second remedy, which can be applied at the same time, consists of increasing the volume of antigen solution introduced into the well, and if necessary, increasing the dimensions of the well. If such steps are taken, it is important that the volumes of the standard solutions and the sizes of the wells containing them, be increased in similar fashion, since omission of this precaution may be a source of errors.[8]

In a trial experiment with albumin, and using antigen wells of 2 mm diameter filled with 2 μl of antigen solution, it was found that rabbit antiserum could be diluted with nonimmune rabbit serum up to a point where the smallest readable ring corresponded to an absolute amount of antigen of about 0.0025 μg, which was equivalent to a concentration of 1.25 μg/ml.

(b) *Disc Interference.* If a precipitin ring grows so large that it reaches the vicinity of a neighboring precipitate, both rings will bulge out toward each other as a prelude to their fusion. This is due to the fact that each ring tends to deplete the antiserum from the zone of gel surrounding its boundaries (Fig. 3). In practice one, therefore, will have to dilute the samples up to a point where their rings cannot interfere with each other.

(c) *Salt Concentration.* Care should also be taken not to compare samples dissolved in media showing great differences in osmotic pressure, as may happen when working with solutions that have been concentrated by freezing-and-thawing or lyophilization without prior removal of the salts.

(d) *Temperature.* Temperature changes during the incubation have no discernible effect upon the final size of the precipitates,[8] although they markedly influence the progress of diffusion; which is one more reason to defer measurements until completion of the diffusion.

ii. Problems Arising from the Antigenic Constitution of the Sample

(a) *Heterogeneous Antigen Solutions.* It will often prove difficult to obtain an antiserum completely specific for the desired antigen in a complex mixture. Each antigen will react with its corresponding antibodies from the antiserum-gel and give rise to a separate precipitin ring. The problem is then to identify the ring belonging to the appropriate component. This may occasionally be achieved by applying a specific staining after termination of the diffusion period, e.g., in the case of lipoproteins, or the hemoglobin–haptoglobin complex, or with enzymes lending themselves to histochemical reactions (see Section 14.E.1.d.).

More general methods of identification can be applied if one has access to a preparation of the desired antigen—even a crude one—provided the antigen in question predominates over other constituents. One may, for instance, set up each sample in duplicate, with one well receiving the sample as such, and the twin well the same volume of sample plus an addition

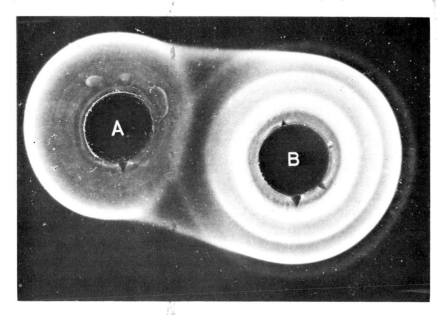

Fig. 5. Illustration of the use of complex antisera. This antiserum gave four major precipitin disks when tested against whole human serum (B). The disk corresponding to β_{1A}-globulin was identified by applying a purified solution of the latter antigen in a neighboring well (A) and observing the fusion of the corresponding precipitate.

of purified antigen. The ring belonging to the desired antigen will then betray its identity by being greater in size around the mixture well. Alternatively, one may provide three wells for each sample: one well receiving the reference antigen; the second, which is close to the first, re-receiving the sample; the third, spaced farther apart, also receiving the sample. The rings given by the desired antigen around the reference well and the nearby sample well are thus made to merge (Fig. 5); the corresponding ring around the more distant sample well, about whose identity there should then remain no doubt, can be used for the actual measurement.

(b) *Mixture of Related Antigens.* This situation is typified by the case of the immunoglobulins. If an antiserum is made against purified human IgG, it is usually found to cross-react with IgA and IgM, on account of the presence in the latter of kappa- and lambda-type light chains, which were also present in the original antigen molecule. Absorption with IgA and IgM will remove these cross-reacting antibodies. Still, more often than not, the resulting antiserum will fail to give a sharp precipitin ring when tested against whole human serum. Multiple rings or a single ring with hazy contour are the usual outcome of the reaction. This is due to the fact that the gamma-type heavy chains, with which the antiserum reacts, are themselves a mixture of at least four subclasses of related molecules. There appears to be no other remedy but to test several antisera until one is found that happens to produce sharp rings, presumably because it reacts with only one of the gamma-chain subclasses. One out of six anti-IgG antisera tested by Laterre *et al.*[10] proved to have this quality.

(c) *Polymerization of Reactants.* It would seem that an appreciable proportion of the antigenic determinants becomes hidden when protein molecules combine with each other to form polymers. We have observed, for instance, that the precipitin areas given by the 7 S form and the 17 S form of the same IgA myeloma protein were very different, the latter being much smaller than the former.[10a] This difference was of a purely quantitative kind, since no spur was noted upon comparison in Ouchterlony plates, and since either of the two antigens was able to remove all antibodies reacting with the other antigen. Presumably, differences in diffusion coefficient also played a role in this discrepancy, though measurements were made after termination of the diffusion. The situation here described, therefore, is not to be compared to a similar observation by Fahey and McKelvey,[6] who measured the diameters of the rings after one night of incubation.

One may conclude that polymer mixtures, such as haptoglobins of types 2-1 and 2-2, or IgA-immunoglobulins (especially those of many myeloma sera and in exocrine secretions) require the use of standards of similar molecular size and heterogeneity. For instance, serious errors would arise if it were attempted to quantitate a predominantly 9 S IgA-myeloma globulin by using as a standard IgA from normal serum (most of which is 7 S); or Hp 1-1 with Hp 2-2 as a standard. A solution to this problem, which is being tried out at the author's laboratory, may consist of

[10] E. C. Laterre, H. Heulle, G. Mancini, and J. F. Heremans, *in* "Protides of the Biological Fluids" (H. Peeters, ed.), Vol.11, pp. 227–230. Elsevier, Amsterdam, 1966.

[10a] J. P. Vaerman and J. F. Heremans, unpublished observations (1968).

depolymerizing both the sample and the standard by means of cysteine or some other thiol, and preventing repolymerization by means of iodoacetamide. Such a treatment would of course be effective only with proteins whose polymerization depends upon disulfide bridges (which is the case with haptoglobins and serum IgA, but presumably not with exocrine IgA).

(d) *Denaturation of Sample or Standard.* When solutions of purified proteins are stored at 4° for prolonged periods, as is likely to happen with reference reagents, there will occur two types of changes, both of which decrease the precipitin areas given by such preparations. One source of loss of antigenic determinants is due to enzymatic cleavage. This is particularly the case with samples of serum proteins, which are likely to contain trace amounts of proteolytic enzymes such as plasmin. The author has experienced this type of trouble with purified preparations of IgA and IgM isolated from normal serum and stored under sterile conditions. The second type of change, which consists in the formation of molecular aggregates, also entails a pronounced decrease in the antigen titer of the solution, presumably because antigenic determinants become hidden by the same mechanism that operates during polymerization. We have noted that aggregation is particularly prone to occur in solutions of serum albumin, and, therefore, have made it a standard practice to free such preparations from high molecular weight components by passing them through a Sephadex G-200 column before using them as references. It should also be noted that the method of preparation is of paramount importance to the stability of proteins during storage. For instance, preparations of albumin prepared by the use of cold ethanol (Cohn fraction V) are unsuitable for this type of work.

It should be stressed that the types of alterations cited here cannot be detected by assaying the protein content of the standard solution by chemical or physical means. Such changes may lead, on the other hand, to considerable overestimations in the measurement of the sample solutions. It is also important to note that concentrated mixtures, such as whole serum, display considerably greater stability than dilute solutions of isolated proteins. We therefore believe it preferable to prepare and use the purified antigen only for the purpose of standardizing a large batch of pooled human serum. This standard serum is then distributed among a number of small plastic tubes that are kept frozen until use.

It should also be mentioned that new antigenic determinants may be revealed, and formerly existing determinants destroyed, by such procedures as reducing the disulfide bridges of a protein, or exposing it to denaturing agents.

(e) *Interference by Rheumatoid Factor(s)*. Owing to the fact that the anti-serum has been heated during preparation of the gel, some or all of its IgG-immunoglobulin may have been converted to aggregates liable to react with rheumatoid factor(s). If such factor(s) are contained in the sample, a spurious precipitin ring may be generated which may occasionally mimic the antigen–antibody precipitin ring to be assessed. A still more serious difficulty is encountered when IgM is the antigen to be measured. Since rheumatoid factor is itself of IgM nature, part of the latter protein may precipitate in the gel by acting as an antigen, and part by functioning as an antibody to the aggregated immunoglobulins of the gel. If much of the latter is present in aggregated form, a large proportion of the sample IgM may be precipitated around the rim of the sample well, and perhaps no precipitin ring will be visible at all. It has been the author's experience that this situation is a serious obstacle to the measurement of the IgM titer in rheumatoid sera by immunodiffusion methods.[11] Depolymerization by disulfide-splitting agents may possibly provide a solution to this problem.

d. Recent Applications

The applicability of the method has been extended in various directions. Increased sensitivity has been achieved through the use of radioactively labeled antibodies[12] as well as by increasing the density of the precipitate by means of antiserum reacting with the antibodies.[13] Cellulose acetate has been proposed as a substitute for agar or agarose gels.[14] A "reversed" version of the method (antigen in the gel; antibody in the wells) has been applied to the titration of antibodies.[15,16] The method has also been adapted to the qualitative[17] and quantitative[18] analysis of antigenic relationships between different substances, and a system has been described by which an antigen related to the immunizing antigen can be titrated without the requirement of a separate calibration curve.[18]

[11] J. F. Heremans, "Les globulines sériques du système gamma." Arscia, Brussels, and Masson, Paris, 1960.

[12] D. S. Rowe, *Bull. Wld. Hlth Org.* **40**, 613–616 (1969).

[13] P. Rümke and J. C. Breekveldt-Kielich, *Vox Sang.* **16**, 486–490 (1969).

[14] C. Vergani, R. Stabilini, and A. Agostoni, *Immunochemistry* **4**, 233–237 (1967).

[15] J. P. Vaerman, A. M. Lebacq-Verheyden, L. Scolari, and J. F. Heremans, *Immunochemistry* **6**, 279–285 (1969).

[16] J. P. Vaerman, A. M. Lebacq-Verheyden, L. Scolari, and J. F. Heremans, *Immunochemistry* **6**, 287–293 (1969).

[17] G. Mancini, D. R. Nash, and J. F. Heremans, *Immunochemistry* **7**, 261–264 (1970).

[18] D. R. Nash, L. Scolari, and J. F. Heremans, *Immunochemistry* **7**, 265–274 (1970).

7. DETERMINATION OF RELATIVE ANTIGEN AND ANTIBODY CONCENTRATIONS IN TUBES*

a. GENERAL PRINCIPLES

i. Simple Diffusion

Technical details for the preparation of tubes for simple diffusion and the measurement of the position of the precipitate are given in Section 14.B.1. It was demonstrated also that if the progressive position of the leading edge of a zone of precipitation in a simple diffusion tube is plotted against the square root of time, the points fall on a straight line whose slope, k, characterizes the rate of advance of the zone of precipitation. With a constant concentration of serum, the greater the antigen concentration, the greater the value of k, and a plot of k against the logarithm of the relative concentration of antigen gives a straight-line function except for very high antigen concentrations.[1] Such a curve may be used as a standard to which k values of unknown antigen concentrations may be referred in order to determine their concentrations in relative units.

Similarly, if a constant antigen concentration is diffused against serial dilutions of serum and k values are computed, k may be plotted against relative serum concentration on a logarithmic scale. The resulting curve is also a straight line except for extreme antigen–antibody ratios, and may be used as a standard curve to which k values of unknown antibody concentrations may be referred in order to determine their concentrations relative to the standard.

ii. Double Diffusion

The preparation of agar tubes for double diffusion is described in Section 14.B.2. As in simple diffusion, the quantitative method depends on accurate measurement of the band position. The band position, p, is taken as the distance from the antigen–agar interface to the center of the region of maximum band intensity, divided by the total agar length. The greater the antigen concentration, the greater will be the value of p, provided the same serum concentration is used in all tubes. Although most p values change slowly with time, at any specific time, for a given antigen dilution series, a plot of p versus the logarithm of the relative antigen concentration yields a straight line.[2] Such a line may be used as a standard curve to which the p values of unknowns may be referred.

* Section 14.C.7 was contributed by John R. Preer, Jr.

[1] J. Oudin, *Compt. Rend.* **228**, 1890 (1949).
[2] J. R. Preer, *J. Immunol.* **77**, 52 (1956).

Likewise, if the antigen concentration is held constant in a series of tubes in which a serum dilution series is used, p will be smaller for higher antibody concentrations. A plot of p at any given time versus relative antibody concentration on a logarithmic scale is also linear and may be used as a standard curve to determine the relative antibody concentration of unknowns.

iii. Comparison of Methods

In our hands simple diffusion has proved slightly more sensitive in detecting dilute antibody, while double diffusion is much more sensitive in detecting dilute antigens. For quantitative purposes, however, single diffusion is more precise; that is, values for p have a larger standard error than k. This is due in part to the facts that in simple diffusion the position of the sharp leading edges of zones of precipitation may be determined with relatively greater precision and that in double diffusion the distances involved are relatively small.

b. General Technique

The first step is the preparation of standard curves relating k or p to concentration in arbitrary units. Convenient dilutions are $1:2$, $1:4$, $1:8$, etc. It is important that dilutions of both antigen and antibody used to prepare standard curves be made in medium as closely as possible approximating that of the unknown solutions to be tested later. Molar concentration differences of 0.2 or more between standards and unknowns are sure to produce measurable errors, as indicated above. Normal serum is a useful diluent for antiserum in antibody assays. In the event that unknowns are suspected of having large variations in density from one to the other, then one of the devices suggested earlier should be used to avoid differences in convection, such as the solidification of aqueous layers with gel. Satisfactory gel formulas and general techniques used in setting tubes and reading band position in simple and double diffusion are described in Section 14.B.2.b. It is advisable to prepare tubes in duplicate, and standard errors may be reduced further by using several replicate tubes. Once set, tubes should be placed at constant temperature and moved as infrequently as possible. Standard curves are constructed by plotting k or p against the logarithm of concentration in arbitrary units. Generally it will be found that the points are best fitted by a straight line.

In the case of simple diffusion, if tubes are set in the afternoon of the first day, they may be read on the mornings of the second, third, and fifth days to yield three well-spaced points on a plot of band position against the square root of time. This procedure enables one to obtain two determinations of k and ascertain whether k is remaining constant, as it should.

In the case of double diffusion, tubes may be read on the following day. It is desirable that gel lengths between the reactants in double diffusion be made no longer than 5 mm. Greater lengths result in too great a loss in sensitivity. With an agar length of 5 mm, most antigen–antibody systems show a decrease in p of approximately 0.07 for each halving in antibody concentration. Longer agar lengths yield smaller changes in p, and longer times yield greater changes in p. In the author's experience, spurious band splittings and other artifacts, sometimes seen in double diffusion, are minimized by keeping tubes for only 24-hours, or at most 3 days.

Unknowns are treated as nearly as possible like standards, and simply referred to the standard curves for determination of concentration in relative units.

c. Control of the Effects of Nonreacting Substances

Certain effects on k and p result from the behavior of nonreacting components of the system; in quantitative work they must be controlled. The major factors known to be important are as follows.

i. Convection

If simple and double diffusion tubes are kept vertical with antigen on top, gravity-induced convection will occur in the liquid antigen layer if it is more dense than the liquid making up the gel layer, but will not occur if the liquid has the same or a lower density. An increase in protein of as little as 10 mg/ml can change a nonconvective system into a convective system. Since convection results in higher concentrations of antigen at the antigen–gel boundary than in nonconvective systems, higher k and p values will result.[3] The effect is large, amounting to as much as an apparent doubling in concentration. It is of little importance whether convection occurs or not, but convection induced by nonreacting substances must be the same in all tubes used to make standard curves or assay for unknowns.

Several ways of repressing convection are available. The addition of agar to liquid layers, of course, completely eliminates convection. The use of small-diameter tubes (2 mm and less) and their storage in a horizontal position reduces the magnitude of the convective effect. Conversely, convection may be induced in the antigen layer in all tubes routinely by adding extra protein (e.g., bovine serum albumin to a concentration of 3%) to all tubes and storing them vertically with the antigen on top (or prevented by storing them with the antigen on the bottom). The convective system is roughly twice as sensitive as the nonconvective.

[3] J. R. Preer and W. H. Telfer, *J. Immunol.* **79,** 288 (1957).

ii. Viscosity

Variations in viscosity of the fluid incorporated into the gel layer have been found to affect k in simple diffusion tests,[4] and a similar effect on p in double diffusion might be expected. k is inversely proportional to the square root of viscosity. The viscosity effect seems to be important only in the case of antibody assays in simple diffusion, for in other cases the composition of the gel layer is kept constant. Variations may be avoided by making the serum dilutions in normal serum.

iii. Concentration Gradients

Increases in k in simple diffusion and p in double diffusion are brought about by additions of substances (sucrose, for example) to the antigen layer in concentrations greater than 0.2 M. Corresponding additions to the serum containing gel in simple diffusion lower the values of k and p, while additions to both serum and antigen layers produce no effect.[3] Although this effect has not been given a satisfactory theoretical explanation it appears to be nonspecific and occurs whenever there are large differences in molar concentrations of nonreacting components in the different layers. In most immunological applications the nonspecific concentration gradient effect is not a serious factor, for such large molar concentration differences between unknown and standard samples either do not exist, or are known and can be controlled. Large molecules such as proteins do not produce the nonspecific concentration gradient effect because sufficiently high molar concentrations cannot be obtained. If it is necessary to work with samples containing high concentrations of nonspecific substances, a standard reference curve should be constructed from tubes set under the specified conditions.

iv. Agar

Neff and Becker[4] found that k in simple diffusion is affected by the number of times agar has been melted. It is therefore advisable to make up a large batch of agar, dispense it into many small tubes, and use each batch of agar only once before discarding.

d. Effects of Variation in Properties of Reactants

It is clear that a direct proportionality between the number of molecules of the reactant being assayed and the relative concentrations which we determine by assay is to be desired. Ideally, we can expect this relation

[4] J. C. Neff and E. L. Becker, *J. Immunol.* **78**, 5 (1957).

to be fulfilled in the case of antigens so long as the properties of the reactants are constant. This simple relation will not hold if the properties are not constant—if, for example, samples come from differing strains of organisms which produce genetically different but cross-reacting antigens, or if an antigen dissociates under certain conditions, or if it may take several forms with differing distributions of the various forms among samples. The requirement for constancy is not peculiar to gel diffusion or any other serological method; it is of importance in all quantitative measurements. Constancy is especially important in serological methods, however, due to their great sensitivity to molecular conformation.

In the case of the measurement of relative antibody concentration, the criterion of homogeneity and constancy of distribution of molecular species from one serum to another is not met.[5] Hence a measurement of antibody concentration has no real meaning except in terms of the method used to measure it. Thus "univalent" antibody (nonprecipitating) might be measured by special absorption techniques and might be expected to have a large effect on k and p, but it would not be adequately measured by the usual precipitation tests in liquid medium. Even if all the antibody were precipitable, there is no assurance that quantitative precipitation would give measurements of relative antibody concentration identical to those obtained from k and p, but under most circumstances a good correlation is to be expected.

In conclusion, there is no *a priori* reason why the gel diffusion methods are in any way less desirable or useful than other procedures; hence they are just as highly recommended from a theoretical point of view.

[5] W. C. Boyd, "Fundamentals of Immunology," 3rd ed. Wiley (Interscience), New York, 1956.

8. DETERMINATION OF ANTIGEN AND ANTIBODY CONCENTRATIONS IN ABSOLUTE WEIGHT UNITS*

a. INTRODUCTION

Finger and Kabat[1] have described a method for roughly estimating the concentration of antibody in absolute weight units. In principle, at least, it should also be capable of giving the order of magnitude of antigen concentrations. It is relatively simple in application, and particularly in questions dealing with the homogeneity of antigen–antibody systems it could and should be much more widely used than it has been so far.

* Section 14.C.8 was contributed by Elmer L. Becker.

[1] I. H. Finger and E. A. Kabat, *J. Exptl. Med.* **108**, 453 (1958).

Becker[2] has described a method utilizing the Oudin technique which combines measurements of band density* and the rate of band movement. It is capable of greater accuracy than that of Finger and Kabat at the cost of increased experimental and computational complexity.

In addition, Smith et al.[3] have described a general method for putting upper limits to the amount of antigenic impurities remaining after extensive purification of antigens. Although it will not be described here, anyone engaged in purification of antigens should be aware of the availability of such a procedure.

b. Method of Finger and Kabat Utilizing the Preer Technique†

Finger and Kabat[1] showed that when antigen and antibody are present in equivalent concentrations as determined by the quantitative precipitin reaction in liquid media, the sensitivity of detection of antibody in the Preer technique was about 3 to 9 μg of antibody nitrogen per milliliter and about 1 to 12 μg of antigen per milliliter. The upper limits for antigen detection should undoubtedly be increased for very high molecular weight, slowly diffusing antigens (cf. Finger and Kabat).[1] The concentration of a given antibody is estimated by diluting the antiserum until the band just disappears when tested in the Preer technique with the equivalence concentration of antigen. The dilution of antiserum multiplied by 3 to 9 μg of antibody nitrogen per milliliter gives the estimate of the antibody content per milliliter of the undiluted antiserum. Since the antigen and antiserum are both diluted so as to maintain the equivalence ratio, finding the limiting dilution of antibody gives at the same time the limiting dilution of antigen. The concentration of antigen in the stock solution is found by multiplying 1 to 9 μg of antigen per milliliter by the limiting dilution of antigen.

It is obvious that, even at best, the antibody content will be known over a threefold range of concentration. However, for many purposes this range of uncertainty can be borne resignedly if not gladly. The range of uncertainty in antigen concentration is at least ninefold, so that the technique is useful only for determining the order of magnitude of the antigen.

In finding the ratio of antigen to antibody and equivalence, Finger and Heller[4] add varying amounts of antigen to a constant volume of antiserum in a total constant volume of 0.6 ml or less. The stoppered tubes are incu-

---

[2] E. L. Becker, Arch. Biochem. Biophys. **93**, 617 (1961).
* When the terms band density, density, or optical density are used, it is the optical density of the leading edge of the precipitate band which is meant.
[3] H. Smith, K. Sargeant, and J. L. Stanley, J. Gen. Microbiol. **26**, 63 (1961).
† Preer technique of double diffusion in tubes is described in Section 14.C.2.
[4] I. H. Finger and C. Heller, J. Immunol. **85**, 332 (1960).

bated at 37° for 1 hour and then kept at 4° for 18 to 48 hours. The supernatants are centrifuged off and tested for the presence of the given antigen and antibody by double diffusion (tubes). Equivalence is given by the antigen concentration at which neither antigen nor antibody is found in the supernatant.

c. THE BAND DENSITY METHOD

i. Introduction

This gel precipitin method has been demonstrated to be valid only for rabbit antibodies to protein antigens.[2] Whether it is also applicable to nonprotein antigens and to antibodies from animals other than the rabbit has still to be investigated. The measurement of the antibody nitrogen content of rabbit antisera is relatively simple and straightforward, and is capable under favorable circumstances of giving results that agree very well with quantitative precipitin measurements in liquid media.[5] However, the determination of antigen nitrogen is more laborious and subject to distinctly greater sources of error.

ii. Materials

Reaction tubes 7.0 ± 0.25 mm o.d., 5 mm i.d., and 84 mm long are used routinely. They are obtainable from Corning Glass Works, Corning, New York, or Scientific Glass Apparatus Co., Bloomfield, New Jersey. When antigen or antiserum is scarce, we have used tubes 4.0 mm o.d. and 40 mm long. There is a loss of sensitivity with the use of the thinner tubes, but they are otherwise satisfactory. The tubes are coated and stored as described in Section 14.B.1.a. The other reactants—agar, diluent, etc.—are as also described in the same section.

For determining the optical density the antigen solution in agar is usually employed at a final concentration of about 1.0% in 0.3% agar. The exact concentration is not critical however, as long as it is high enough so that the resulting band density is independent of time and antigen concentration.[5] Usually three concentrations of antiserum are employed. These dilutions should be made as accurately as possible. Final concentrations in the Oudin tube of 0.01 to 0.05 mg of antibody nitrogen per milliliter are employed; a final concentration of 0.1 mg AbN/ml or above usually requires too high a concentration of antigen to be practical.

iii. Filling of Tubes

The tubes are filled as described in Section 14.B.1.a. However, because heating the antisera may affect the optical density of the band (A. Hay-

[5] A. R. Hayden and E. L. Becker, *Arch. Biochem. Biophys.* **93,** 631 (1961).

den, unpublished observations) the temperature should be more carefully controlled than when only qualitative observations are to be made. The diluted antisera are kept at 53° for only 30 seconds before being mixed with an equal volume of 0.6% agar which is also at 53°. Immediately after mixing, the antiserum–agar is added to the tube with a Pasteur pipet, and the tube is placed in a constant-temperature bath. After gelling, the antigen–agar is added to the upper layer, and the tubes are capped. Unless the antigen is particularly heat labile, no more than ordinary precautions with regard to temperature are required when filling the tube with the agar–antigen mixture.

iv. Reading of Optical Densities

After approximately 20 hours of incubation at 25°, the readings of the optical density of the leading edge of each band are made. Any densitometer of sufficient sensitivity and stability which permits the manual or automatic scanning of the tube will serve for this purpose.*

In scanning the tubes, the optical density just in front of the fastest moving band is set at zero. When more than one band is present, the optical density of the leading edge of each band in back of the fastest moving band is obtained by difference. The greater the distance between bands the more accurate such determinations will be.

Plotting the optical densities of a given band against the percent antiserum should give a straight line. This is both the necessary and sufficient condition for validly relating optical density to precipitate nitrogen. Experience has convinced us that it is not necessary that the line extrapolate through the origin as was previously stated.[2] If the line is not straight, the antiserum must be diluted further, or antigen concentration be raised, or both. One can correct for a straight line not going through the origin by drawing a line through the origin parallel to the experimental line.

v. Preparation of Standard Curve

So far as our present experience shows, any protein–rabbit antiprotein system can serve for determining the standard curve relating optical density to total nitrogen precipitated at equivalence. Once determined, such a standard curve will serve for any other protein–rabbit antiprotein

---

* We have found the Bausch & Lomb densitometer (No. 33-84-91) Bausch & Lomb Co., Rochester, New York, the Automatic Recording Microdensitometer Model MF 111C, Joyce-Loebl & Co., Ltd., A 8 Princeway, Team Valley, Gateshead, England, and the Fluoro-Microphotometer No. 4-7102, with scanning attachment No. 47331, American Instrument Co., Silver Spring, Maryland, all satisfactory. The last has only 60% of the sensitivity of the other two, but it is only one-third to one-fourth the price. With the American Instrument Co. and Bausch & Lomb instruments, attaching an automatic recorder is advantageous.

system. A reasonably homogeneous antiserum being used, the total nitrogen per milliliter of antiprotein precipitated at equivalence in liquid media is measured. One then determines the optical density of the band given by three or more antiserum dilutions, as described above. The optical densities are plotted against the total nitrogen precipitated at equivalence for each dilution, and the resulting straight line is the standard curve.

vi. Determination of Antibody Nitrogen

The total amount of precipitate, per milliliter of antiserum, T, at equivalence is equal to the amount of antigen added, Ag_e, and the amount of antibody, Ab, precipitated, i.e.,

$$T = Ab + Ag_e = Ab\,(1 + 1/R) = Ag_e\,(1 + R) \qquad (1)$$

where R is the ratio of antibody to antigen at equivalence. In order to use Eq. (1) it is necessary to know R in absolute units for the given antigen antibody system. T is then found from measurements of optical density by means the standard curve relating optical density to total nitrogen per milliliter of antiserum precipitated at equivalence. The antibody per milliliter of antiserum corresponding to the antigen–antibody system producing the band in question is then calculated from Eq. (1).

If R is not known, one may estimate it from the diffusion coefficient of the antigen and the curve of Fig. 1 relating the diffusion coefficient to R (note that R is in units of antibody and antigen nitrogen). The diffusion coefficient of the antigen, if not known, may be determined by any of the methods of Section 14.D.1 that are applicable.

vii. Determination of Antigen Concentration

Knowing T and R (absolute), the antigen precipitated at equivalence, Ag_e is calculated from Eq. (1). The nitrogen of the stock antigen solution referable to this specific antigen is calculated from Ag_e and R (relative). R (relative) may be determined directly in a fashion similar to that described by Finger and Heller,[4] and given in Section 14.C.2. R (relative) may also be calculated from R_0, the immobilization ratio of the band by means of Eq. (2).

$$R = \frac{D_2}{R_0 D_1} \qquad (2)$$

We find it convenient to calculate R_0 as the milliliters of undiluted stock antigen solution which has to be added to 1 ml of antiserum to give no movement of the band. R_0 may be determined in the process of determining the diffusion coefficient of the antigen, D_1, using Eq. (1), Section 14.D.1. It may also be determined by extrapolating the straight line ob-

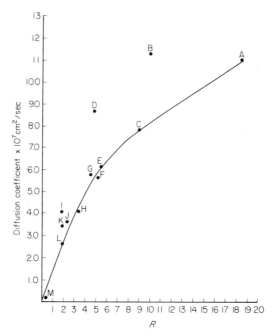

FIG. 1. The relationship between, R, the ratio of antibody nitrogen to antigen nitrogen in the precipitate at equivalence, and D_1, the diffusion coefficient of the antigen.

tained by plotting the distance, x, the band moves in some given time, t, against the logarithm of the antigen concentration. This straight line relation holds when the ratio of antibody in the lower layer to antigen in the upper layer of the tube is sufficiently high.[6] It is necessary, here, also to have the antigen as well as antiserum in agar.

R (*relative*), the milliliters of undiluted stock antigen which must be added to 1 ml of antiserum to bring the system to equivalence, contains Ag_e.

[6] E. L. Becker and J. C. Neff, *J. Immunol.* **83,** 571 (1960).

D. Immunoelectrophoretic Analysis (IEA)

1. INTRODUCTION*

Zone electrophoresis of proteins in agar gels as performed by Gordon *et al.*[1] suggested the possibility of combining the resolving power of this

* Section 14.D.1 was contributed by Curtis A. Williams.

[1] A. H. Gordon, B. Keil, and K. Sebesta, *Nature* **164,** 498 (1949).

technique with the sensitivity and specificity of immunochemical analysis by double diffusion in gels. Immunoelectrophretic analysis (IEA) as described by Grabar and Williams[2, 3] was the application of these parameters to a simple two-step procedure in a layer of agar gel.

Many refinements have been introduced, usually in the context of special requirements of a given research problem. Scheidegger adapted IEA to microscope slides,[4] which permitted great economy of materials and time, but not without some loss of detail. These methods are described in Section 14.D.2.

Immunoelectroosmophoresis (IEOP), described in Section 14.D.3.c, permits rapid development of precipitates in gels by placing both antigen and antibody in the electric field so that they migrate toward one another.

Agar gels are the most widely used, and only these will be discussed in detail; but other gels have been employed for IEA. Pectin produces a rather viscous gel, but it is possible to perform IEA in it.[5] The major disadvantage is that it is difficult to control the gel properties. Even gelatin can be used if all procedures are carried out under refrigeration.[6] Being protein, gelatin will carry a charge varying with the pH of the solvent buffer. If gelatin is firmly fixed to the support, however, adjustment of pH would be a means to regulate electroosomotic flow (see discussion in Section 14.D.2) of the solvent phase toward the cathode. Acrylamide gels are very clear, virtually without electric charge,[7] and by varying the gel concentration its resolving power by molecular sieving can be manipulated. Because of the low porosity of the acrylamide gel matrix at gelling concentrations, however, diffusion is slowed and pattern development is significantly retarded. Silica gel is unsuitable for almost any antigen–antibody diffusion technique since proteins adsorb to it.

IEA on cellulose acetate strips, which would also qualify as a micromethod, was developed by Kohn.[8] With this technique, precipitates must be stained before they can be seen; thus it must be known in advance how long a diffusion period is required for the pattern to develop. This difficulty is overcome by transferring the acetate strip to agar after electrophoresis, adding antiserum to the agar layer, and allowing diffusion and precipitation to proceed in the transparent agar. These modifications are described in Section 14.D.3.

[2] P. Grabar and C. A. Williams, *Biochim. Biophys. Acta* **10**, 193 (1953).

[3] P. Grabar and C. A. Williams, *Biochim. Biophys. Acta* **17**, 67 (1955).

[4] J. J. Scheidegger, *Intern. Arch. Allergy Appl. Immunol.* **7**, 103 (1955).

[5] P. Grabar, W. W. Nowinski, and B. D. Genereaux, *Nature* **178**, 430 (1956).

[6] A. J. Crowle, "Immunodiffusion." Academic Press, New York, 1961.

[7] B. Antoine, *Science* **138**, 977 (1962).

[8] J. Kohn, *in* "Chromatographic and Electrophoretic Techniques" (I. Smith, ed.), Vol. 2, 2nd Ed., pp. 84–146. Wiley (Interscience), New York, 1968.

Another transfer method which takes advantage of the sieving properties of hydrolyzed starch gels is described by Poulik in Section 14.D.4. The original transfer technique was done with filter paper electrophoresis strips.[9] More recently transfer methods employing acrylamide gels[10] and Sephadex thin layers[11] have been described. These modifications may prove useful for special purposes.

IEA is primarily a qualitative tool, but experienced investigators can make discriminating judgments about the amounts of certain antigens represented by an IEA pattern. There have been some efforts to develop a quantitative method by formalizing the several parameters or by comparing reactions with those of known solutions.[12] The most promising modification for quantitation of components in complex mixtures is the two-dimensional "crossed" immunoelectrophoresis developed by Laurell[13] and described by Clarke in Section 14.D.5. It depends on standardized antisera and the data obtained are relative to known antigen concentrations, but the method should find broad application.

There are important considerations common to all techniques of immunoelectrophoretic analyses. All methods depend on precipitating antibodies present in quantities sufficient to detect the antigens of interest so the investigator; and it must be realized that all antisera differ from all others in some way. This is particularly troublesome when commercial sources of antisera are employed, and long-range experiments or screening programs are foreseen.

Selection of antisera are considered in the contexts of specific applications in Section 14.D.2. If it is necessary or desirable to produce one's own antisera, the reader should consult Volume I, Chapter 2. Another consideration is the great variety of apparatus available commercially, of which one may be better adapted to a given purpose than others. This is primarily of concern in laboratories where several different lines of research or analysis are being pursued. In general the authors have described the procedures and apparatus which they have devised for their own work. These particular conditions, therefore, may not prove to be optimal with other antigens or antisera.

In summary, IEA is a principle, not a technique. We try here to demonstrate several ways in which the principle may be adapted and examples of the many experimental problems to which it can be applied. If the investigator encounters difficulties in applying the methods as described,

[9] M. D. Poulik, *Can. J. Med. Sci.* **30**, 417 (1952).

[10] K. Felgenhauer, *Biochim. Biophys. Acta* **160**, 268 (1968).

[11] L. A. Hanson, B. G. Johansson, and L. Rymo, *Clin. Chim. Acta* **14**, 391 (1966).

[12] O. Ouchterlony, *Acta Pathol. Microbiol. Scand.* Suppl. 154, 252 (1962).

[13] C. B. Laurell, *Anal. Biochem.* **10**, 358 (1965).

he would do well to consult other technical reviews[6, 14–18] in which somewhat different procedures may have been emphasized. Some reviews call attention to specific applications such as normal and pathological plasma protein patterns,[15–22] immunoglobulins,[18, 22, 23] antigen structure and fragmentation, [23, 24] and composition of biological fluids and extracts.[6, 16, 18, 20] These reviews should be consulted for references that may be helpful. In addition there are published classified bibliographies including all diffusion methods: up to 1962,[25] 1962 to 1968.[26] A volume of abstracts on electrophoresis including IEA[27] has also become available.

[14] P. Grabar, *Methods Biochem. Anal.* **7**, 1 (1959).

[15] C. Wunderly, *Advan. Clin. Chem.* **4**, 207 (1961).

[16] P. Grabar and P. Burtin, eds., "Immunoelectrophoretic Analysis." Masson, Paris, 1960, and Elsevier, Amsterdam, 1964.

[17] P. Burtin and P. Grabar, *in* "Electrophoresis" (M. Bier, ed.), Vol. 2, pp. 109–156. Academic Press, New York, 1967.

[18] L. P. Cawley, "Electrophoresis and Immunoelectrophoresis." Little, Brown, Boston, Massachusetts, 1969.

[19] F. Scheiffarth and H. Götz, *Intern. Arch. Allergy Appl. Immunol.* **16**, 61 (1960).

[20] J. Clausen, *Sci. Tools* **10**, 29 (1963).

[21] F. Peetoom, "The Agar Precipitation Technique and its Application as a Diagnostic and Analytical Method" Thomas, Springfield, Illinois, 1963.

[22] S. E. Ritzmann and W. C. Levin, *in* "Lab Synopsis" Vol. 2, 2nd Ed. Behring Diagnostics Inc., Woodbury, New York, 1969.

[23] J. Heremans, "Les globulines seriques du system gamma." Masson, Paris, 1960.

[24] M. Kaminski, *Progr. Allergy* **9**, 79 (1965).

[25] O. Ouchterlony, "Handbook of Immunodiffusion and Immunoelectrophoresis." Ann Arbor Sci. Publ., Ann Arbor, Michigan, 1968.

[26] G. Schwick, K. Storiko, and W. Becker, *in* "Lab Synopsis" Vol. 1, revised Ed. Behring Diagnostics Inc., Woodbury, New York, 1969.

[27] B. J. Haywood, "Electrophoresis Technical Applications." Ann Arbor Sci. Publ., Ann Arbor, Michigan, 1969.

2. IMMUNOELECTROPHORETIC ANALYSIS IN AGAR GELS*

a. GENERAL CONSIDERATIONS

Although many modifications of immunoelectrophoretic analysis (IEA) have been introduced, the most widely used is that described by Grabar and Williams[1] in which all operations are performed in a single layer of gel. When IEA is employed for routine screening, for the study of major components of antigen mixtures, or for analysis of precious materials the microtechnique first described by Scheidegger[2] is generally preferred. For detection and study of less prominent antigens, particularly in more com-

* Section 14.D.2 was contributed by Curtis A. Williams.

[1] P. Grabar and C. A. Williams, *Biochim. Biophys. Acta* **10**, 193 (1953); **17**, 67 (1955).

[2] J. J. Scheidegger, *Intern. Arch. Allergy Appl. Immunol.* **7**, 103 (1955).

plex mixtures or when greater resolution is required, larger plates must be used. The difference in the size of the plate imposes certain differences in technique and procedure which will be outlined in Section e below. The basic principles described below, however, and much of the apparatus and materials (discussed in Section b) are common to the macrotechnique and the microtechnique.

An antigen solution is placed in a vertical starting well in a layer of agar gel containing an electrolyte buffer. The several components of the

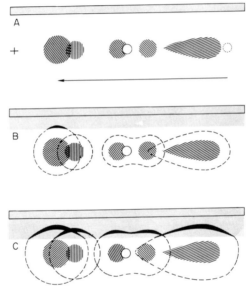

Fig. 1. Schematic diagrams of immunoelectrophoretic principles. (A) Antibody is added to lateral trough following zone electrophoresis; the individual proteins are shown in their positions resulting from electrophoresis, with early diffusion occurring during electrophoretic separation. (B) Early diffusion stage with first precipitate forming. (C) Late diffusion stage with pattern complete. See text for details.

mixture are separated electrophoretically by passing direct current through the gel. The gel plate is removed, and a lateral trough parallel to the axis of electrophoretic migration is filled with an antiserum. Figure 1A illustrates this stage of the procedure for a hypothetical mixture of five antigens. The starting well is represented by the small circle in the middle of the plate. The anode is at the left, and the arrow indicates the direction and distance of electrophoretic migration of the "fastest" component. At the mildly alkaline buffer pH generally employed, agar carries a net negative charge due to the ionization of inorganic acid groups. This fixed charge is balanced by H_3O^+ which moves toward the cathode.

H_3O^+, of course, is the solvent itself; thus the entire fluid phase and all its solutes have a net cathodic flow (to the right in Fig. 1A) called electroosmosis. The true starting *point* for electrophoresis has therefore shifted after the fact and is indicated by the small dotted circle—the starting *well* is now merely a blemish in the gel. Antiserum is represented by the gray shading in the lateral trough. Figure 1B illustrates the initial diffusion stage and first precipitate forming as the antigen diffusion fronts (dotted lines) intersect the antibody diffusion front (shaded area). The antigen component to the right is shown with a skewed charge distribution such as is found with γG immunoglobulin. The two smaller components in the middle of the plate are shown to be immunochemically related or identical in Fig. 1C, their arcs joining in a continuous reaction. This type of pattern is seen with genetically variant forms of a protein in heterozygotes. Transferrin sometimes shows this property. It is also characteristic of the pattern seen when the active and inactive forms of the third component of complement (C3) are both present in a serum. The arcs of precipitate of unrelated antigens form independently and cross, each unaffected by the other. Antibody not precipitated by its specific antigen continues to diffuse along a linear front.

IEA has been used to enumerate antigenic components in mixtures, to detect impurities, and to monitor purifications; to analyze soluble tissue antigens of animals and plants and antigens in extracts of microorganisms and culture media; to study growth, development, and biosynthesis; to detect genetic variants by mobility differences of proteins in blood serum and in microbial extracts; to detect or confirm and monitor pathological conditions reflected in the proteins of body fluids. Many more applications are suggested by the sections on staining (14.E.1), autoradiography (14.E.4), and on the various modifications of IEA (14.D.3–5). Over 80 pertinent articles are abstracted from the 1965–1968 literature in a volume of abstracts on electrophoresis.[3] This reference work is recommended for its scope, rather than its completeness with respect to IEA.

By far the most widely studied antigen mixture is human plasma, or protein fractions thereof. Figure 2 is a composite diagram of IEA precipitates observed with human plasma adapted from a review by Scheiffarth and Götz.[4] No two multispecific antisera are likely to give identical IEA patterns, however, and most will give patterns less complex than that shown here. Moreover, with antisera of high complexity, no two normal plasma samples used as antigen are likely to give identical patterns. Also, because of the variability in the relative positions and visibilities

[3] B. J. Haywood "Electrophoresis Technical Applications," pp. 91–115. Ann Arbor-Humphrey Sci. Publ., Ann Arbor, Michigan, 1969.
[4] F. Scheiffarth and H. Götz, *Intern. Arch. Allergy Appl. Immunol.* **16,** 61 (1960).

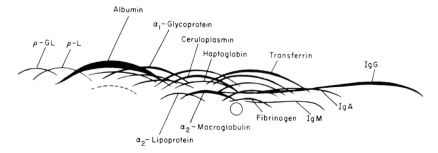

Fig. 2. Composite diagram of immunoelectrophoretic analysis of human plasma proteins. The anode is to the left. "Prealbumins" are labeled ρ-GL (for glycoprotein) and ρ-L (for lipoprotein). The pattern as drawn suggests the approximate relative positions of the more frequently observed precipitation arcs. Modified from Scheiffarth and Götz.[4]

of the arcs under different experimental conditions, only "landmarks" such as albumin and immunoglobulins are identified by observation alone. Most other identifications must be considered tentative when every new antiserum is used or with each change in experimental conditions. A review of the properties and the identification of plasma proteins by IEA[5] will be especially useful in this particular case but will not be emphasized here. More general experimental conditions and variables are described in Section e, and methods of identification are illustrated in Section d.

b. APPARATUS AND MATERIALS

i. Zone Electrophoresis Apparatus

Equipment for gel electrophoresis may be as elaborate as the budget permits or as simple as the principle requires. The only expensive basic requirement is a direct current power supply—unless, of course, the laboratory is equipped with a direct current outlet, in which case only a rheostat is required.

In the latter case a perfectly adequate minimal apparatus may be constructed with plastic storage boxes as buffer reservoirs and graphite pencil cores as electrodes. The gel plates rest on the sides of the buffer reservoirs; electrical contact is made between them and composition sponges, which are immersed on edge in the buffer next to the sides of the reservoir supporting the plates. They should rise slightly above the buffer level. The sponges prevent mixing of the initial buffer, which is in contact with the plates, with buffer of changed composition due to electrolysis at the electrodes. Ideally the electrical contact should be made

[5] P. Burtin and P. Grabar, *in* "Electrophoresis" (M. Bier, ed.), Vol. 2, pp. 109–156. Academic Press, New York, 1967.

with strips of the same agar that is used on the plates, since electroosmotic flow of fluid will then be the same in the contact leads as that on the plate itself. This apparatus may be placed under an inverted plastic box to protect it from dust and to permit the atmosphere to become saturated with moisture.

The improvisation above can be adopted also where direct current is furnished by a power supply, but laboratories engaged in routine or large-scale work, in which reproducibility and control of experimental conditions is essential, will wish to invest in more convenient and more standardized apparatus. Figure 3 illustrates diagrammatically two basic types of such equipment.

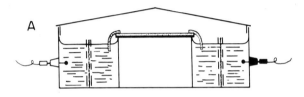

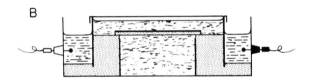

FIG. 3. Diagrams of apparatus for electrophoresis in gels. (A) Adaptation of conventional zone electrophoresis equipment. (B) Inverted gel method of Wieme[6] with agar block buffer reservoirs and cooling fluid. See text for descriptions.

The more frequently encountered apparatus, in which the gel plate rests on the sides of two buffer reservoirs, as described above, is shown in Fig. 3A. Most commercially available equipment is some modification of this design.* The self-contained reservoirs are provided with inbuilt platinum electrodes and jacks, and with convection baffles to retard mixing of electrolysis products with the contact buffer. In the model shown the baffles are perforated slots into which filter paper may be

* National Instrument Laboratories, Washington, D.C.; Gelman Instrument Co., Ann Arbor, Michigan; Buchler Instruments, Fort Lee, New Jersey; Colab Labs, Chicago Heights, Illinois; Behring Diagnostics, Inc., Woodbury, New York; Behringwerke Ag., Marburg, Germany; Kallestad Laboratories Inc., Minneapolis, Minnesota; Shandon Scientific Company, Sewickley, Pennsylvania; Analytical Chemists, Inc., Palo Alto, California; Pfizer Diagnostics, New York, New York.

inserted. A tight-fitting peaked lid maintains the humid atmosphere and prevents the condensed moisture from falling on the plate.

Layers of agar gel about 1 mm thick are usually flexible enough to bend without breaking and are recommended for contact leads between the gel plate and the buffer in the reservoir. Thicker agar leads must be supported by filter paper, gauze, or cellophane. Electrical contact may also be made with filter paper, flannel cloth, chamois leather, or specially designed nylon wicks (Gelman Instrument Company). The disadvantage of all these is that in them the electroosmotic flow is not the same as in agar. If electroosmosis is greater in the lead than in agar, fluid will enter the anodal end of the plate swelling the gel, and there will be a net loss of fluid at the cathodal end. The opposite effect is seen if electroosmosis is greater in the agar than in the leads. The resulting difference in gel cross sections induces a difference in voltage gradient at the two ends of the plate, and therefore in rates of electrophoretic migration. This consideration is more important in the microtechniques where the gel layer on the plates is already relatively thin.

The method developed by Wieme,[6] shown in Fig. 3B, overcomes several difficulties inherent in the more popular method described above. To set up this apparatus, a buffered agar *stage* is poured to brimming and allowed to gel in the proximal chambers of the reservoirs. When solidified, the agar block is raised slightly above the top of the reservoir side and new molten agar is poured into the distal chambers up to the partition. The distal chambers are then filled with buffer to the level of the stage. The gel plate is inverted so that the ends make direct contact with the agar stages. The prepared apparatus may be used for several short electrophoresis runs, the polarity being reversed on each successive run. This refinement also permits the immersion of the plate in an electrically inert and nonmiscible fluid such as high-boiling-point petroleum ether. Fire hazard can be further reduced by use of *n*-heptane (b.p. 98°), although the flash point is −1°. The fluid layer prevents any evaporation from the plate, and it may also be used as a coolant by circulation if desired.

This latter method must be viewed primarily as a precision research tool. For most applications of IEA, this degree of control over conditions is not essential.

In routine IEA it is frequently necessary to run many analyses at once. Commercial equipment usually provides for this, but each has its limitations and drawbacks. In the author's laboratory we have adopted what we consider to be the best features of several systems. Figure 4A is a photo-

[6] R. J. Wieme, "Agar Gel Electrophoresis," pp. 35, 68–77. Elsevier, New York, 1965.

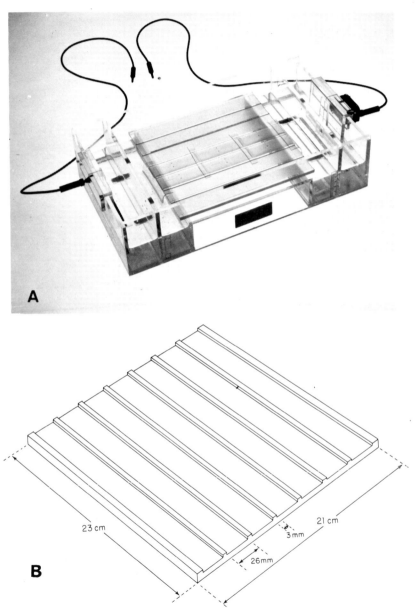

FIG. 4. (A) Tandem stage gel electrophoresis apparatus for 21 microplates. (B) Diagram of removable lucite stage designed by the author. See text for use.

graph of an apparatus that will permit 21 microplates to be run simultaneously. Figure 4B is a diagram of the removable stage of our devising. It makes use of the tandem arrangement introduced by LKB, but it permits independent handling, removal, and substitution of 25 × 75 mm plates (microscope slides). As few as three plates may be run, but even with a full stage, electrical contact is made with a single uniform agar lead at each end. Additional agar strips of uniform thickness and width are laid across the ends of the middle row, connecting all the plates in tandem. The basic apparatus, designed originally for paper electrophoresis,* came equipped with removable electrode carriers with jacks and a safety switch that interrupts the current when the cover is removed.

ii. Power Supply

Any direct current power supply that will deliver voltage to the gel layer sufficient to provide up to 6 volts per centimeter is suitable. The current required will depend on the cross section of the gel and the conductivity of the buffer used. The voltage required at the source will depend on the length of the gel and the loss of potential in the buffer reservoirs and the contact leads to the gel plate.

Commercial suppliers of basic electrophoresis apparatus usually have the appropriate size power supply, but in general a 200 to 300 volt rectifier is ample. Provision for delivery of constant voltage is usually an expensive option and is of little value in gel electrophoresis. Conditions in the fluid and gel phases of the circuit change during any given run, and the full circuit output readings seldom reflect accurately the voltage gradient on the gel plate. This must be measured directly on the plate with a voltmeter. Probes should be inserted through an insulating block which allows a fixed separation between them (e.g., 6 cm). The voltage may be checked and adjustments made periodically during the run. After the initial evaporation, saturation of the atmosphere, and stabilization of temperature, there will be little change on the plate during a 60 to 90 minute run. Therefore, a constant current power supply, after adjustment, at 20 minutes should maintain a fairly uniform voltage gradient. It is recommended that the voltage gradient be checked at 30-minute intervals.

iii. Diffusion Chamber

During the diffusion of antigens and antibody it is important to maintain a humid atmosphere to prevent desiccation of the gel. Of equal

---

* Buchler Instrument Co., Fort Lee, New Jersey. Model is discontinued. The removable Lucite stage pictured in Fig. 4B was designed by the author and milled locally.

importance is a relatively constant temperature. As discussed in Section 14.A.1, sudden changes in temperature during pattern development will produce artifacts.

The simplest solution to these requirements is a sturdy plastic refrigerator storage box with a tight-fitting lid. Humidity can be maintained with a moistened sponge. Developing plates must rest on a level platform (e.g., a plastic test-tube rack), which should be checked with a spirit level. Commercial suppliers have devised chambers that accommodate a variety of diffusion plates, but usually the chambers have been designed with their own system in mind. An LKB-designed chamber is a plastic box type which takes 18 microslides on special carriers; it is highly suitable, but functions as moist chamber best when used in the inverted position.* With macroplates (e.g., 5 × 7 inch or 13 × 18 cm photoplate glass), an upright chamber with plate supports and a hinged door is available.†

The chamber may be placed at any desired temperature from cold room to 37° incubator. If it is to be moved about while fluid is in the wells or troughs, however, care must be taken to avoid spillage, and it must always be placed so that the contained plates are level. There is sometimes good reason to develop a pattern in the cold. If it is wished to study patterns of early development on microplates, which develop rapidly at room temperature, incubation at 2 to 5° overnight may be convenient. Macroplates develop more slowly, and incubation in the cold is recommended only if necessary to control growth of bacteria and molds or to retard the action of proteolytic enzymes that may be present in the antigen mixture. Incubation at 37° will accelerate development, but also it will encourage microbial growth. Preservatives should be included in the agar (e.g., 0.01% Merthiolate, 0.2% sodium azide, or both) if incubation at 37° or at room temperature is to proceed for more than a few hours. Incubation between 20° and 25° is most convenient since observations and photography are usually conducted at these temperatures. Removal of developing plates from low or high temperature to room temperature for observation, even for a short period, will risk precipitation artifacts.

iv. Viewing and Photographic Apparatus

Precipitates in gels are best observed by dark-field illumination. Once a plate is stained, however, it must be studied and photographed against a bright field.

A discussion of viewers and photographic technique is given in Section 14.E.2.

* Gelman Instrument Co., Ann Arbor, Michigan.
† HCS Corporation, Wichita, Kansas.

v. Preparation of Agar

Agar of reasonably high purity is commercially available but rather expensive. Semirefined agar such as Bacto-Agar (Difco) or Agar-Agar (Baltimore Biological Laboratories) is much less expensive but requires repeated washings and filtration. Special preparations such as Ion Agar and agarose generally require no washing, but filtration in fluid state through sintered glass (coarse grade) is recommended since even these highly refined products contain variable amounts of dust. The selection of these gels is usually made on the basis of optical or electrical properties. Agarose, for example, induces less electroosmotic flow (see Fig. 8 in Section c). Agarose is expensive; it may be prepared in the laboratory as described in Section 14.F.2.

Granular products are washed in distilled water until no further color is leached out (changes during 3 days in the cold). The water is then replaced by washing successively with ethanol and acetone, and the agar is collected on a Büchner funnel. The grains may be dried from acetone on the funnel or spread in a thin layer on foil or paper. The residual water content of "dry agar" may be 15 to 30%. (If it is desired to use agar on a dry weight basis—which is recommended, a known hot solution can be precipitated with excess ethyl alcohol, centrifuged, and the precipitate dried to constant weight.) Granular agars, previously washed and dried, are melted directly in buffer and filtered through a coarse sintered-glass funnel under slight negative pressure. When more thorough washing is desired, the procedure used for crude agar can be used.

Crude shredded agar can also be employed if it is properly purified. It must be dissolved and filtered through several layers of gauze, then through coarse fluted papers at 80° to 95°. A 3% solution may be treated in this fashion in the autoclave. A sintered-glass funnel may also be used with more dilute agar solutions, but only after large lumps have been removed. The agar is allowed to gel, then is cut into slivers, allowed to soak in several changes of distilled water and stored as a gel with preservative. The final agar concentration of the gel is determined by drying a sliver to constant weight in an oven.

After initial preparation agar should be melted only once, immediately prior to use; at this time the concentration of agar is adjusted with water and buffer in appropriate amounts.

Various preparations will set to different degrees of firmness. Recommended concentrations for some products are: 1.2 to 2% for Noble Agar (Difco), 1.0 to 1.5% for agarose, and 0.7 to 1.0% for Ion Agar (Oxoid).

For a more complete discussion of the properties and preparation of gels, see Section 14.F.1.

c. EXPERIMENTAL CONDITIONS

The discussion of conditions in the paragraphs below will serve to introduce the wide spectrum of variables which the worker must consider when conducting experiments with IEA. These variables can serve as powerful tools if carefully used, or they can plague one if ignored. For the most part, the illustrations are IEA patterns obtained by the micro-technique. While they are presented for the technical principles under discussion, they demonstrate, as well, some of the many applications of IEA.

When an antigen mixture and complementary antiserum are being used for the first time, it is best to proceed in the simplest possible way, i.e., barbital buffer (pH 8.2 to 8.6, ionic strength below 0.05), 1 to 1.5% agar, 6 volts/cm for 90 minutes; the concentration of the principal expected antigens should each be at least 1 to 5 mg/ml, and the anti-serum should be used undiluted. When the resulting pattern is examined critically, many variations in conditions will suggest themselves.

i. Relative Concentration of Antigen and Antibody

The critical balance of reactant concentrations in gel diffusion analyses has been discussed in several other sections (14.B.2,3; 14.C.1–8). In IEA the important points to remember are that (1) reactions where antibody is in excess are forced toward the center line of the plate and become pro-gressively diffuse with increasing antibody excess; (2) antigen excess reactions move toward the lateral trough, and in extreme antigen excess will migrate out of the field or dissolve except for the tips of the arc, where antigen concentration is minimal (cf. Fig. 14A); (3) equivalence relationships will vary widely from one antiserum to another.

These principles are illustrated in Fig. 5. The IEA pattern of normal human plasma, developed with a commercial goat antiserum, reveals at least twenty reaction systems. Several of these are in antigen excess: prealbumin lipoprotein (extreme left, seen only when the plasma is diluted five times), albumin, three α_2-globulins, transferrin and γG im-munoglobulin (extreme right). Some are near equivalence, as indicated by their sharp and dense precipitates: two α_1-globulins, a β_1-globulin, and γA immunoglobulin (appearing as a spur beneath the γG).

Other patterns have developed in antibody excess and virtually dis-appear on dilution of the antigen. With normal undiluted plasma, γM immunoglobulin appears as a faint diffuse haze extending to the right of the starting well toward the cathode. The γM component could be easily identified with this antiserum by employing 2–3 times more antigen by repeated filling of the center well, as suggested by the bottom panel which is a 5-times diluted plasma from a patient with Waldenström's macroglobulinemia. The γM is quite sharp, as is transferrin at this dilution, while γG is seen in antibody excess. The albumin is still in great antigen excess, however; the plasma must be diluted 20 times to bring the albumin precipitate into equivalence with this antiserum. The third and fourth panels of Fig. 5 are two different γG multiple myeloma plasmas. They are also diluted 5 times, a circumstance that removes the residual

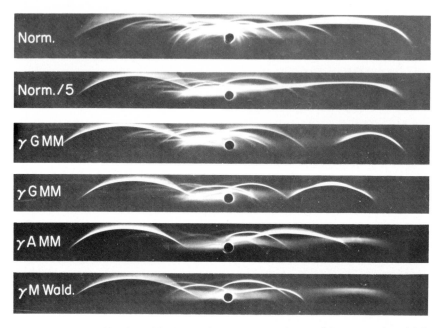

FIG. 5. Effect of antigen dilution on IEA patterns of normal human and multiple myeloma (MM) plasma. Norm./5 indicates five-times diluted antigen. All myeloma plasmas are diluted five times for analysis. γM Wald. indicates Waldenström's macroglobulinemia. Patterns were developed with goat antiserum. See text for discussion.

normal γG reaction and places the paraproteins near equivalence so that their homogeneous electrophoretic dispersions can be demonstrated. The fourth panel is a γA myeloma, which is still in antigen excess after dilution.

Monitoring of procedures aimed at antigen purification is one application of IEA where careful attention to relative amounts of antigen and antiserum employed is of paramount importance. It is axiomatic that neither IEA nor any other immunochemical test can prove purity, since even the most complex antisera may lack sufficient antibody for a given contaminant. Nevertheless, when the relevant antibodies are present, antigenic impurities can be detected if the appropriate amounts of the reactants are used. Figure 6 illustrates this principle. Three different preparations of ragweed antigens are analyzed by the same rabbit antiserum. Microplates B and C clearly demonstrate the importance of using a sufficient quantity of antigen for the evaluation of heterogeneity. On plate C, 4 μg of a highly purified antigen reveals no impurities while

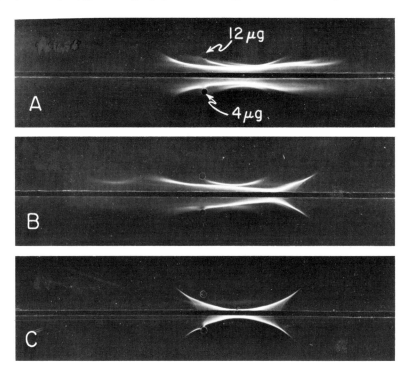

FIG. 6. Detection of heterogeneity in partially purified ragweed antigens by rabbit antiserum against crude pollen extracts. (A and B) Partially purified preparations. (C) Highly purified preparation. Patterns of each preparation were developed by the same rabbit antiserum using 4 and 12 μg of protein, respectively, in the starting wells.

12 μg contains enough of two additional antigens to react visibly with the antiserum.

In the analysis of antigen mixtures, errors of interpretation due to concentration effects are not too frequent because some prior expectation of electrophoretic position exists. The application of IEA to the study of electrophoretic distribution of antibody, on the other hand, may be critically dependent on relative concentration. If antibody to the same antigen occurs in different electrophoretic zones, as it frequently does in horse antisera, there is seldom the same amount of antibody represented in the different zones.

Figure 7 is the IEA pattern of antibody distribution in a hyperimmune horse antiserum against human plasma antigens. The patterns were developed by diffusing Fraction IV-7 of human plasma from the lateral trough on either side of the plate. This fraction is quite rich in transferrin but it contains many other antigens, including albumin and immuno-globulin, in smaller amounts. Development with a 2 mg/ml solution of antigens gives a strong precipitate with antibody located in the γ zone which is continuous with the antibody excess reaction of the same com-

0.5 mg IV-7/ml

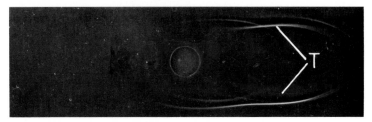

2 mg IV- 7/ml

FIG. 7. Effect of antigen concentration in lateral troughs on detection of classes of antibody in horse antiserum. Hyperimmune horse antibodies against human plasma antigens were resolved electrophoretically on 13 × 18 cm plates in standard barbital buffer at 5 volts/cm for 4 hours. Ethanol fraction IV-7 (transferrin rich) was then added to the lateral troughs, and the pattern was photographed by contact printing (see Section 14.E.2.f) after 3 days' diffusion (C. A. Williams, Ph.D. Thesis, Rutgers University, New Brunswick, New Jersey, 1954). See text for discussion.

ponent in the β zone. The unwary observer might suspect this to be the precipitate of anti-transferrin antibodies. Instead, this is the albumin reaction—the transferrin reaction is the strong precipitate in the γ zone developed on the other side of the plate with a 0.5 mg/ml solution of antigens. With the more concentrated antigen the transferrin reaction is in great antigen excess, faint and nearly dissolved. Also, there is shown to be only traces of antibody to transferrin in the β zone. There are two general rules to remember: First, immunized animals rarely if ever make antibody to components of complex mixtures in amounts proportional to their concentration in the immunogen. Second, a single arbitrary ratio of an antigen mixture to antiserum is seldom satisfactory for more than very few of the reaction systems.

ii. Electroosmosis

Electroosmotic flow of the fluid phase in an agar gel is due to the net negative charge on the agar matrix (see Section a and Fig. 1). For example, β_2-globulins and γ-globulins of serum appear to migrate toward the cathode. Therefore the starting wells should be cut near the middle of the plate. An agarose matrix carries a significantly smaller charge, thus inducing a slower electroosmotic flow. With agarose gels the starting wells may be placed about halfway between the middle and the cathode end of the slide. Figure 8 illustrates the effect of different rates of electro-

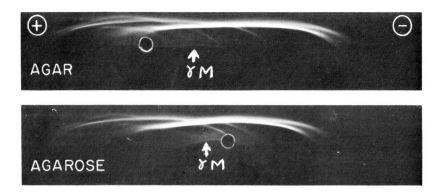

Fig. 8. Patterns of a whole human serum developed with a goat antiserum to immunoglobulins. The different rates of electroosmosis in agar and agarose determine the position of components in relation to the starting well. (For this figure, appropriate sections of the original plates were lined up with respect to corresponding precipitate bands.) See text.

osmosis on the patterns of human immunoglobulins. If agarose is used, the starting well will be located in the midst of the pattern of immunoglobulin precipitates, partially obscuring the γM line. Studies of immunoglobulins of γ and β_2 mobility are therefore best performed in agar. Conversely, antigens with mobilities in the β_1 and α_2 ranges frequently give more legible patterns in agarose.*

iii. Buffer Systems

The selection of the buffer system suitable for a particular analysis can be very important to any electrophoretic procedure. Because of its great

* Prepared agarose layers on flexible plastic supports are available from Analytical Chemists, Inc., Palo Alto, California, and Pfizer Diagnostics, New York, New York.

inherent resolving power, however, less attention has been given to buffer systems in IEA than in other electrophoretic procedures. But even in IEA the antibody precipitates of two components may lie too close to be readily distinguished.

Choosing a pH nearer the isoelectric points of two proteins that migrate close together at pH 8.6 may maximize the effect of any charge difference between them and lead to their separation. The pH ranges for buffer systems often employed are

Sodium acetate*	4.0– 5.5
Sodium phosphate*	6.0– 8.0
Sodium barbital*	8.0– 9.0
Sodium borate*	8.0–10.0

but other systems such as Tris are also satisfactory. Many other buffer systems are given in Appendix II, Volume II.

The choice of buffer anions, however, is often more important than pH to the resolution of complex mixtures. The buffer anion may also affect electroosmotic flow, and the proportion of buffer ions to other electrolytes frequently affects the migration of certain proteins and hence the resolution of mixtures. The IEA patterns in Fig. 9 illustrate several effects to be considered in choosing a buffer system for electrophoresis.

The second and third patterns of Fig. 9 show that changes in pH have little effect on resolution in the pH ranges in which electrophoresis is most commonly performed. Borate buffers at pH 8.0 or pH 8.6 at first glance separate plasma proteins to about the same degree. In the β zone where the pattern most differs from that obtained with phosphate (first pattern), however, differences may be discerned. These differences are probably not due to pH *per se*, but rather to the different concentration of borate affecting proteins differentially according to the relative amounts of carbohydrate associated with them. Borate binds to hydroxyl groups on adjacent carbon atoms and gives sugars and polysaccharides a net charge so that they migrate in an electrical field. It is also probable that this is the reason for the marked increase in electroosmotic flow—since agar is a polysaccharide, it would be expected to have a greater net charge in a borate buffer. This buffer can be useful for study of serum β-globulins since electroosmosis moves them completely away from the starting well and since resolution of these proteins is clearly superior to that obtained in phosphate (first pattern) or barbital (fourth and fifth patterns). The transferrin precipitate in borate, for example, is completely resolved from

* Suitable formulations of these buffers at ionic strengths 0.03 to 0.05 can be planned on the basis of Volume II, Appendix II: acetate, buffers **3** or **4** diluted 1:3 or 1:2; phosphate, buffers **29** or **32** diluted 1:3 or 1:2; barbital, buffers **12** and **13**; borate buffer **18C**.

that of another component partially obscured in the phosphate or barbital patterns.

In phosphate the α_2-globulins can be studied fairly well, but they are not as well separated from the β-globulins as they are seen to be in the barbital-chloride buffer (fourth pattern). When no chloride is added (fifth pattern) the slower globulins are poorly resolved but the α_1-globulins

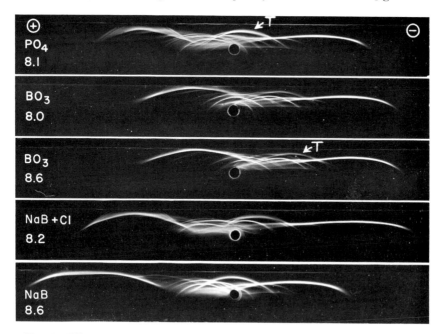

FIG. 9. Effect of varying pH and buffer anions on electrophoretic resolution of human plasma proteins by IEA (T = transferrin). Electrophoresis was performed at 5 volts/cm for 90 minutes. Antigens of human serum are developed by a commercial goat antiserum. All buffers were adjusted to equal specific conductance (approximately 3×10^{-4} mho at 0°). The cation was sodium in all cases. Buffer compositions were as follows. PO_4, pH 8.1: 0.0024 M NaH_2PO_4, 0.04 M Na_2HPO_4 (ionic strength 0.12); BO_3, pH 8.0: 0.10 M NaOH, 0.50 M H_3BO_3 (ionic strength 0.10); BO_3, pH 8.6: 0.10 M NaOH, 0.30 M H_3BO_3 (ionic strength 0.10), NaB + Cl, pH 8.2: 0.026 M NaOH, 0.04 M diethylbarbituric acid, 0.04 M NaCl (ionic strength 0.066); NaB, pH 8.6: 0.1 M NaOH, 0.12 M diethylbarbituric acid (ionic strength 0.10).

and the albumin are well separated. To study the α_1-globulins this buffer should be considered, and for additional visibility of α_1-globulins anti-albumin antibodies should be removed from the antiserum by absorption with purified albumin at the equivalence point (see Chapter 13.A.3.a).

One of the simplest barbital buffers, giving a pH about 8.2, is used routinely in the author's laboratory. It is prepared as follows: 0.1 M

barbital sodium (20.6 gm/liter), 770 ml; 0.1 N HCl, 230 ml. The ionic strength of this buffer is 0.077, i.e., the molar concentration of the Na⁺, and it is diluted with an equal volume of water for use in agar gels ($\Gamma/2$ = 0.038, specific conductance = 3×10^{-3} mho at 25°). We shall refer to this as the *standard barbital buffer*. This buffer system is tabulated in Volume II, Appendix II.8.B (No. 12), but if another pH is chosen, note that the ionic strength and the conductance change with the Na⁺ concentration (cf. buffer No. 7).

Some premixed buffer salts are commercially available. One* is based on the barbital–acetate–HCl buffer of Michaelis (Volume II, Appendix II.8.B, Nos. **8** and **11B**).

iv. Buffer Concentration

Varying the ionic strength at constant current has two effects. The voltage gradient is increased with less electrolyte, thus increasing effective migration rates. This also affects the potential migration rate of the agar, however, and thereby increases electroosmosis. This is illustrated in Fig. 10. The γG immunoglobulin has moved proportionately farther toward the cathode than the albumin has moved toward the anode. Adjustment of ionic strength, therefore, may facilitate resolution and possibly visualization if the precipitate in question is moved farther away from the starting well.

* Gelman Instrument Co., Ann Arbor, Michigan.

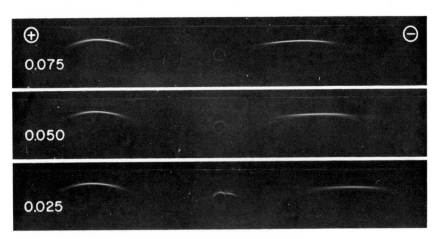

FIG. 10. Effect of varying ionic strength on the separation of serum albumin (left) and γG immunoglobulin (right). Both antigens are applied as solutions at 2 mg/ml. Goat antiserum against whole human serum was used. Ionic strengths shown (0.075, 0.050, 0.025) were prepared by dilution of standard barbital buffer (see text). Electrophoresis was carried out for 90 minutes. Three plates (75 × 25 mm) were run in tandem to assure equal current.

Ionic strengths between 0.025 and 0.05 have proved most satisfactory for electrophoresis in agar. This will vary somewhat, however, with the buffer system. Voltage gradients of 5 to 7 volts/cm are practical limits for good agar electrophoresis without special provisions for cooling. In this context gel thickness also becomes a variable to consider.

Using 1.5% Noble Agar, as purchased, in the standard barbital buffer at ionic strength 0.038 as a 1.3-mm layer, 16 ma/cm² cross section (5.5 ma per microplate) gives a voltage gradient of 6 volts/cm. Under

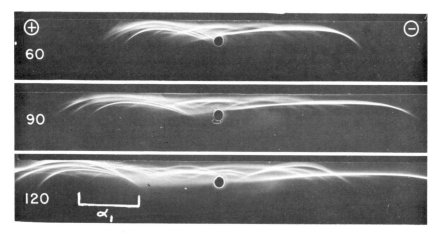

Fig. 11. Effect of duration of electrophoresis on resolution of IEA patterns. Rat serum antigens were electrophoresed in standard barbital buffer on microplates for 60, 90, and 120 minutes at 6 volts per centimeter. Patterns were developed with specific rabbit antisera. Twice-concentrated antiserum was used on the 120-minute plate.

these conditions albumin and γG immunoglobulin are separated by 25 to 30 mm in 90 minutes.

v. Duration of Electrophoresis

If varying the buffer formulation fails to resolve components of interest, prolonging electrophoresis may help. Two factors are involved. Obviously, one is the greater separation of components with time. A more subtle factor depends in part on the first—more antibody can be employed so that fewer components are in great antigen excess. Without greater electrophoretic dispersion, addition of more antibody might obscure more than it would reveal, since denser precipitates generally result and since precipitates of minor components formed in greater antibody excess would increase the background haze.

Figure 11 shows the effect of prolonging electrophoresis on microplates up to 2 hours. The antigen mixture is rat serum and the pattern is developed with a rabbit antiserum. Note the extraordinary complexity of the albumin–α_1 zone and its partial resolution at 120 minutes. Only the slow α_1-globulins are electrophoretically resolved from the albumin precipitate, but sharpening the precipitates in that zone by the addition of more antiserum reveals the great complexity. The importance of carefully adjusted reactant concentration is stressed above in Section c.i.

Prolonging electrophoresis is not without physical effects on the system, but if the voltage is adjusted each 30 minutes, the average voltage gradient can be maintained. Under these conditions, Fig. 12 shows that

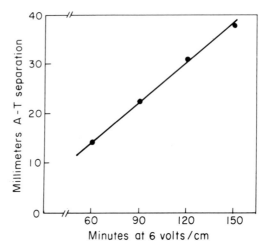

FIG. 12. Electrophoretic separation of rat albumin (A) and rat transferrin (T) as a function of time at a voltage gradient of 6 volts/cm. See text for discussion.

there is a regular rate of electrophoretic separation with time. A-T separation—the measured distance between the albumin and transferrin concentration maxima—is an arbitrary estimate of electrophoretic migration.*

vi. Diffusion Distance

The distance between the lateral trough and the starting well is an experimental condition that can greatly affect the IEA pattern. Increas-

---

* Both albumin and transferrin are highly soluble and stable and of similar molecular size; they are major components in nearly all IEA patterns of plasma proteins. Because their independent dispersion patterns are symmetrical, their points of maximum dispersion patterns are symmetrical, their points of maximum concentration are unambiguous—being essentially the peak of the arc. An alternative measure would be the migration of albumin from an inert marker (glycogen or a neutral dye) which would accurately reflect the electroosmotic displacement of the starting point.

ing this distance has two consequences: (1) Precipitates of major reactions are sharper with less severe effects of antigen or antibody excesses. (2) Minor reaction systems take longer to develop and may never appear sufficiently dense for adequate study. Basically, these are concentration effects not unlike those discussed in Section i, and therefore this variable must be manipulated in concert with concentration and development time. Figure 13 compares two patterns of rat serum antigens obtained with all variables identical except for the diffusion distance. Note that several reactions, clearly visible in the upper pattern (2.6 mm), have not developed in the lower pattern (4.6 mm). Note also that the background haze in the α and β zones of the 2.6-mm pattern is absent from the 4.6-mm diffusion field. This is due to the failure of many minor reactions

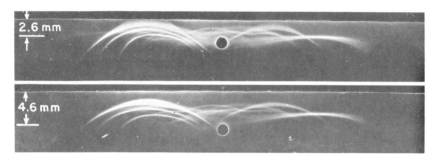

Fig. 13. Effect of diffusion distance on IEA patterns of rat serum antigens (2.6 vs. 4.6 mm). All conditions, including amounts of antigen in wells and rabbit antibody in lateral troughs, and diffusion time were identical. See text for discussion.

in antibody excess to develop, making observation of the major reactions somewhat easier.

vii. Source of Antiserum

Not only do antibodies from different species have different physico-chemical properties, they also combine with antigen under different optimal conditions. Many of these variables are discussed in Section 13.A.1,2.

Hyperimmune horse antibodies against many protein antigens form precipitates which are soluble in both antigen and antibody excess. Precipitation in gels, therefore, produces lines that are quite sharp but which tend to dissolve readily in antigen excess. Earlier bleedings of immunized horses contain relatively more of the γ-zone antibody and the precipitates resemble more the patterns developed by rabbit or goat antiserum. Figure 14 compares patterns developed with antisera from horse, goat, and rabbit.

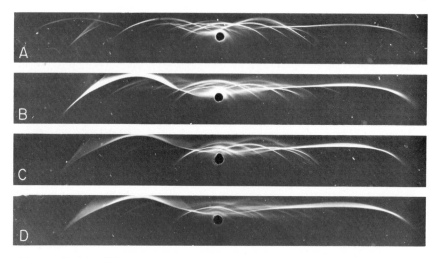

FIG. 14. Species differences among antisera. IEA patterns of same human plasma sample developed with four commercial antisera. A and B |are| horse antiserum patterns; A shows a prealbumin and many α- and β-globulin reactions at or near equivalence, but the albumin precipitate, except for its left-hand tip, is dissolved in antigen excess. C is a goat antiserum pattern. D is a rabbit antiserum pattern. Most of the differences are due to variability in relative concentrations of antibodies with corresponding specificity. The unusual clarity of the reactions in pattern A is due to the high solubility of precipitates in antigen- and antibody-excess with antisera containing greater amounts of β-zone antibody to several antigens. See text for discussion.

If fowl antisera are employed it may be necessary to dialyze the antiserum against 10% NaCl prior to use or to fill the trough a second time with 10% NaCl. Chicken antibodies exhibit optimal serological precipitation in a high salt medium (see Section 13.A.2.c and Vol. I, Section 2.B.3).

viii. Recording Results

The best records for all gel diffusion experiments are photographs. Good drawings are acceptable when it is desirable to omit precipitates that partially obscure the experimental purpose or to generalize a phenomenon from several experimental plates. Drawings are necessary when the eye can detect faint reactions that only heroic photographic technique would capture. When interim stages of pattern development are needed without disturbing the plate, drawings or very rapid photographic procedures are recommended. Photographic procedures are described in Section 14.E.2 and will not be dealt with here.

Plate preparation for photography, however, is important. Most of the IEA patterns illustrating this section are photographs made from micro-

plates, washed, and dried as outlined below in Section e.ii.(e). The plates
were stained and placed in an enlarger, and the patterns were projected
onto printing paper. If this technique is selected, then the choice of dye
should be considered carefully. Figure 15 compares two identical plates,
one stained with bromophenol blue, the other with Ponceau red. The
latter dye stains heavily and will permit registry of very faint precipitates. Only a small amount of red color will suffice, even if the precipitate
is nearly transparent, since bromide printing paper is red blind. Bromophenol blue, on the other hand, stains less heavily and projects blue light
—which readily exposes the printing paper—from faint precipitates and
background. A sharper pattern is obtained, but faint precipitates may be
lost in printing. Bromophenol blue is an indicator dye, however, which
changes through green to yellow at acid reactions. If the stained slide is

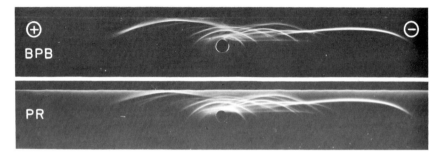

FIG. 15. Comparison of two stains on identical IEA patterns. BPB, bromophenol
blue; PR, Ponceau red. The BPB microplate is also shown in Fig. 9, second panel;
the bottom panel of Fig. 9 is a plate stained with PR.

washed in dilute acetic acid, sufficient yellow is produced in the faint
precipitates to permit their registry. Bromide printing paper is also
yellow blind.

A difficulty frequently encountered with antigenic extracts from
tissues and microorganisms is the presence of nonantigenic substances
having limited solubility or some binding affinity for the agar matrix.
Dyes that stain proteins bind to this material, producing a distracting
image on the photograph. This is seen in Fig. 16A, the upper pattern.
The lower pattern of Fig. 16A is the same slide photographed wet (i.e.,
before drying and staining) in the same enlarger on the same printing
paper (Section 14.E.2.d). The nonspecific blemish (and the unsightly
evidence of overflow of antigen in the starting well) are not recorded.
Otherwise however, the two methods gave equivalent results.

If reaction precipitates are weak then neither the stained nor wet
mount projection technique will register a suitable record. Figure 16B

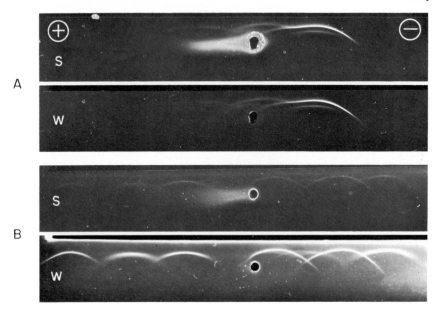

Fig. 16. Methods of photography of microplates. (A) Partially purified yeast antigen developed with rabbit antiserum. S, dried, stained plate photographed by projection. W, same plate photographed wet by projection prior to drying and staining. (B) Rat cerebral cortex antigens developed with unabsorbed rabbit antiserum (second reaction from left is plasma albumin). Stained plate was photographed as in (A); wet plate was photographed by camera with dark-field illumination. See text for discussion.

illustrates such a case. The upper pattern is a projection of the stained preparation. The lower pattern is the same slide, before drying and staining, but in this case it was possible to capture the record by intense oblique lighting and photography on film.

d. IDENTIFICATION OF ANTIGENS

It is clear from Fig. 14 that identification of the majority of antigen–antibody reactions in a complex pattern is not possible from observation alone, even if their position were known in a pattern obtained with another antiserum. Additional tests must be performed. Often an antigen in a precipitate retains a specific chemical property, such as an enzyme activity or a nonprotein moiety, which may be detected by color reactions. These methods are presented in Section 14.E.1. Certain antigens bind small molecules or metals, and their identification can sometimes be made by exchange with radioactive ligands and autoradiography of IEA patterns as described in Section 14.E.4.

Only methods of immunochemical identification will be covered in this section. There are two general approaches. One approach relies at some point on a purified antigen (or in certain special cases a mixture of antigens of a defined nature). The other approach may be called "pattern interaction."

i. Use of Purified Antigens

IEA patterns of a hypothetical mixture containing antigens a, b, and c are shown in Fig. 17. The objective is to identify antigen b.

(a) *Production of Specific Antiserum.* If an antigen is highly purified, if it is scarce, and if continued need for identification is anticipated, the immunization of an animal may be justified. Sometimes as little as 1 mg

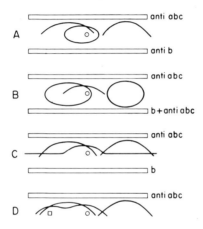

Fig. 17. Methods of identification of antigens in complex mixtures subjected to electrophoresis. (A) Monospecific antiserum, anti b, is applied to one lateral trough. (B) Absorbed multispecific antiserum, b + anti abc, is applied to one lateral trough. (C) Purified antigen, b, is applied to one lateral trough. (D) Antigen b is applied to plate in a small deposit after electrophoresis. See text for discussion.

of antigen is sufficient if the appropriate methods are employed (see Chapter 2, Volume I). Figure 17A illustrates schematically the use of a specific antiserum in the lateral trough opposite the one with the multi-specific antiserum. The arc of precipitate formed produces an ellipse with the corresponding reaction in the complex pattern.

(b) *"Absorption" of Antiserum.* If the purified antigen contains highly immunogenic impurities, making the foregoing procedure unsatisfactory, and if a generous supply is at hand, anti-b antibodies usually can be neutralized (or removed) preferentially by adding antigen b to the antiserum.* The b precipitate will not form on the side developed by the absorbed antiserum (b + *anti abc* in Fig. 17B). If the amounts of impurities are significant in the purified antigen preparation, other antibodies may be reduced below the concentration needed for good reaction proportions. With appropriate antigen mixtures or fractions, it is theoretically possible to absorb out all antibodies but one, giving a monospecific antiserum to be used as shown in Fig. 17A. More frequently, however, complex absorptions are performed with mixtures of antigens representing different tissues, species, genetic mutants, embryological stages, tumors, etc. The antibodies remaining acquire some definition by this procedure, as do those that are removed. But these antisera cannot be used as shown in Fig. 17B, since there are nearly always excesses of some antigens present after absorption with complex mixtures. These excess antigens will behave as shown in Fig. 17C, forming long lines of precipitate interacting with the complete pattern. The results are usually too confusing to be helpful.

(c) *Pattern Distortion by Supplementary Antigen.* Figures 17C and 17D illustrate two ways to use purified antigen directly on the plate. In Fig. 17C antigen b is added to the lateral trough opposite the antiserum. This would ordinarily form a long straight line of precipitate with anti-b antibodies diffusing from the antiserum trough. Antigen b localized electrophoretically on the plate, however, had already precipitated the antibody in that region, and the straight line of precipitate is deflected into the b arc of the IEA pattern.

A more economical method can be used if the purified antigen is precious. The square in Fig. 17D represents a small deposit of antigen b; a few micrograms are sufficient on microplates. The supplementary antigen can be added to another well cut in the agar, to a small piece of filter paper or cellulose acetate membrane that is then placed on the agar surface, or it can be applied as a small drop (1 μl) directly to the gel surface by means of a micropipet. The arc formed by the added antigen will join the b arc of the IEA pattern.

(d) *Pattern Interactions.* There are a number of instances when variations in the relative amounts of an antigen or in its mobility make identification by observation impossible even though a well characterized antiserum is employed. This might be the situation with proteolytic split products, fetal variants, genetic variants, inactivated enzymes or

---

* Absorption of antiserum refers to the specific removal of antibody to a given antigen. This procedure is best performed at antigen–antibody equivalence if that quantitative relationship is either known or readily determined (see Sections 13.A.3.a.iv., 13.E., and 14.C.5.c). Alternatively antigen is added in small increments and precipitate is removed after each addition until no further reaction can be detected.

enzyme precursors, and induced components, such as "acute phase" serum proteins.

Such problems can be approached by the methods illustrated above if the purified antigen is available. Often, however, the identification can be readily made by one of two methods shown in Fig. 18. A hypothetical antigen mixture abc gives a familiar pattern with an antiserum, but

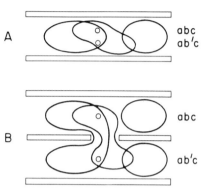

FIG. 18. Identification of antigens by pattern interactions. (A) Adjacent well method. (B) Interrupted trough method. Variant antigen, b', is shown to be immunochemically similar to b by allowing patterns developed by same antiserum to form continuous precipitates. See text for discussion.

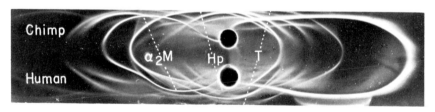

FIG. 19. Interaction pattern of chimpanzee and human serum samples in adjacent wells. Chimp transferrin (T) has lower mobility than human transferrin; chimp haptoglobin (Hp) has higher mobility and is greatly elevated due to recent infection; chimp α_2-macroglobulin has much higher mobility than the human homolog [C. A. Williams and C. T. Wemyss, Ann. N.Y. Acad. Sci. **94**, 77 (1961)]. See text for discussion.

another antigen preparation does not—antigen b is altered and is designated b'.

In Fig. 18A, abc and ab'c are placed in adjacent wells. The wells are spaced far enough apart so that the upper and lower patterns develop independently without initial interference. As diffusion and precipitation is extended, b and b' are shown to be immunochemically similar although their mobilities differ. Figure 19 demonstrates the application of the adjacent-well method to the identification of some of the components of chimpanzee serum. A known human serum pattern is used for the interaction. Antigenic similarities are great between close phylogenetic relatives even though concentrations and mobilities of antigens can vary markedly.

Figure 18B illustrates a plate on which the two antigen mixtures are separated by a lateral trough that is discontinuous. The patterns interact through a "diffusion window."

ii. Nomenclature of New Components

With antigen mixtures as well systematized as blood plasma, nomenclature of components presents only slight difficulty. This is the source of a major problem, however, since any investigator can name an antigen according to its general electrophoretic mobility, add a suffix numeral or letter and claim the identification. This practice has been a source of confusion since it has no relationship to the biological function or biochemical properties of the antigen which would serve to relate it to its homolog in, for example, the plasma of another species or another genetic strain of the same species. While it is often necessary to follow this practice for experimental records in laboratory notebooks, investigators are urged not to permit their laboratory jargon to become part of the published literature.

The temptation to name components is particularly strong when antigen mixtures from microbiological or tissue extracts are being studied by IEA, since frequently there will have been no previous analysis. Here again general restraint is urged, but a particular appeal is made to investigators not to use α, β, or γ notations for electrophoretically distinct components of mixtures other than vertebrate blood plasmas. This system of Greek letters was introduced by Tiselius[7] to identify concentration maxima of horse plasma proteins in moving-boundary electrophoresis (see Chapter 6, Volume II).

iii. Arbitrary Electrophoretic Mobility

An ingenious solution to the problem of nomenclature and identification has been described by Aoki et al.[8] Lactic dehydrogenase (LDH) isoenzymes give five almost equally spaced bands upon electrophoresis in agar. Arbitrary electrophoretic mobility (AEM) values of 20, 40, 60, 80, and 100 were assigned to these bands, and these values were used as a standard scale to assign AEM values to all components of a complex mixture detected by IEA. These authors were able to give relative

[7] A. Tiselius, *Biochem. J.* **31**, 1464 (1937).

[8] T. Aoki, D. Parker, and J. L. Turk, *Immunology* **16**, 485 (1969).

mobility designations to fifteen antigenic components of guinea pig epidermis. The most rapidly migrating antigen, which was numbered 1 as a notebook label, has an AEM of 122; the slowest, antigen 15, had an AEM of 7.

A method such as this could be of great assistance in comparing IEA patterns obtained with different antisera or results obtained by other laboratories or with other buffer systems.

e. TECHNIQUE AND PROCEDURES

The standard IEA method as developed by Grabar and Williams[1] is recommended for occasional application to research problems where maximum resolution of complex systems is desirable. The superior resolution results mainly from the greater electrophoretic separation and from the much greater visibility of minor reactions because of increased depth of the agar layer and larger amounts of reactants. This method is referred to below as the *macrotechnique*. No commercial equipment has been specifically developed for the macrotechnique because it is expensive in materials, and it is otherwise inconvenient for routine laboratory analyses where instrumentation is most helpful.

The *microtechnique* is widely used, on the other hand, and a broad selection of apparatus is offered commercially. Each of these is supplied with a set of specific instructions along with a general outline of principles. Each has its strong points and its weak points which have different relative importance in the context of the specific applications. It is inappropriate to discuss them in detail in the procedures below since the investigator must make his selections on the basis of the experimental conditions illustrated above in Section c, and with careful consideration of his present and his possible future experimental objectives.

i. Macrotechnique

(a) *Preparation of Plates.* Any clear glass plate may be used. Photoplate glass has several advantages: it is thin, optically uniform, and available precut in convenient sizes.* The most frequently used size is 13 × 18 cm (5 × 7 inches), but 8 × 10 cm (3¼ × 4 inches) lantern slide cover glasses are also suitable for smaller patterns.

Plates should be carefully washed in hot detergent and rinsed thoroughly with water and then with alcohol–diethyl ether (1:1). Avoid scratching the surface. After each use, plates should be brought to boiling to remove all adherent agar.

* Lantern slide cover glasses are usually stock items with photography supply houses. Larger plates can be obtained from Eastman Kodak, Rochester, New York, on special order.

An agar coating ("subbing") is applied and dried on one surface to serve as an anchor for the experimental gel layer. If the plate is clean, a hot solution of 0.2% agar in water can be evenly applied with a large artist's brush. When gelled or tacky the layer is dried to a transparent film in an oven at 100° to 110° for 5 minutes. (If the plates are heated more than recommended, the agar coat will turn brown and opaque.) Inspect plates carefully for scratches, dust specks, etc., and store in a dustfree box with lintless paper spacers, preferably within a polyethylene sac as a barrier to grease in the air.

(b) *Experimental Agar Layer.* Agar is washed and mixed with buffer and preservative as described above in Section b.v. Plates must be absolutely level to ensure uniform thickness. There are two main methods for accomplishing this.

A leveling stage may be improvised with a piece of 5-mm plate glass and modeling clay (e.g., plasticene). The clay is modeled into 2-cm balls and placed at the corners of the stage as feet. A machinist's spirit level is needed for precision leveling (small centering-type spirit levels may be used for initial crude leveling). Place plates on stage and recheck level. Rapidly pour a measured amount of agar at 70 to 80° onto the plate from about 2 cm height, avoiding formation of bubbles. If bubbles are present, break them by flaming quickly with a fleeting pass of a Bunsen burner. For a layer 3 mm thick on a 13 × 18 cm plate, use 70 ml of molten agar, or 16 ml for a 2 mm layer on the 8 × 10 cm plate. Draw the molten agar to the edges of the plate with the lip of the pouring vessel or a warmed stirring rod. Surface tension will contain the layer on the plate if the stage is level and the agar is not too hot when poured. Devise a dust cover, for example, one made with aluminum foil, and allow gel to solidify for at least one hour. If this method is employed, leads for electrical contact must be applied as discussed in Section b.i. Alternatively, the plates may be inverted on an apparatus like that shown in Fig. 3B.

The second method is less convenient but has the advantage of forming the experimental layer and the contact leads at the same time. A standard rectangular Pyrex baking dish (e.g., 8 × 12 inches, about 1.5 inches deep) is set on a firm surface and fixed in place with modeling clay. A 1-cm layer of 2 to 3% agar is poured in the bottom of the dish to provide the level surface. When hardened a 13 × 18 cm plate is placed on the base agar and 3 × 13 cm strips of glass are butted to the ends of the plate. Strips of filter paper, 4 × 13 cm, are laid on these so that they overlap the experimental plate by about 1 cm. These papers will support the contact leads and should be fixed in place on the glass with a few drops of hot buffered agar. The volume of buffered agar required to give a layer of the desired thickness is calculated simply: dish dimensions times the combined thickness of the layer and the glass, less the volume of the glass. If the dimensions cited above are used and the experimental layer is to be 3 mm and the glass is 1.5 mm thick, the volume of agar required is about 235 ml. When the gel has set, cut around the three-section plate with a scalpel or sharp spatula and carefully lift the preparation out of the dish. Separate the end glasses from the filter-paper supports, using the spatula if necessary, and make a straight transverse cut in the agar layer directly over each end of the plate. Bend the leads down at right angles and fill the gap in the layer with molten agar.

Starting wells should be cut in the gel at carefully planned intervals so that when the lateral troughs are cut, *after electrophoresis*, the desired diffusion distance is achieved. It is a good practice to have several standard patterns drawn on cards or on other glass plates to be placed under the IEA plate when cutting the starting wells and troughs. Round starting wells are most commonly used, and these may be cut with common cork borers. Diameters up to 6 mm are recommended for troughs on 25-mm centers, and up to 8 mm for troughs on 30-mm centers. With larger plates than these, good resolution may require a considerably longer electrophoresis time (4 to 6 hours). A slit-shaped starting well may be preferable when long periods are allowed for electrophoresis.

(c) *Application of Sample.* The dialyzed sample is warmed in a water bath at 54° to 58°, and buffered double-strength agar is melted at 100° and then brought to the same water bath. Equal volumes are mixed thoroughly in the water bath. With a warmed pipet the mixture is introduced into the starting well. It is important that the sample mixture bond to the agar layer. This may be facilitated by softening the inside of the well with a piping-hot water rinse or by passing a hot stirring rod over the inner surface before adding the sample. Any separation which may occur during electrophoresis must be sealed immediately with hot agar. Figure 7 illustrates a macroplate prepared in this manner.

If the sample cannot withstand heating at 50° to 60°, several alternatives are available.

1. Agar "plugs" cut with a smaller borer cutter can be placed in the dialyzed sample allowing the antigens and buffer to diffuse into the plug overnight. The plug is placed in the well, and the gap is sealed with hot agar.

2. The sample may be added directly to the well. Immediately a calculated amount of dry dextran gel (Sephadex) is slowly added to the sample in the well. It is best to use a small-pore gel (G-25), which will exclude all macromolecules. Sephadex G-25 takes up 2.5 times its weight in fluid. The final volume of the mixture should not exceed the well volume. This two-phase bed is topped and sealed with hot agar.

3. A narrow (1 × 8 mm) slit may be cut in the agar layer. The sample is added as fluid, which is quickly imbibed into the agar. This may be repeated with about 25 μl at each application. After two applications the uptake of fluid is very slow. The slit is then filled with hot agar.

4. A filter paper strip (3 mm wide) may be dipped in the sample and applied on the uncut surface of the gel. It can be removed before electrophoresis, but if this is done at least 30 minutes should be allowed for the sample to be absorbed into the gel.

5. Concentrated samples may also be applied directly to the surface with a micropipet. More than 5 μl applied as a droplet spreads too widely, however. More sample may be applied by waiting and repeating. Application in a thin line gives excellent resolution.[9]

(d) *Electrophoresis.* At 6 volts/cm at room temperature or 8 volts/cm at 5° in barbital buffer at pH 8.2, ionic strength 0.038, separation of serum albumin and transferrin occurs at a rate of about 15 mm/hour (see Fig. 12). Albumin and a low mobility γG myeloma protein (which should remain near the true starting point—see Fig. 5) would separate at twice that rate. In 3 hours the full spectrum of serum proteins, including prealbumin, should cover 10 to 12 cm. The IEA precipitation pattern may extend over 14 cm.

Check the voltage at least twice during the run, first about 20 minutes after the start, and adjust to the preselected voltage gradient (see Section b.ii). At room temperature it may be desirable to use a lower voltage (e.g., 4 volts/cm) and run the experiment longer. There should be less evaporation due to heating if this precaution is adopted.

(e) *Application of Antiserum.* When the plate is removed from the electrophoresis apparatus, the contact leads are cut away and the pattern to be followed is placed under the plate. A sharp knife and a straight edge are essential. Troughs of uniform width may be cut with an improvised double-bladed cutter. Two single-edged razor blades can be bolted together with machine screws across a spacer of metal or plastic. Several different sizes of trough are possible depending on the size of the spacer; 3 to 4 mm is customary for troughs on 25 to 30 mm centers.

The dried adhesion layer on the glass sometimes makes removal of the agar from the cut trough difficult. Take care not to damage the walls of the trough. The bottom of the trough can be resealed by rapidly passing a No. 2 brush, dipped in hot agar, down the trough. This precaution will also improve the optical quality of the plate for photography later on.

The amount of serum added to the trough should be carefully measured

---

[9] P. Goullet, *Experimentia* **20**, 49 (1964).

as a condition of the experiment. If it is thought that less antiserum should be used, the trough should be narrowed. For more antiserum, the immunoglobulin fraction should be concentrated [see Volume I, Chapters 2.C.2 (Fig. 1 and text) and 3.A.2].

On macroplates it is sometimes advantageous to mix the antiserum with agar at 50° to 60° and add the gelling mixture to a wide trough (e.g., 1 cm). Development of the IEA pattern is slower, but handling the plate during the first few days is easier since it does not have to be level. Also in cases where antigen is in great excess (see Section c.i), the precipitate will continue to form in the antiserum-agar zone, rather than disappear into an empty trough. This is a bothersome refinement, however, and it is recommended that it be used only when required.

Development time of the IEA pattern, other conditions being equal, depends on the diffusion distances and the quantities of antigen and antibody used. The pattern will continue to "mature," however, revealing the minor systems well after the principal components are visible. For example, if a pattern with troughs on 18 to 20 mm centers (e.g., on 8 × 10 cm plates) shows the major systems in 2 days, it should be kept under observation for 5 to 6 days. Beyond that time any new development should be viewed with suspicion.

Note that it is during this period that beautiful experiments are ruined for photographic recording because of bacterial and fungal growth. Use preservatives.

ii. Microtechnique

The general procedures for the microtechnique derive from those described above for the macrotechnique. Section i should be read first, since only the major variations imposed by miniaturization are detailed below. As mentioned, most commercial suppliers furnish adequate specific instructions to conduct IEA with their equipment.

All but one (Fig. 7) of the figures illustrating experimental conditions in Section c are microplates, thus readers may use these as technical guides.

(a) *Preparation of Plates.* Microscope slides (25 × 75 mm or 1 × 3 inches) are the most convenient readily available support. Lantern slide cover glasses are also useful since several samples can be run on the same support, or an intermediate-size experiment can be run in the long direction. Slides are cleaned and an adhesion coat of dilute agar is brushed on with a No. 6 artist's brush. The coat is dried for 5 minutes in a 100° oven. When dry, the slides should be returned to their box with the coated surfaces oriented in the same way, indicated by an arrow on the box. Much time will be saved by coating a whole box of slides (50 to 100) at once. Some workers omit the adhesion coat, relying on scrupulously clean slides for good adhesion. This is not recommended if slides are later to be washed on edge in slotted staining dishes or jars. In large-scale routine work, repeating an analysis may be simpler and cheaper than the coating procedure; but gel-bearing slides should be washed in a horizontal position if the subcoat is not employed.

The experimental buffered agar, cooled to 70° to 80°, is rapidly pipetted onto the leveled slides from a warmed measuring pipet. For individual slides, 2.5 ml is added to each from a 5-ml pipet. Three to four slides can be prepared with each filling (2.5 ml gives a layer about 1.3 mm thick). The tip of the empty pipet is used to draw the warm agar to the edges of the slide before it becomes tacky. Prepared slides are best used after 12 to 24 hours of storage in a humid box in the cold room.

Agar contact leads should be prepared with the same agar. An *uncoated* glass plate (e.g., 20 × 25 cm) is placed on the leveling stage, and a volume of hot agar is applied to give a layer 1.0 to 1.3 mm thick. A thickness which is flexible but not brittle must be determined for the type and concentration of agar employed. When thoroughly gelled, and preferably aged for at least 12 hours in a humid storage box, this layer may be cut in convenient strips to make contact between slides and the buffer (see Figs. 3A and 4A). The plate with the unused portion of agar may be held for future use in the refrigerator in a moist chamber or plastic sac for several days. The distance from the end of the slide to the buffer must be short (1.0 to 1.5 cm) if unreinforced leads are to be used without great risk of breaking. The lead should lap the end of the plate not more than 5 mm.

(*b*) *Cutting the Pattern.* Except for the very occasional pilot study when freehand cutting may be acceptable, the microtechnique requires some sort of standard pattern cutter. Otherwise the process is too time consuming, imprecise, and accident prone. There are several models available commercially and, while they are generally supplied as accessories to a complete set-up, they may be purchased separately.* A reasonable variety of well sizes, trough widths and lengths, and diffusion distances may be selected. Some have more flexibility than others, but often such a feature is more expensive than valuable once a standard pattern is worked out.

A satisfactory and inexpensive trough cutter can be devised with a pair of single-edge razor blades bolted together across metal spacers with machine screws. Excellent well cutters are made by cutting off the point

* Combinations of components from different supplies may prove best. In the author's laboratory the Gelman-LKB cutter is used with their plastic frame as a guide and a storage tray, but slides are all prepared individually, not according to the LKB-Gelman system (Gelman Instrument Co., Ann Arbor, Michigan).

of a hypodermic needle and sharpening the cut end on the *inside* surface. A 19-gauge needle is used to produce a 1-mm well, a 13-gauge needle a 2-mm well. The well cutters may be mounted integrally with the trough-cutting blades, as in several commercial devices. The simple, spaced razor blades described above can have well cutters mounted on them by using a larger machine screw and adding two outer 5-mm blocks through each of which a 19-gauge well cutter is inserted 2.5 mm from its adjacent blade. Two blades separated 1 mm apart and provided with 19-gauge needles would produce a pattern similar to that shown in Fig. 6. In Figs. 8 through 11 the wells pictured are 1.2 mm in diameter and the troughs are 1.0 mm wide.

Note that the wells *and* the troughs are cut before electrophoresis, but that the agar is not removed from the troughs until antiserum is to be added. The cut well plugs are removed from the holes by suction. Suitable orifices for the suction tip are narrow-tipped Pasteur pipets (drawn down to 0.5 mm), or the shaft of hypodermic needles cut square across, or stainless steel tubing of 1.2 mm (1/16-inch) o.d. The suction tube is joined by a short length of narrow flexible tubing to larger tubing such as 1/4-inch bore, 1/8-inch wall "gas tubing," which leads to the side arm of a filter flask. The latter serves as trap to receive bits of agar and rinse water, protecting vacuum line or aspirator pump. The suction line is left on and is interrupted by the fingers, a pinchcock or a Pratt T-clamp. With suction interrupted, the narrow tip is brought vertically over the agar plug with illumination provided by low oblique light in a darkened area on a sheet of black paper. The clamp is relaxed momentarily and the plug will enter the tip and be carried upward. At intervals the suction tip and narrow tubing are flushed by drawing up some distilled water.

(c) *Application of Sample.* The simplest applicator is a melting-point capillary tube (1.0 to 1.5 mm, i.d.) drawn to a fine tip in a pilot flame. It can be filled at an angle near the horizontal, and it will discharge its contents to the starting well when the tip is touched to the well at a steeper angle. If the well is filled to just brimming, the volume of the sample applied is easily determined. For rapid filling of larger wells (e.g., 2 mm diameter, 4 μl capacity) a disposable Pasteur pipet may be drawn to a fine tip; but volumetric micropipets may provide greater precision.

Wells may be filled more than once if more antigen is needed, but each filling is imbibed into the agar at a much slower rate. When 1 μl of solution contains sufficient antigen, some workers prefer to apply it directly to the surface. When done with care this is quite satisfactory, but precise placement is difficult and requires a steady hand.

(d) *Application of Antiserum.* After electrophoresis (see Section c.iv for duration) cut the ends of the troughs with a small sharp instrument and lift out the agar with the flat end of a toothpick. The use of sharp or over-size instruments risks damage to the walls of the trough. A break, crack, or gouge will cause an irregular diffusion front and a distorted precipitation pattern in the vicinity.

Troughs may be filled with a volumetric micropipet if less antiserum than the trough capacity is to be used. If the capacity volume is desired, fill to brimming with a Pasteur pipet drawn to a fine tip. Add antiserum slowly from one end of the trough so that if an overflow accident should occur it would have minimal effect on the precipitation pattern.

Troughs may be filled twice if the second filling is made as soon as the trough is empty. It is preferable, however, to concentrate the antiserum* or to prepare a concentrated immunoglobulin fraction (see Volume I, Chapter 3, Section A.2).

Precipitation patterns are well developed after diffusion overnight at room temperature. They will mature further for 2 or 3 days; although antigen-excess reactions may become obscure, minor equivalence reactions will become visible as patterns mature. Many minor antibody-excess reactions will produce a background of poorly defined precipitate, which may make study of even the prominent reactions difficult.

(e) *Washing, Drying, and Staining.* As discussed above in Section c.viii, it may be best to photograph slides periodically during development, and also finally in the wet state. But if the reactions are to be stopped at a given time, the only way is to diffuse all reactants out of the gel. Slides are placed in slotted jars or dishes and covered with a 2% NaCl solution. A wash of 2 to 4 hours is sufficient to *stop the reaction*, but if slides are to be dried and stained, washing is continued for at least 48 hours with several changes of 2% NaCl solution made up in 0.05 M phosphate buffer at pH 8.0 (0.375 gm of KH_2PO_4 and 12.6 gm of $Na_2HPO_4 \cdot 7H_2O$ per liter). The salt solution is replaced with water for 1 day.

To dry the slides, place them on a holder or tray and fill all wells and troughs with water. Cover with a soaking-wet sheet of filter paper, being careful not to trap air bubbles in the wells and troughs. Tilt the tray to drain off excess water. The slides are dried in an incubator, or at room temperature by directing a fan on the tray. In this manner the original dimensions of the wells and troughs are preserved and the gel layer is dried to a transparent film on the slide. Lint from the filter

---

* In the author's laboratory antisera are concentrated twofold by fluid absorption with dry porous gels such as Sephadex G-25 or Lyphogel (a polyacrylamide product from Gelman Instrument Co., Ann Arbor, Michigan). A six- to eightfold concentration can be effected by the method described in Volume I, Chapter 2, Section C.1 (Fig. 1 and text).

paper may be removed from dried slides by gently rubbing with the finger under a running tap. At this point, the slides may be dried in air for storage or placed directly in a staining solution. Staining procedures and color reactions are described in detail in Section 14.E.1. Photography is discussed above in Section c.viii, and methods are presented in Section 14.E.2.

3. IMMUNOELECTROPHORETIC ANALYSIS ON CELLULOSE ACETATE MEMBRANES*

Cellulose acetate membranes (CAM) may be used in the place of gels for a modification of the classical Graber-Williams immunoelectrophoresis (IEA). Both the electrophoretic separation and the subsequent diffusion take place in the membrane. The antiserum is applied to the electrophoretic strip in the form of impregnated filter paper strips. Diffusion takes place in a specially designed moist chamber. The precipitation pattern is revealed by staining after elution of the soluble nonprecipitated reactants.[1-3]. The apparatus is the same as that described for CAM electrophoresis in Chapter 6.C.2, Volume II.

a. PROCEDURE

i. Preparation of Strips

The CAM strips should be somewhat longer than for simple electrophoresis to allow for diffusion of the most rapidly and the most slowly migrating fractions. For small-scale IEA 7 to 5 cm by 3 to 5 cm is a suitable size. (A microtechnique can also be used; it gives satisfactory and more rapid results with consequent economy of materials.) For multiple patterns, wider strips are employed. Buffer impregnation, blotting, and placing in position are as described for CAM electrophoresis. A preservative should be added to the buffer solutions to inhibit growth during the diffusion period.

ii. Application of Sample and Electrophoresis

The antigen is applied in the form of a drop or a short streak according to the desired pattern. The position of application is as for CAM electrophoresis. The optimal volume depends on the concentration and nature of

* Section 14.D.3 was contributed by J. Kohn.

[1] J. Kohn, in "Chromatographic and Electrophoretic Techniques" (I. Smith, ed.), Vol. 2., pp. 120–137. Heinemann, London, 1968.

[2] J. Kohn, in "Protides of the Biological Fluids" (H. Peeters, ed.), pp. 120–121. Elsevier, Amsterdam, 1961.

[3] B. Laurent, Scand. J. Clin. & Lab. Invest. 15, 98 (1963).

the sample and the width of the strip. For serum electrophoresis 0.5 to 2 μl is adequate. The addition of bromophenol blue to serum samples is strongly recommended as this indicates the diffusion and migration of the applied sample during the electrophoresis period enabling termination at the most suitable distance and time.

As for CAM electrophoresis, care should be taken that at least 15 mm are left clear between the ends of the separation pattern and the edges of the strip supports. This can be judged by watching the migration of the colored albumin or by correct timing, established by previous experience.

iii. Application of Antiserum

After the electrophoretic separation has been completed the CAM strip is removed and placed on a moist pad inside a diffusion chamber similar to that described for double diffusion (Section 14.B.5.c.i), with a rectangular well of the required size, e.g., 3 to 4 $\times$ 6 to 8 cm cut out to accommodate the CAM strip. The CAM strip is thus supported only by its edges, which should overlap the support by about 5 mm.[4]

Filter paper strips (Whatman No. 1) approximately 1 to 2 mm wide are impregnated with the antiserum and are placed gently on the strip according to the desired pattern, i.e., one antigen against two antisera or vice versa. The impregnation of the filter paper strips with antiserum is best carried out by running a Pasteur pipet down the strips while held vertically. The appropriate amount of antiserum and the optimal diffusion distance has to be determined by experience for each antigen–antibody system. Essentially the same principles apply as for IEA in gels. For IEA of serum proteins by the commonly available antisera, an antigen–antiserum ratio of 1:25, which corresponds to about 40 to 50 μl of antiserum per strip, is usually satisfactory. If specific antisera are used the length of the antiserum strip need only be slightly longer than the expected electrophoretic position of the antigen. This results in economy of antiserum. As the thin filter paper strips can only hold part of the amount of antiserum required, the remaining volume is added after the impregnated antiserum strip has been placed in position on the electrophoretic strip. Care should be taken that the antiserum does not spill beyond the filter paper strip. The diffusion distance between the margins of the applied sample and the antiserum strip may vary from 3 to 6 mm or proportionately less for microtechniques. Situating the antiserum strip and the subsequent additional applications of antiserum must be performed gently without pressing the strip down or otherwise distorting the membrane.

Alternatively, the antiserum is applied with the electrophoretic strips

[4] J. Kohn, *Nature* **217**, 1261–1262 (1968).

still in a position in the tank. This technique is used if the diffusion is taking place under oil.

iv. Diffusion

The principle and technique are the same as for double diffusion (Section 14.B.5.c). The optimal diffusion time is best established by preliminary experiment, as the precipitation lines only become visible after staining. For most IEA of serum proteins, a period from 18 to 48 hours at room temperature is adequate.

v. Elution, Washing, Staining, Drying, and Clearing

After the diffusion is considered to be completed, the antiserum strips are lifted from the CAM which is then processed as described for double diffusion (Section 14.B.5.iv).

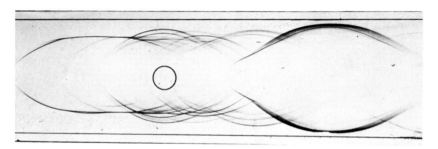

FIG. 20. Immunoelectrophoresis on 12 × 2.5 cm CAM strips. 2 μl human serum, application site indicated by circle. Position of antiserum strips is shown by parallel lines. Two different antisera were employed. Diffusion time 36 hours.

Staining, drying, and clearing of the eluted CAM strip follows the rules recommended for simple CAM electrophoresis. Ponceau S is recommended if strong precipitation lines are expected, and Nigrosin for weak precipitates and low concentration of reactants (Chapter 6, Section C.2, Volume II). For special staining techniques see Section 14.E.1. Photographic records may be made by incident or transmitted light. Figure 20 is an example of IEA patterns on CAM.

b. TRANSFER METHOD

This technique while based on the same principles, consists of electrophoretic separation on a CAM strip and diffusion in agar gel. This is achieved by transferring the electrophoretic strip or sections of it onto the surface of an agar gel and applying antiserum-impregnated filter paper strips at a suitable distance and position on the agar.

Agar and agar plates are prepared as described in Section 14.D.2. If 1% sodium azide gel is used, no buffer is required as the azide is an electrolyte as well as an antibacterial agent. Lantern slide cover plates (8 × 10 cm) are particularly convenient as they are suitable for projection and for multiple patterns. Recommended thickness of gel layer is approximately 1.0 mm.

i. Preparation of CAM

The CAM strip should be somewhat longer than for ordinary electrophoresis, e.g., 12 cm × 2.5 cm, in order to accommodate all the fractions and allow for diffusion. The strip is marked lengthwise by two parallel lines about 8 to 10 mm apart (3 to 5 mm each side of the center). This will permit a strip of appropriate width to be cut out accurately and with straight edges. Alternatively, the electrophoretic separation is performed on a 5 to 10 mm-wide CAM strip, which is then applied to the gel plate without any cutting. If this technique is adopted, the sample should be applied across almost the entire width of the strip. The buffer impregnation, blotting, application of sample and the electrophoretic run is as described in Chapter 6, Section C.2. of Volume II. The optimal volume varies, but much larger samples can be applied than for ordinary electrophoresis. For small-scale IEA of serum (12 × 2.5 cm strip) and a 10 cm bridge gap, 3 to 4 μl can be safely applied. The volume of the sample, however, is not critical and will vary with the circumstances, depending on the resolution required. The addition of bromophenol blue to the sample is recommended.

ii. Transfer of the Electrophoretic Strip

After the separation is completed the current is switched off and the strips are removed from the tank. A section is cut out along the marked parallel lines by means of long-bladed scissors or a sharp cutting edge. The electrophoretic strip is placed gently on the surface of the gel in a position indicated by a previously prepared pattern drawn on white paper and placed under the gel plate; care should be taken to avoid air bubbles.

iii. Application of Antiserum

The antiserum strip is prepared as described in Section 3.a.iii. above, but thicker filter paper is used (e.g., Whatman No. 3). The optimal volume of antiserum to be applied is best determined for each system by experiment. For human serum and with commonly available antisera, a ratio of 1:25 or 1:30 appears to give satisfactory results. As the fluid holding capacity of the filter paper strips is limited, one impregnation may not be sufficient and more antiserum has to be applied. This is done with the antiserum strips in position on the gel plate. For IEA of serum a distance of 3 to 5 mm between the electrophoretic and antiserum strips is recommended. The ends of the strips overlapping the gel plate are cut off.

After the electrophoretic strips and the antiserum strip have been applied, the gel plate is placed in a moist chamber and left there for the immunodiffusion to take place. The conditions are the same as for IEA in gels, and the precipitation lines become clearly visible.

iv. Drying and Staining

When the precipitation pattern is considered to be satisfactory, the gel plate is taken out and the CAM and filter paper strips are lifted or floated off by a gentle stream of water. The plate can now be photographed; but with the transfer technique, staining of the dried plate is simpler and

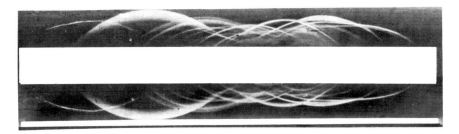

Fig. 21. Transfer method. Human serum separated on CAM (center strip) transferred to agar slide. Patterns developed by horse antiserum applied on filter paper strips (top and bottom). Diffusion 36 hours.

more practical, as no preliminary washing is necessary. The procedure is the same as recommended for IEA in gels (see Section 14.D.2). For protein staining, Ponceau S is recommended and gives excellent results. The stained plates are rapidly washed in 5% acetic acid; there should be hardly any background staining (see Fig. 21).

c. Immunoelectroosmophoresis (IEOP)

This ingenious, elegant and very useful technique is based on the differential migration rate of antigen and antibody on electrophoresis. Filter paper was used first as a support, but the method was applied with even greater success to agar[5] and cellulose acetate.[1, 6] These latter two media are particularly suitable for the purpose as the γ-globulins can be made to migrate toward the cathode, whereas many antigens have an

[5] A. Bussard, *Biochim. Biophys. Acta* **34**, 258 (1959).
[6] J. E. Webster, *J. Med. Lab. Technol.* **22**, 10–11 (1965).

anodic mobility. Thus, by placing the antibody-containing specimen on the anode side, and the antigen on the cathode side, 5 to 10 mm away on the same electrophoretic axis, the reactants will move toward each other and form a precipitation line at equivalent proportions. Conditions of the electrophoretic run are similar to those for ordinary protein separation. After the run is completed (15 to 60 minutes), the strip is eluted and stained in the usual manner as recommended for CAM immunodiffusion. Optimal conditions, i.e., position of application sites and distances, are found by experience for each antigen–antibody system.

This technique has proved most useful for the demonstration of precipitating autoantibodies in Hashimoto's disease.[6] The method in agar, also called "transmigration"[7] or cross-over[8] electrophoresis has been used for rapid forensic identifications,[9] detection of antibody to *T. polyspora* in "farmer's lung" disease,[10] and detection of hepatitis antigen.[11]

d. DISCUSSION

The CAM technique is particularly useful in laboratories in which gel methods are not routinely employed. The CAM method is also very suitable for IEA of isotope-labeled substances.

The transfer technique combines the clear and sharp separation of cellulose acetate electrophoresis with the advantages of diffusion in gels, avoiding some of the inconveniences and drawbacks of electrophoresis in agar gel. As the electrophoresis is not carried out in the gel, very thin gel layers can be used, greatly increasing the sensitivity and the sharpness of the precipitation lines. Electrophoretic separation can be performed at any pH. The continuity of the gel is not interrupted by grooves and wells, and there is no need for special cutting devices and techniques.

A most useful modification consists in carrying out the electrophoresis on a wider strip and applying the sample as a 1.5 to 2 cm line across the width of the strip. After separation of the fraction is completed, the strip is cut into three parallel lengths. The central part, about 5 to 8 mm wide, is placed in a moist chamber on a suitable support, while one or both of the marginal lengths are immediately stained and washed. The central part of the strip is then removed from the moist chamber and is placed in juxtaposition to the stained control, so that the exact location of the fractions can be established and appropriately marked. The sections corresponding to individual fractions, or any desired segments of the pattern are cut out and transferred onto an agar gel plate, separated from each

[7] N. Lang, *Klin. Wochschr.* **33**, 29–30 (1955).
[8] S. Nakamura and T. Ueta, *Nature* **182**, 875 (1958).
[9] B. J. Culliford, *Nature* **201**, 1092 (1964).
[10] J. G. Jameson, *J. Clin. Pathol.* **21**, 376 (1968).
[11] A. M. Prince and K. Burke, *Science* **169**, 593 (1970).

other by 3 to 5 mm. The rest of the procedure is as described above. This modification has been found to be particularly useful for the light chain typing of paraproteins.

It is sometimes convenient to place the cleared strips between glass plates, e.g., lantern slides, to project them to a size more suitable for detailed analysis as well as for demonstration and lectures. This saves a photographic procedure.

The more common errors include careless handling, delay in application of antiserum strips after current has been switched off, uneven application of antiserum to filter paper strips, suboptimal antigen–antibody ratios (usually insufficient volume of antiserum), and poor electrophoretic technique with distortion of the separation pattern. In the transfer method there exists some risk of drying out due to delay in applying the electrophoretic strip. This is particularly dangerous when the electrophoretic strip is cut and applied in sections.

4. IMMUNOELECTROPHORETIC ANALYSIS BY TRANSFER FROM HYDROLYZED STARCH GEL*, †

a. INTRODUCTION

The general principles of immunoelectrophoresis are discussed in Section 14.D.2. The techniques presented here depart from those principles in that the two fundamental steps of immunoelectrophoresis techniques— (1) electrophoresis, and (2) immunoanalysis—are not performed in the same medium. The antigen(s) are separated first on filter paper,[1] starch gel,[2] or acrylamide,[3] and are then transferred and embedded in a transparent gelled medium, such as agar or acrylamide, for immunoanalysis. A transfer method employing cellulose acetate membranes is described in Section 14.D.3.b. In spite of the additional step (transfer) required by these methods, they are easy to perform and they are desirable when a better resolution of the antigens is demanded or where antigen–antibody reactions are to be performed in different buffer (e.g., high salt concentration). The high resolving power of starch gel or acrylamide electrophoresis provides a distinct advantage over cellulose acetate membranes or agar

* Section 14.D.4 was contributed by M. D. Poulik.

† Supported in parts by grants from the National Institutes of Health, AI 05785 from the National Institute of Allergy and Infectious Diseases, and HE 07495 from the National Heart Institute, and in part by the Children's Leukemia Foundation of Michigan.
[1] M. D. Poulik, Can. J. Med. Sci. **30**, 417 (1952).
[2] M. D. Poulik, J. Immunol. **82**, 502 (1959).
[3] J. T. Seto, and Y. Hokama, Ann. N.Y. Acad. Sci. **121**, 640 (1964).

when sufficient material is available. This is especially true of proteins which polymerize naturally (e.g., γA myeloma proteins) or in which the polymerization may be induced by the method of preparation (e.g., albumin, ceruloplasmin). Furthermore, the feasibility of separation of the subunits of proteins (polypeptide chains) in starch gel prepared in buffers containing dissociating and/or reducing agents extends their usefulness for structural investigations. Such methods have been developed[4] and applied in studies on human γ-globulins.[5, 6] Immunoanalysis of two-dimensional zone electrophoresis, which is the method of choice in the author's laboratory, will be described in detail. Adaption of conventional (vertical) starch gel techniques and urea starch gel electrohoresis (see Volume II, Chapter 6, Section C.3) will also be considered. Similar immunoanalytic procedures are applicable to most of these techniques.

b. Two-Dimensional Zone Electrophoresis[7]

The principle of the method is as follows. The antigens under study are first separated by electrophoresis in filter paper (first dimension) and transferred (with the filter paper) into a starch gel (second dimension). Electrophoresis is conducted in this medium at 90 degrees to the direction of the first electrophoresis.

i. Filter Paper Electrophoresis—First Dimension

(a) Equipment and Materials. Lucite or plastic chambers of several styles are available commercially and may be used. Whatman filter paper No. 3MM is used as the supporting medium for the electrophoresis. A pipette delivering 0.1 ml of material is used for application of the sample. The apparatus employed in the author's laboratory will accommodate paper strips 40 × 4 cm.

The buffer used for filter paper electrophoresis is pH 8.55 and is composed of 0.048 M sodium acetate, 0.48 M sodium barbital, and 0.0073 M hydrochloric acid. A very useful buffer can also be prepared by dissolving 2.5 gm of sodium acetate and 7.36 gm of sodium barbital in 1 liter of distilled water. The pH is adjusted by adding glacial acetic acid to achieve a final pH of 8.9.

(b) Procedure. The filter paper strips are soaked in the buffer and dried off quickly on a sheet of filter paper (Fisher 9-800) until they lose their sheen. They are then placed on the supporting frame and the overhanging

[4] M. D. Poulik, in "Protides of the Biological Fluids" (H. Peeters, ed.), p. 399. Elsevier, Amsterdam, 1964.
[5] M. D. Poulik, Nature 202, 1174 (1964).
[6] M. D. Poulik, Ann. N.Y. Acad. Sci. 121, 470 (1964).
[7] M. D. Poulik, and O. Smithies, Biochem. J. 68, 636 (1958).

paper is introduced into the electrode vessels filled with the buffer to complete the circuit. The filter paper strips become "equilibrated" with the buffer of the electrode vessels upon standing for 10 to 20 minutes. The material to be analyzed (0.1 ml) is then carefully applied to the filter paper at a predetermined place close to the cathode. Precaution is taken not to apply the material too close to the edges of the filter paper to avoid smearing of the protein bands by diffusion of the serum around the edges of the filter paper. The electrophoretic chamber is then closed and placed in a room or a hood where the chamber temperature can be maintained relatively constant between 27° and 29°. A voltage of 120 to 130 volts is applied across the electrodes (1.2 ma per filter paper strip). The run is terminated after 16 to 18 hours. The buffer in the electrode vessels is used for 2 to 3 runs, and the electrode vessels are rotated after each run to prevent pH change of the buffer. After termination of the run, the filter papers are dried in a horizontal position for 10 to 15 minutes. A narrow strip (0.5 × 15 cm) is cut off from one edge of each filter paper and stained rapidly in bromophenol blue (e.g., 100 mg dye per liter 0.002 M HgCl$_2$ in 0.02 M acetic acid) to localize the bands and to determine the quality of the separation. If the separation is adequate, another filter paper strip is cut off (1 × 14 cm) from the unstained semidry filter paper strip and transferred into the gel. As experience is gained, one can omit the staining step since albumin, transferrin, and haptoglobins can be easily localized by their characteristic color, and consequently the quality of separation can be readily determined.

ii. Starch Gel Electrophoresis—Second Dimension

(a) Equipment and Materials. A special electrophoresis tray consists of a Plexiglas base (16 × 14 × 0.6 cm i.d.) and four Plexiglas frames fastened to each other with metal or plastic pins. All frames are 3 mm thick. Constructional details are shown in Fig. 22A. It is necessary to coat the base and the frames with a thin layer of mineral oil before the hot starch is poured into the tray. The tray described holds 320 to 340 ml of starch. The electrode vessels, electrodes, and power supply are the same dimensions and type as described in Volume II, Chapter 6, Section C.3.

The discontinuous system of buffers[8] are most convenient for this procedure since the duration of the experiment does not exceed 4 hours. The procedure for preparation of the gel is the same as described in Volume II, Chapter 6, Section C.3. In this laboratory, usually 4 gels are prepared each day. To save time, enough starch is prepared to fill two trays at one time (750 ml). After the hot starch has been poured into the

[8] M. D. Poulik, Nature 180, 1477 (1957).

trays, they are covered with plastic sheets of slightly larger size than the base of the tray. The gels are used after standing overnight at room temperature.

(b) *Procedure.* After completion of the filter paper electrophoresis run, as described above in Section i, a filter paper strip bearing the antigens is transferred into the starch gel. In order to complete this step successfully, it is necessary to make a place in the starch gel for the introduction of the filter paper strip. A cut is made across the 14-cm dimension of the gel with a dermatome knife (14 cm long) about 1 cm from the cathode end

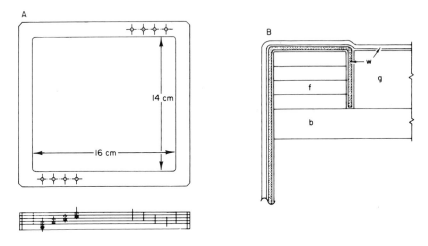

FIG. 22. (A) Construction details of starch gel electrophoresis tray (see text). (B) Arrangement of paper wicks: b, base; f, frames; w, paper wicks; g, starch gel. One paper wick set (stippled) is fitted tightly behind the starch gel. The second set is to be applied to the top of the gel.

of the gel. The resulting narrow block of gel is removed and saved. Then a second cut is made across the gel 2 to 3 cm from the first cut, and this section of the gel is pushed back with the aid of the dermatome knife until it touches the cathode end of the tray. Thus, a 1-cm wide slot is provided which facilitates the insertion of the filter paper strip bearing the antigens. Precaution is taken not to entrap bubbles between the cut surface of the gel and the filter paper, and also not to rub the filter paper over the cut surface. This operation requires some experience in order to accomplish it in one step. The slot in the gel is closed by replacing the displaced gel and the removed block into their original positions. The gel is covered with Saran Wrap, except for narrow sections (1.5 cm) at each electrode to which the paper wicks will be applied (Fig. 22B). Because of the considerable thickness of the gel (1.2 cm), provisions are made to allow adequate contact with the buffer in the electrode vessels (see Fig. 22B). To save material and time, two gels are usually run in tandem as shown in Fig. 23. A voltage of 400 volts is applied across the electrodes for 4 to 5 hours. If the gels are overheating (which may occur after 1 to 2 hours), the voltage is cut back to 250 to 300 volts. Since a "brown line" is moving through the gel in this system in front of all the proteins, it provides a convenient means of locating the components at any time.

After termination of the experiment the gels are cooled at 4° to 6° for 30 minutes prior to slicing. The filter paper used in transfer is removed so that unobstructed slicing may proceed. The first frame is then removed and a heavy plastic sheet is placed on the gel to prevent buckling during the slicing. Using the second frame as a guide, the first gel layer is sliced and placed onto a staining dish, stained with Amido Black 10B and

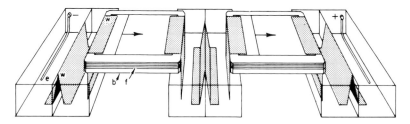

Fig. 23. Arrangement of the two-dimensional zone electrophoresis with two starch gels run in tandem.

decolorized (for procedure see Volume II, Chapter 6, Section C.3). Within 15 to 20 minutes, the major protein zones are visible and this gel layer can be then used as a guide for localization of the proteins to be investigated by immunological methods. It must be realized, however, that the gel shrinks upon decolorization. Consequently the position of identical zones will be slightly different in the *unstained* gel layer which will be dissected for immunological analysis. To avoid error, holes 5 mm apart are punched through the whole thickness of the unsliced gel at the anode portion and along the right side of the gel. The holes serve as guides in the stained and unstained starch gel layers for subsequent dissection of the gel block(s) bearing the antigens.

When the bands are adequately localized, the second frame is removed and a second layer of the gel is sliced using the third frame as a guide. This layer is removed and is ready to be used for the immunoanalysis. Two additional gel layers are still available for further analysis if so desired.

c. IMMUNOANALYTICAL PROCEDURES

i. Equipment and Materials

1. Microscope slide
2. Two-bladed cutter
3. Antiserum–trough cutter (adjustable drawing pen)
4. Moisture chamber (any Plexiglas box fitted with tight lid to prevent evaporation)
5. Bacto-Noble Agar (1%) (Difco, Detroit), containing 0.1% sodium azide
6. Antiserum
7. Immunocells (see reference 2 for detailed description)

ii. Dissection and Transfer of the Gels

The general procedure described here in connection with the two-dimensional starch gel electrophoresis may also be employed with both the conventional starch gel electrophoresis and the urea or urea mercaptoethanol starch gel electrophoresis (Volume II, Chapter 6). Special considerations are mentioned for these several methods:

(a) *Two-Dimensional Gel.* With a cutter (7 cm long), a starch strip which bears a presumptive antigen is dissected from the second gel layer parallel to the direction of migration. The starch strip (7 × 0.5 × 0.3 cm) is transferred onto the microscopic slide and covered with warm agar; the agar is allowed to solidify. Then with an adjustable drawing pen, two narrow antibody troughs are cut about 10 to 15 mm from and parallel to the starch strip. The troughs are filled with the appropriate antisera, a Pasteur pipet being used, and the slide is placed into the moist chamber. Whenever necessary, e.g., in comparative studies, several starch strips can be placed on a larger glass plate, either parallel to each other or at different angles, whatever the need may be. Antibody troughs are cut out between the starch strips in a manner similar to that described above. The diffusion proceeds at room temperature.

It may be necessary to transfer agar gel or filter paper with the separated antigens for immunoanalytical analysis. For such work an immunocell consisting of a plunger, a glass-walled cell, and a cover is very useful. The medium containing the separated antigens is placed on the Lucite plunger and lowered with it into the immunocell. Warm agar is poured over the medium bearing the antigens to a height of about 1 cm and allowed to solidify. Antiserum is then evenly applied over the solid agar. The cell is tightly closed and let stand at room temperature. The cell is observed from its side. This modification seemed advantageous when buffers containing high amounts of salt (4 to 14%) are needed (e.g., chicken antisera).

(b) *Conventional Starch Gel Electrophoresis.* After electrophoresis the gel is sliced into two halves, one of which is stained and decolorized immediately. This gel layer serves as a guide for localization of the proteins to be studied. Subsequent operations are the same as those described in the preceding section.

(c) *Urea and Urea–Mercaptoethanol Starch Gel.* The procedures are the same whether the vertical gels or the two-dimensional gels are used. After the gels have been sliced into halves, one half is stained and decolorized immediately and the other is placed in a suitable container and washed under cold tap water. Washing may continue for 3 to 4 hours in order to completely remove urea or urea and mercaptoethanol. Subsequent operations are the same as outlined above for two-dimensional gels.

Two-dimensional urea–starch gel immunoelectrophoretic analysis has been applied to the study of the papain digest of γG-immunoglobulins. The unstained layer of the gel was first exhaustively washed (4 hours) in cold running water. Starch strips a–k were selected for the immunoanalysis based on the gel layer stained with Amido Black 10B; after removal of the strips, the gel remaining is also stained (Fig. 24A). It is seen that the washing procedure (which removed urea) did not greatly diminish the amount of protein, thus sufficient protein should be available in the dissected, unstained starch strips for immunological reactions.

The starch strips were subjected to immunoanalysis using antiserum specific for light chain determinants (kappa and lambda) and antiserum specific for the heavy chains determinants, respectively. Drawings of the precipitin arcs developed (Fig. 24B) are correlated with the positions of the separated subunits of the Fab, Fc, and F′c fragments (see Vol. I, Chapter 3.A.1, for nomenclature and Chapter 5 for immunoglobulin structure).

The vertical lines, a–j, represent the starch strips used for the immunodiffusion experiment. Precipitate arcs drawn to the left of these lines were developed with the anti-light chain antiserum, and precipitin lines drawn to the right of the lines were developed with the anti-heavy chain antiserum. The figure shows that the major protein zone of the Fab fragment (strips a–f) react with this anti-light chain antiserum and that additional faster migrating subunits also afford precipitin arcs (strips a–c). The two major subunits of the Fc fragment (strips e–j) yield precipitin lines. However, additional faster migrating subunits are also detected (strips f, g, and h). The F′c subunits (strip j) are shown by a strong precipitin arc. All the subunits of the Fc and F′c fragments separated by two-dimensional electrophoresis in urea–mercaptoethanol starch gel afford characteristic, strong precipitin arcs. However, those of the Fab fragment are found not to be reactive. These results indicate refolding to the proper tertiary structure after removal of the urea and/or mercaptoethanol or

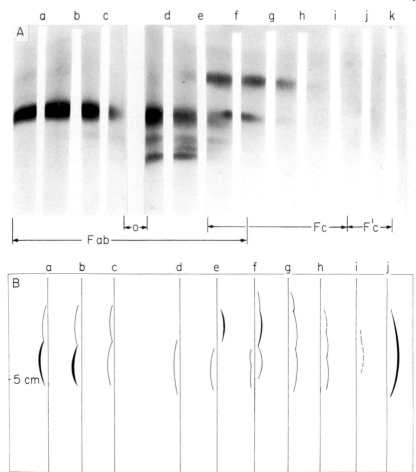

FIG. 24. Immunoelectrophoretic analysis of the papain-digested γG immunoglobulins. (A) Photograph of the two-dimensional subunit map after electrophoresis in urea–starch gel. a–j, Dissected starch blocks used for the immunoanalysis. (B) Drawing of the precipitin arcs developed with specific antisera. For further details see text.

that the integrity of most of antigenic determinant(s) does not depend on the tertiary structure of the separated subunits.

iii. Recording of Results

The formation of the precipitin bands is observed at regular intervals (8, 16, 24, 36 hours, etc.) and their positions are noted and accurately drawn. Contact photography may be used to secure permanent records. Both slides and the immunocells can be handled in a similar fashion.

Slides may also be processed to obtain a permanent record of stained precipitin arcs. The starch strip is carefully removed from the surrounding agar gel after termination of the experiment. The gap is filled with warm agar (1%), allowed to solidify, and placed in a container containing 0.9% sodium chloride and 0.1% sodium azide for 24 hours. After this period of time the slides are removed and covered with wet Whatman No. 1 filter paper and dried at room temperature. The dried slides are then washed in distilled water and placed in Amido Black 10B solution and stained for 5 minutes. The stained slides are decolorized in a solution of 50% methanol and 10% acetic acid. After drying at room temperature, slides are ready to be photographed. Staining procedures are described in Section 14.E.1. Techniques of photography are described in Section 14.E.2.

5. TWO-DIMENSIONAL (LAURELL) IMMUNOELECTRO-PHORESIS FOR ESTIMATION OF ANTIGENS IN RELATIVE UNITS*

The value of immunoelectrophoresis, introduced by Grabar and Williams,[1] is often limited because results are not quantitative and their interpretation requires great skill and experience. Ressler showed that antigens could be forced by an electric current into a bed containing antiserum, thus producing a number of superimposed curves.[2] Laurell combined these methods so that the peaks formed were no longer superimposed, but separated according to the mobility of the various proteins in agar.[3]

The method described here is a modification of Laurell's technique, adapted to give quantitative data on a large number of antigens simultaneously.[4,5] Such information should be of considerable value, and while the technique as described has been developed for the estimation of plasma proteins in pathological conditions, it is obvious that it can be applied to any proteins normally studied by conventional immunoelectrophoresis. Several clinical studies are reported, including hemochromatosis,[6] the measurement of thyroxine-binding,[7] protein concentra-

---

* Section 14.D.5 was contributed by H. G. Minchin Clarke.

[1] P. Grabar, and C. A. Williams, Jr., *Biochim. Biophys. Acta* **10**, 193 (1953).
[2] N. Ressler, *Clin. Chim. Acta* **5**, 795 (1960).
[3] C.-B. Laurell, *Anal. Biochem.* **10**, 358 (1965).
[4] H. G. Minchin Clarke and T. Freeman, *Clin. Sci.* **35**, 403 (1968).
[5] H. G. Minchin Clarke and T. Freeman, *Protides Biol. Fluids* **14**, 504 (1966).
[6] A. H. Amin, H. G. Minchin Clarke, T. Freeman, J. M. Murray Lyon, P. M. Smith, and R. Williams, *Clin. Sci.* **38**, 613 (1970).
[7] D. Pearson and T. Freeman, *Clin. Chim. Acta* **26**, 365 (1969).

tion in schizophrenia and epilepsy,[8] protein concentrations in normal children,[9] in normal adults,[6] tuberculosis and sarcoidosis,[10] Still's disease, gout and rheumatoid arthritis,[11] multiple sclerosis,[12] pregnancy and pre-eclampsia.[13]

a. PRINCIPLE

The technique depends on the migration of antigens into a bed of antibody globulin. After a simple electrophoresis of the antigens in agar, a strip of gel containing the separated proteins is transferred to a second glass plate. Agarose containing antiserum is poured over the remainder of the plate. The antigens are forced into the antibody-containing gel by an electric field placed at right angles to the initial separation. The antigens migrate into the gel until they are all precipitated by the antiserum. Provided that the current is applied until no further migration occurs, the area under any protein peak is directly proportional to the concentration of that protein in the human serum, and inversely proportional to the concentration of antibody to that protein in the animal antiserum.

The application of "crossed electrophoresis" is obviously limited to antigens whose electrophoretic mobility differs significantly from the antibody under the conditions of the second, right-angle migration. For example, this limitation would preclude the accurate determination of immunoglobulins in serum samples.

b. METHOD

i. Antiserum

Rabbit, sheep, and goat antisera have proved satisfactory, but horse antiserum cannot be used because the precipitates are soluble in antibody excess. Rabbit or sheep antisera are preferable because the gel can usually be washed completely free of unprecipitated antiserum to give a clear background whereas goat serum contains a component which appears to be bound to the agarose. However, goat anti-human whole serum,

[8] H. G. M. Clarke, T. Freeman, and W. Pryse-Phillips, J. Neurol. Neurosurg. Psychiat. (1970).

[9] B. Abrams and T. Freeman, Clin. Sci. **37**, 575 (1969).

[10] H. G. M. Clarke, T. Freeman, and W. Pryse-Phillips, Thorax **25**, 423 (1970).

[11] H. G. M. Clarke, T. Freeman, and W. Pryse-Phillips, Brit. J. Exptl. Path. **51** (1970).

[12] H. G. M. Clarke, T. Freeman, and W. Pryse-Phillips, Clin. Chim. Acta. (1970).

[13] H. G. M. Clarke, T. Freeman, and W. Pryse-Phillips, submitted for publication (1970).

produced in our laboratory, was used in the studies illustrated here. To reduce background staining the goat whole-antiserum was precipitated first with 1.8 M (45% saturated at 20°) and then 1.6 M (40% saturated) ammonium sulfate, the final precipitate being dialized against 0.06 M barbital buffer. At this stage the antibody can be concentrated by dissolving the ammonium sulfate precipitate in a volume less than that of the original serum.

ii. Technique

There are two electrophoretic stages: first and second dimension.

(a) *First Dimension—Separation*. Simple zone electrophoresis is run in agarose. A thin glass plate (8 cm × 10 cm) is covered to a depth of about 0.15 cm with an agarose gel. This is made up by mixing equal volumes

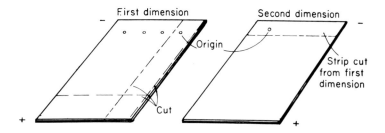

FIG. 25. Diagram of first and second dimension gels.

of 2% agarose and barbital buffer (15.5 gm of barbital sodium, 0.77 gm of calcium lactate with HCl added to give pH 8.6). Sodium azide (1/10,000) is added to limit bacterial growth. A hole 2 mm in diameter is made in the gel with a metal punch, 2.5 cm from the negative end; it is filled with 6 μl of serum from a microburet. Four such holes will fit conveniently on each first-dimension plate (Fig. 25). Electrophoresis is best carried out on a water-cooled surface, with 10 to 15 volts/cm for 60 minutes. (Separations can be obtained without cooling by using a lower voltage for a longer time; but greater diffusion results in broader and flatter arcs in the subsequent second dimension.) A longitudinal strip 1.5 cm wide, containing all the separated proteins, is cut from the first-dimension gel and transferred to a second glass plate (8 cm × 10 cm). Transfer is best effected by means of a long razor blade in order to minimize distortion of the first-dimension gel. The distance from the origin hole to the cut edges of the strip should be kept constant.

(b) *Second Dimension—Precipitation.* The remainder of the second plate is then covered with agarose and barbital buffer in the concentration of the first dimension but containing, in addition, by substitution for part of the barbital buffer, enough antiserum (0.5 to 5 ml depending on titre) to whole human serum to precipitate the human serum fractions on the surface of the plate. This mixture should meet the edge of, but not run over, the first dimension strip already on the plate. The antiserum should not be heated above 50°. Electrophoresis is carried out on a cooled surface using 2 to 2.5 volts/cm for 22 hours. Absorbent cloth, paper, or sponge wicks are used, elevated from the cooled surface by strips of Perspex; the plates are laid gel downward on the wicks. This minimizes distortion of the peaks by condensation. The antigens migrate until they are totally precipitated by their corresponding antibodies to form a number of discrete but overlapping precipitation peaks. The gel is then washed in 0.9% saline to remove unwanted antiserum and dried in an oven at 37°. Staining may be by any of the techniques used for conventional electrophoresis.

The volume of antiserum to be added to each plate is independently determined for every fresh pool of antiserum by running a series of gels containing increasing quantities of antiserum. The total volume of the gel is maintained by altering the volume of barbital buffer. Because the antiserum has been dialyzed against a 0.06 M barbital buffer, the final pH and molarity are not affected. A brief examination of these plates will show the optimum volume of antiserum.

The areas beneath the peaks are measured by projecting the plate onto white card (using a photographic enlarger) and drawing, cutting out, and weighing each area. This has proved more accurate than planimetry and less tedious than counting squares; an alternative method for measuring areas by means of an electronic integrating device* has been found satisfactory.[4]

c. IDENTIFICATION

As in many immunochemical methods, identification is the most difficult aspect of the technique. The following human serum proteins have been identified in the pattern shown in Fig. 26: albumin, α_1-lipoprotein, α_1-antitrypsin, orosmomucoid, ceruloplasmin, α_2-macroglobulin, haptoglobin, β_1-lipoprotein, cholinesterase, transferrin, hemopexin and $\beta_{1A\text{-}C}$-globulin. The photograph (Fig. 26) shows the proteins that have been identified with certainty, together with some presumptive identifications.

The problem has been approached in a number of different ways.

* Designed by J. Lewin, and manufactured by Chemical Electronics Co., C.W.S. Hall, Durham Road, Birtley Co., Durham, England.

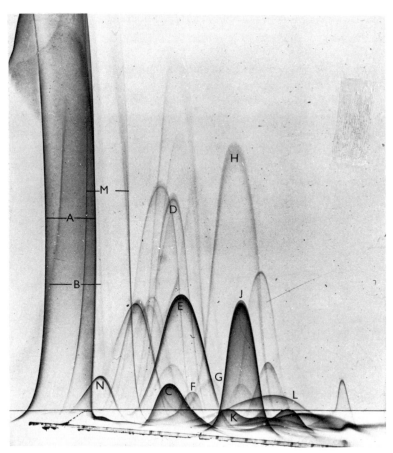

FIG. 26. Photograph of a stained plate made with human serum and goat antiserum to whole human serum. A strip of agarose containing electrophoretically resolved serum proteins is placed along one edge of the plate (bottom of figure) and molten agarose containing antiserum is poured over the rest of the plate. When the plate has gelled, the antigens are forced into antibody layer by electrophoresis (mode at top of figure). Migration is continued until all of each antigen is precipitated by its specific antibody. On this plate, 37 precipitation zones can be seen. Those identified with certainty are: A, albumin; B, α_1-lipoprotein; C, α_2-macroglobulin; D, ceruloplasmin; E, haptoglobin; F, β-lipoprotein; G, pseudocholinesterase; H, hemopexin; J, transferrin; K, β_{-1A-C}; L, γ-globulin (part of γ complex); M, orosomucoid; N, α_1-antitrypsin.

1. Where pure protein fractions were available, these were mixed with normal serum and an increase in size of one peak was noted.

2. Specific antisera added to the human serum prior to the initial electrophoresis resulted in a decrease in size of the appropriate peak.

3. Haptoglobin and other proteins with a specific binding function were identified by the addition of the appropriate materials.

4. Specific staining procedures are available for some proteins: e.g., ceruloplasmin, hemopexin, cholinesterase, lipoprotein (see Section 14.E.1).

5. The difficulties of identification encountered using an antiserum against whole human serum suggests the use of antisera against subfractions of human sera. Sephadex gel filtration is helpful in separating the serum proteins according to molecular size. Preliminary work using antisera generated against the three main Sephadex G-150 fractions shows that the antisera against the two fractions containing the larger components contains few enough proteins so that identification is simplified. Fractions so obtained can be mixed with normal serum and the resulting plates compared to those run with normal serum alone.

d. RESULTS

The basic data obtained from this type of analysis are area measurements for each protein. Where pure protein fractions are available, it is

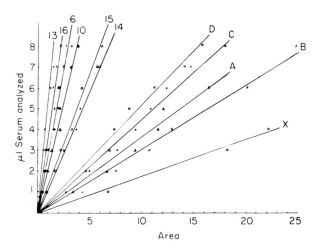

FIG. 27. Areas of several different proteins obtained after separation of increasing volumes of serum.

possible to express results in absolute terms. For instance, if 6 μl of a 2 mg/ml standard shows an area of 10 units and the unknown serum gives an area of 15 units, then the concentration of that protein in the unknown serum is 3 mg/ml. Unfortunately few pure proteins are available, and for the majority of proteins it is necessary to express results in relation to a standard normal serum. The area produced by either pure

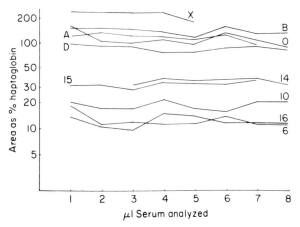

FIG. 28. The same data as in Fig. 26, but areas are expressed as a percentage of one protein (haptoglobin).

standards or standard normal serum has to be calculated for each new pool of antiserum.

The results obtained from single analyses of 1, 2, 3, . . . 8 μl of normal serum are shown in Figs. 27 and 28. The basic linearity in these plots demonstrates that, for a given pool of antiserum, area is propositional to concentration. The scatter shown represents the error for a single analysis. This error, calculated by repeated estimation (by cutting and weighing)

TABLE I
QUANTITATIVE ELECTROPHORESIS[a]

Protein	Mean percent area	Standard deviation	Coefficient of variation
6	87.0	6.9	0.08
7	203.1	11.4	0.06
8	505.5	48.8	0.10
9	489.7	44.8	0.09
10	76.9	8.2	0.10
11	79.9	9.6	0.12
12	100.0	—	—
14	118.6	6.7	0.06
16	465.5	52.4	0.11
17	45.3	5.4	0.11
18	202.0	38.3	0.19
19	76.4	11.2	0.15

[a] Expected error on one estimation of serum, calculated from 15 areas expressed as percent transferrin.

of areas from a single serum is shown in Table I. These figures represent chiefly the errors inherent in the drawing, cutting, and weighing method of estimation and can be reduced either by repeated estimations or by the use of an electronic device for measuring areas.

E. Characterization of Precipitates in Gels

1. COLOR REACTIONS FOR THE IDENTIFICATION OF ANTIGEN–ANTIBODY PRECIPITATES IN GELS*

* Section 14.E.1 was contributed by José Uriel.

a. INTRODUCTION AND PRINCIPLES

The increased resolution of immunochemical precipitates by diffusion in gels, and in particular by immunoelectrophoresis, does not by itself assure the identification of a given antigen. There are several technical difficulties that increase with the complexity of the immunochemical system under investigation. Certain antigen–antibody complexes may form diffuse precipitates difficult to be resolved or too faint to be seen. With complex mixture of antigens, such as body fluids or tissue extracts, the close proximity of the precipitation lines in double diffusion or similar electrophoretic mobilities of components often make their individual recognition very difficult. Moreover, the position of the precipitation zone depends on the relative concentrations of antigen and antibody. It is easy to understand, therefore, that the position of a line can be altered when the concentration of either the antigen or the antibody are changed.

These difficulties often can be overcome by the use of characterization reactions without resort to monospecific antisera or purified antigens required for immunochemical identifications. Staining techniques of antigen–antibody precipitates in double diffusion were introduced by Bjorklund[1] and in immunoelectrophoresis by Uriel and Grabar.[2] Characterization reactions of antigens in immune precipitates in gels have been developed to provide additional information about the nature of the immunochemical precipitates, thus facilitating their identification.[3, 4a]

The characterization of antigens in antigen–antibody complexes utilizes reactions that permit the visualization of the constituents being studied on the basis of a given chemical or biological property. In order to allow a precise localization, it is preferable that the reaction products formed be insoluble and colored. Nevertheless, these two conditions are not indispensable, and the identification can be accomplished on the basis of other properties, such as radioactivity, fluorescence, gas liberation, or

[1] B. Bjorklund, *Proc. Soc. Exptl. Biol. Med.* **79**, 324 (1952).
[2] J. Uriel and P. Grabar, *Ann. Inst. Pasteur* **90**, 427 (1956).
[3] J. Uriel, *in* "L'analyse immunoélectrophorétique; ses applications aux liquides biologiques humains" (P. Grabar and P. Burtin, eds.), p. 33. Masson, Paris, 1960.
[4a] J. Uriel, *Ann. N.Y. Acad. Sci.* **103**, 956 (1963).

by physiochemical changes in the reagents, as is the case with certain enzymatic reactions. The characterization of immunochemical complexes with fluorescent labels will not be discussed here.

For convenience, we consider that there are two types of characterization reactions, *generic* and *specific*. The former allow the demonstration of antigens exhibiting certain properties in common. These properties may be related to the presence of functional groups characteristic of proteins, lipids, carbohydrates, and nucleic acids. The specific characterization reactions permit the identification of an individual antigen and depend upon a specific or reactive group on the antigen molecule which remains available in the antigen–antibody complex.

Unless otherwise indicated all the techniques described below have been subjected to trial in this laboratory. When the same antigenic constituents have been identified by different authors, only the most reliable techniques (in the experience of the author) are detailed.

While the investigator may be able to use these techniques as described, they should also be understood as "type reactions" serving as a guide to the development of the specific tests required.

b. GENERAL PREPARATIONS

i. Choice and Preparation of Gel Media

Agar or agarose gel plates are, at the present time, the best supporting media for the immunodiffusion assays and the subsequent characterization reactions, although the principles are equally applicable to membrane diffusion techniques. Changes in the electrophoretic and diffusion properties of certain proteins (lysozyme, trypsin, macroglobulins, lipoproteins) have been observed in agar but not in agarose gels. These have been explained as being due to interactions with acidic polysaccharides present in varying concentrations in agar preparations. Agarose, a desulfated agar derivative, contains essentially only neutral polysaccharides. On the other hand, the treatment followed for the purification of agarose from agar also removes other impurities, such as traces of heavy metals and pigments, which often are present in commercial preparations of agar. Agarose gels are particularly recommended when enzyme characterization reactions are to be carried out.[4b]

Melted solutions of agar or agarose* in appropriate buffers are poured on glass slides and permitted to gel at room temperature. The immuno-

---

[4b] J. Uriel, S. Avrameas, and P. Grabar, *Protides Biol. Fluids, Proc. Colloq.* **11**, 355. Elsevier, Amsterdam, (1964).

* Noble agar (Difco, Detroit, Michigan) and agarose I.B.F. Industrie Biologique Française (Gennevilliers, Seine, France) can be used without any prior purification.

diffusion assays are then carried out in the usual manner (see respective sections for details). There are no special conditions needed for characterization reactions of antigen–antibody precipitates in gel diffusion media. The original techniques of double diffusion and of immunoelectrophoresis as well as any of their multiple variations can serve for that purpose. In general, micro or semimicro methods are advisable in order to avoid the use of large volumes of reagents. In this laboratory 45 × 110 mm plates are used for immunoelectrophoretic analysis and characterization reactions, but 25 × 75 mm microscope slides are also suitable for most applications.

ii. Washing and Drying the Plate

After the development of the antigen–antibody precipitates, the gels must be washed with buffered saline (pH 7.4 to 8.0) to remove the soluble nonreacting constituents. The washing time depends on the thickness of the gel layer and the volume of the washing solution. As a general rule, one day of washing per millimeter of gel layer in a generous volume of washing solution will be adequate. If continuous mechanical stirring of the solution is used, the washing time can be considerably reduced.

The drying of the plates reduces the gel layer (usually 2 to 5 mm thick) to a thin transparent film. This is accomplished by placing a sheet of good quality filter paper over the surface of the gel plate, which is then placed in an oven at 37° or exposed to a current of air until dry. The filter paper is then removed, and the plate is cleaned for a few seconds in running tap water.[2, 5] The drying serves three purposes: (1) to increase the sensitivity of the chemical reactions after the concentration of the antigen–antibody precipitates on the dried gel; (2) to reduce the time of penetration and removal of the reagents in multistep reactions; and (3) to allow reactions to occur in nonaqueous solvents.

c. STAINING REACTIONS TO DETERMINE THE CHEMICAL NATURE OF PRECIPITATES

i. Proteins

A large number of acidic staining reagents can be used for the characterization of proteins in immunochemical precipitates. Several that have been used successfully are Amido Black, azocarmine, nigrosine, coomasie blue, bromophenol blue, Ponceau red, and light green. They have been used in organic solvents and in aqueous solutions. Aqueous solutions of these dyes possess certain advantages: the solutions keep well in the acid

[5] J. Uriel and J. J. Scheidegger, *Bull. Soc. Chim. Biol.* **37**, 165 (1955).

pH range and at low ionic strength; they yield distinct and easily reproducible colorations, and they do not overstain.

The choice of stain will depend on several factors. If photographic
records are to be made by transmitted light to photographic paper, a green
(yellow) or red dye will reveal the faint reactions somewhat better than
the blue dyes since the emulsion is not exposed by yellow or red light.
Also, when color photography is to be used to contrast the total pattern
of precipitates with that of a specific component, e.g., lipoprotein, enzyme,
a counterstain for protein is selected which gives a different and somewhat
weaker color.

Reagents
  Staining solution:
    Amido Black, nigrosine, azocarmine, Ponceau red, or light
      green, 1 gm
    Acetic acid, 1 M, 425 ml
    Sodium acetate, 0.1 M, 425 ml
    Glycerol, 150 ml

Procedure
Step 1. Immerse the dried plates in the selected stain for about 2 hours.
Since there is no danger of overstaining, a longer period (24 hours) is
not harmful.

Step 2. Wash in aqueous 2% acetic acid containing 15% glycerol until
the gel background is decolorized.

Step 3. Dry in air. If desired the film of gel may be stripped from its
glass support. Since storage of smaller plates does not present a problem,
stripping may be unnecessary and glycerol can be omitted from reagents.
If prolonged storage is anticipated, it is best to expose plates briefly to
ammonia. This will neutralize traces of acid and help prevent breakdown
of the agar film.

Step 4. The use of bromophenol blue with a discussion of its advantage
and disadvantages is given in Section 14.D.2.c.*viii.* Figure 1A is an example of a pattern stained with bromophenol blue and photographed using
the slide as a negative plate in a photoenlarger (see Section 14.E.2).

ii. Lipoproteins

Various dyestuffs of the Sudan series have been employed for the
characterization of lipid constituents in agar.[2] Since all of these are insoluble in water, it is essential that the plates be perfectly dry.

Reagents

Staining solutions: Oil Red O, Scarlet R, Geigy, Sudan IV or Sudan
Black as saturated solutions in 60% ethanol (1 gm of dye per liter of alco-

hol solution). Saturation is accomplished in an oven at 37°, with occasional stirring over a period of 16–24 hours. After the suspensions have reached room temperature, they are filtered and stored in colored glass bottles.

Procedure

Step 1. Immerse the plates for 2 hours in the Sudan Black reagent,* or for 16 hours in the other Sudan solutions. To minimize evaporation, place the stains in covered trays or operate as follows: the glass plate is turned so that the film of agar is on the under side; the ends of the glass

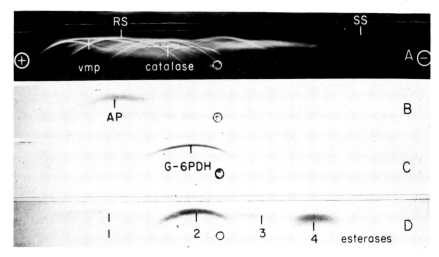

FIG. 1. Immunoelectrophoretic patterns of soluble proteins of *Neurospora crassa*. (A) Dried 75 × 25-mm slide developed for catalase in 3% H_2O_2 by procedure ii.(c).(2), then counterstained for protein with bromophenol blue. (B) Similar slide developed for alkaline phosphatase by procedure iii.(b).(1). (C) Similar slide developed for glucose-6-phosphate dehydrogenase by procedure ii.(a).(3). (D) Similar slide developed for carboxylesterases by procedure iii.(a).(1). Adapted from C. A. Williams and E. L. Tatum, *J. Gen. Microbiol.* **44**, 59 (1966).

plate are supported by two thin strips of wood (approximately 1 mm thick) placed on the bottom of a porcelain tray. The staining solution is poured into the free space between the surface of the agar and the bottom of the tray. This procedure is indicated in all cases where it is desirable to economize on reagents, or where there is the possibility of loss of volatile solvents.

Step 2. Wash in two successive baths of 50% alcohol until background is decolorized. Dry the plates in air.

* Just before use, 0.1 ml of 30% sodium hydroxide is added to 160 ml of the reagent. Nonspecific staining is thus avoided.

Step 3 (optional). Immerse the stained plates for 4 hours in a 15% water solution of glycerol containing 2% of acetic acid and dry again in air. The gel film then will be easily detached from its glass support.

Remarks. Double lipid–protein staining may be accomplished simultaneously[5] or, better, successively with the same plate. In the latter case, the lipid constituents are stained first by the procedure outlined above and then the protein constituents are stained as above.

The combinations Oil Red O–azocarmine and Sudan Black–light green yield the best contrasting colors.

iii. Glycoproteins and Polysaccharides

Periodic acid, an oxidant for determining glycols, combined with the sulfited fuchsin–Schiff reagent has been used for the histochemical demonstration of a variety of constituents containing polysaccharides.[6, 7] This reagent also has been employed for the characterization of glycoproteins after electrophoresis on paper[8] and in agar.[2] The techniques described below are based on the same principle except that two different color reagents for aldehydes are employed.

(a) Periodic Acid–Nadi Reaction. The oxidation of *p*-phenylenediamine with hydrogen peroxide is catalytically activated by aldehydes.[9] A spot test based on this reaction has been developed for the detection of aldehydes.[10] Aldehydes likewise catalyze the oxidation by hydrogen peroxide of an equimolar mixture of *p*-phenylenediamine and α-naphthol(Nadi reagent) to yield a quinoid dye, namely indophenol blue.[11] This oxidation of Nadi is a more sensitive reaction for aldehydes than that of *p*-phenylenediamine alone; in addition, the resulting indophenol blue lends itself better to photometric measurements.

Combined with a preliminary oxidation by periodic acid of the bonds of 1,2-glycols, the reaction has been adapted to the characterization of carbohydrate constituents in agar.

Reagents
a. Periodic acid: 1% solution in 0.2 M sodium acetate
b. Hydroxylamine-HCl: 10% solution in acetate buffer, pH 4.7, 0.2 M.
    The buffer solution consists of equal volumes of 0.4 M sodium acetate and 0.4 M acetic acid.

[6] J. F. A. McMannus, *Nature* **158**, 202 (1946).
[7] R. D. A. Hotchkiss, *Arch. Biochem.* **16**, 131 (1948).
[8] E. Koiw and A. Gronwall, *Scand. J. Clin & Lab. Invest.* **4**, 244 (1952).
[9] G. Worker, *Chem. Ber.* **47**, 1024 (1914).
[10] F. Feigl, *in* "Spot Tests in Organic Analysis" (F. Feigl, ed.), p. 214. Elsevier, Amsterdam, 1956.
[11] J. Uriel, *Clin. Lab. (Zaragoza) (Spain)* **65**, 87 (1958).

c. *H₂O₂-Nadi reagent:* Just before use mix equal volumes of fresh 0.01 M solutions of α-naphthol (144 mg/100 ml) and p-phenylenediamine (216 mg/100 ml), each in 10^{-4} M neutralized solution of EDTA. (The solution of α-naphthol should be heated progressively until dissolution of the α-naphthol is complete). Add one-fifth volume of 0.1 M hydrogen peroxide (commercial 3% solutions may be used).

Procedure
Step 1. Treat the plates as follows:

Hydroxylamine hydrochloride (optional)	45 min
Washing with running water (optional)	15 min
Periodic acid	10 min
Running water wash	10 min
H₂O₂–Nadi reagent	5–10 min
Running water wash	5–10 min

Step 2. Dry the plates in air.
Specific precipitates containing 1,2-glycol bonds stain blue-violet.

(b) *Periodic Acid–Formazan Reaction.* The aldehyde-arylhydrazones from glycoproteins oxidized by the action of periodic acid are coupled with a diazonium salt to produce the corresponding formazan derivatives. The principle of this reaction has been employed in the analytical chemistry of sugars[12] and for the characterization of glycoproteins following electrophoresis in agar.[13]

The series of steps involved in this technique can be presented schematically (reactions 1–4).

$$\text{Glycoprotein + periodic acid} \rightarrow \text{oxidized glycoprotein} \qquad (1)$$

$$\text{Oxidized glycoprotein + phenylhydrazine} \xrightarrow{\text{acetate}}$$
$$\text{oxyglycoprotein-aldehyde-phenylhydrazone} \quad (2)$$

$$\text{Oxyglycoprotein-aldehyde-phenylhydrazone} + o\text{-dianisidine (tetrazotized)} \xrightarrow{\text{acetate}}$$
$$o\text{-dianisidine-4,4'-bis(3-oxidized glycoprotein-5-phenylformazan)} \quad (3)$$
$$(3) + \text{Cu}^{2+} \rightarrow \text{copper complex of formazan derivative} \qquad (4)$$

The complex produced in reaction (4) is a stable and highly colored complex.

Reagents
a. *Periodic acid*: 1% solution in 0.2 M sodium acetate
b. *Phenylhydrazine·HCl:* 0.05% solution in an acetate buffer at pH 4 (equal parts of 0.2 M sodium acetate and 0.8 M acetic acid). The solution of phenylhydrazine should be made fresh each day.
c. *Buffer solution:* Sodium acetate–acetic acid, 0.1 M, pH 4.0

[12] L. Mester, *Advan. Carbohydrate Chem.* **13**, 105 (1958).
[13] J. Uriel and P. Grabar, *Anal. Biochem.* **2**, 80 (1961).

d. Diazo Blue B (*o*-dianisidine tetrazotized): 0.1% solution in 1 *M* sodium acetate. Prepare the solution immediately before use.

e. Cupric acetate: saturated solution in 1 *M* sodium acetate

Procedure

Step 1. Immerse the plates in reagent (a) for 10 minutes.*

Step 2. Wash for about 10 minutes in running water.

Step 3. Put the plates in a bath of reagent *b* for 5 minutes at 60 to 70°.

Step 4. Wash in reagent *c* for 10 minutes to remove the excess of phenylhydrazine.

Step 5. Immerse for 10 minutes in reagent *d*, and wash in running water for an additional 10 minutes.

Step 6. The plates are treated with reagent *e* during 5 minutes to obtain the copper complex of the formazan derivative and washed in running water (10 to 20 minutes).

Antigen–antibody precipitates containing polysaccharides are stained blue-violet.

Remarks on Reactions A and B: The hydroxylamine-HCl, a blocking agent for aldehydes, is used in the event that carbonyl groups are non-specifically liberated by the action of oxygen during the desiccation of the plates. Its use is optional, therefore, if the absence of nonspecific oxidations has been established.

The specificity of the color reactions for glycoproteins and polysaccharides which have been described should be considered from two points of view. On the one hand, there is a preliminary oxidation by periodic acid which seems to be specific for the 1,2-glycols and leads to the liberation of the active carbonyl groups. On the other hand, the specificity is linked to the colorimetric detection of these carbonyl groups by means of suitable reagents. The final result is, therefore, determined primarily by the extent of the periodic acid oxidation.

Among the noncarbohydrate substances susceptible to oxidation by periodic acid, hydroxyamino acids, and lipids should be considered. The former fit into constitution of protein molecules, but they enter into the reaction with aldehyde reagents to only a negligible extent.[13] Active carbonyl groups are split off from unsaturated lipids and phosphatides when oxidized by periodic acid. It has been verified that the serum lipoproteins react with Schiff reagent, Nadi, and phenylhydrazine.[3]

The three methods for the demonstration of glycoproteins and polysaccharides give similar results. The oxidation of Nadi by hydrogen peroxide is catalyzed by the aldehydes and by certain heavy metals. The

---

* Duration of the oxidation for serum glycoproteins. For dextrans, oxidation in reagent *a* must be prolonged for 3 hours. In general, the time necessary for the oxidation of unknown constituents must be established experimentally.

Schiff reagent and phenylhydrazine may react with aldehydes or with ketones. The phenylhydrazine reaction includes a third step, namely, the formation of a formazan derivative. But a necessary condition for the coupling of an arylhydrazine with a diazonium salt is the presence of a functional group of the —CH=N— type. This condition is satisfied in the aldehydephenylhydrazones, but not for the ketophenylhydrazones. The periodic acid-formazan reaction is therefore more specific. The Nadi reaction has the advantage of its technical simplicity.

iv. Nucleoproteins and Nucleic Acids

The techniques described below allow the staining of free nucleic acids (DNA and RNA) or nucleoproteins (NP) in antigen–antibody complexes.

(a) *Staining by Pyronine Y.* The procedure is an adaptation to gel immunodiffusion of the technique used for the histochemical characterization of tissue polynucleotides.[14]

Reagents

Pyronine. 2% aqueous solution: Dissolve the dye in water and purify by repeated extractions with chloroform. The impurities are soluble in the organic phase. Gurr's Pyronine Y (G. Gurr, Ltd. London) gives the most satisfactory results. Store the pyronine solution in colored glass bottles.

Just before use, dilute tenfold the 2% aqueous pyronine in acetate buffer, 0.1 M, pH 4.7.

Procedure. Immerse the plates in the pyronine-buffer reagent for 30 to 60 minutes. Wash in running water until the gel background is decolorized. Dry the plates for several minutes in an oven at 80° to 90°.

Remarks. Pyronine is a general stain for polymerized nucleic acids (DNA or RNA).

The polynucleotide-containing precipitates are stained red.

(b) *Staining by the Feulgen–Formazan Reaction.* The hydrolysis of polynucleotides in hot hydrochloric acid for the purpose of freeing the aldehydes from the deoxypentoses present in certain nucleic acids was introduced by Feulgen. It has been widely used since then in methods for the characterization of deoxyribonucleic acids.

The acid hydrolysis combined with the formazan reaction for aldehydes is the principle of the technique for DNA characterization in agar or agarose gels.[15] Antigen–antibody precipitates containing DNA stain blue-violet.

Reagents. (a) 1 N HCl; (b) phenylhydrazine-HCl; and (c) tetrazotized-o-dianisidine and (d) cupric acetate reagents prepared as described in Section iii.b.

[14] J. Brachet, *Compt. Rend.* **133**, 8 (1940).
[15] J. Uriel and S. Avrameas, *Compt. Rend.* **252**, 1524 (1961).

Procedure. The plates are treated in the following way:

Reagent *a*, 45° to 50°	15 min
Reagent *b*, 60° to 70°	5 min
Running water	10 min
Reagent *c*	5 min
Running water	10 min
Reagent *d*	5 min
Running water	10 min

v. Metalloproteins

Many reagents for metal identification have been developed in analytical chemistry. However, the characterization of metal-binding proteins in gels is limited as follows: (a) in order to avoid hydrolysis of the gel support, the reaction should take place under relatively mild conditions; (b) reactions in acid pH are preferable because in this range the bound metal is split off without simultaneous solubilization of the protein carrier; (c) fast-trapping reactions are needed to ensure a precise localization; (d) the reagents selected should attain a sensitivity below the microgram level.

(*a*) *Staining of Copper-Binding Proteins.* Alizarin Blue S forms a blue lake with cupric ion which is insoluble in either strong acids or acetic anhydride. It was first introduced as a spot test reagent[16] and adapted later for the staining of copper proteins in gels.[17]

Reagent

Alizarin Blue S: saturated solution in concentrated acetic acid

Procedure

Step 1. Just before use, dilute the alizarin reagent ten times with 9 volumes of 70% acetic acid.

Step 2. Immerse the plates for 30 minutes in the staining solution and wash for another 30 minutes in 70% acetic acid.

The copper-containing specific precipitates are stained blue. Under the conditions of the experiment the reaction is specific for Cu^{2+}.

(*b*) *Staining of Iron-Binding Proteins.* The bathophenanthroline (4,7-diphenyl-1,10-phenanthroline) is a sensitive reagent for iron.[18] Its ferrous complex is colored and poorly soluble in aqueous solutions. Iron proteins such as ferritin and transferrin can be identified by this reagent.[19]

Reagents

a. *Bathophenanthroline:* 0.01% solution of bathophenanthroline, sulfonated, sodium salt. Dissolve 2 mg of the iron-reagent in 2

---

[16] F. Feigl and A. Caldas, *Anal. Chim. Acta* **8**, 117 (1953).

[17] J. Uriel, H. Gotz, and P. Grabar, *J. Med. Suisse* **87**, Suppl. 14, 258 (1957).

[18] H. Diehl and G. Frederick Smith, "The Iron Reagents: Bathophenanthromine; 2,4,6-Tripyridyl-*s*-triazine, Phenyl-2-Pyridyl Ketoxime." G. Frederick Smith Chem. Co., Columbus, Ohio, 1960.

[19] J. Uriel and S. Chuilon, unpublished results (1965).

ml of demineralized water. Add 18 ml of 0.02 M sodium acetate. Use at once.

b. Thioglycolic acid

Procedure. Immerse the plates for 1 to 2 hours in the bathophenanthroline reagent. Add 0.1 ml of reagent *b*. After a few minutes, remove the iron-reagent and wash the plates in several baths (15 minutes each) of 2% acetic acid.

Iron-binding antigen–antibody complexes stain red.

Remarks. High quality, iron-free, chemicals and solvents must be used in all the operations, beginning with the washing in buffered saline of the immunodiffusion plates.

d. Specific Reactions for Characterizing Enzymes

i. General Procedures and Applications

The possibility of demonstrating in gel diffusion media the catalytic properties of an enzyme complexed with antibody[20,4a] has permitted the identification of enzymes in crude mixture of antigens.

For antibodies to enzymes allowed to react in the conventional tube method, varying degrees of inhibition of activity have been reported. However, in the experience acquired with immunodiffusion methods, more than twenty-five different enzyme–antibody complexes have been shown to possess sufficient catalytic activity to allow their identification. The disparity in results obtained with these two immunological methods has been discussed elsewhere.[4a, 21]

Substrates and methods of reactions. Synthetic substrates, chromogenic and nonchromogenic, can be used for the identification of enzymes in immunodiffusion precipitates. In the first case, the substrates *per se*, are uncolored or slightly colored solutions. Through the catalytic activity of an enzyme, either the entire substrate is transformed to a colored and insoluble product (see model reaction A, Fig. 2), or the chromogenic moiety split off by the enzyme interacts with a "coupler" present in the reaction milieu to give a final colored and insoluble compound (see model reaction B, Fig. 2). In the case of nonchromogenic substrates, an auxiliary chromogenic system is linked to the former in order to visualize the enzymic reaction. This is generally obtained with the aid of an electron transfer chain in which the final step is a colored product (see model reactions, Fig. 3). The electron chain may be coupled to the primary enzyme–substrate pair through an intermediate enzyme which utilizes as substrate one of the reaction products split from the primary system (see model

[20] J. Uriel, *Bull. Soc. Chim. Biol.* **39**, Suppl. No. 1, 105 (1957).
[21] J. Uriel, *in* "Antibodies to Biological Active Molecules" (E. Cinader, ed.), p. 181. Pergamon Press, Oxford, 1967.

reaction B, Fig. 3). The synthetic substrates used are those that have been developed in the analytical chemistry of enzymes or for histochemical purposes.

In addition to synthetic substrates, natural substrates, such as proteins, carbohydrates, and nucleic acids, can serve for the identification of enzymes in enzyme–antibody precipitates. Changes in the physiochemical properties (solubility, staining capacity) of these substrates after enzymatic action are utilized for enzyme identification.

Specific inhibitors to differentiate enzymes with similar catalytic properties can be employed on the same basis as those used conventionally in the analytical chemistry of enzymes.

(A) 3 p-Phenylenediamine $+ 3 O_2 \xrightarrow{\text{ceruloplasmin}}$ Quinoid derivative (colored and insoluble) $+ 6 H_2O$

(B)   2-Napthyl acetate $+ H_2O \xrightarrow[\text{esterase}]{\text{carboxylic}}$ Acetic acid

2-Naphthol diazonium salt

azo coupling

Azo dye

Fɪɢ. 2. Models of characterization reactions with chromogenic substrates: (A) identification of ceruloplasmin; (B) identification of carboxylic esterases.

Applications. The development of characterization reactions for enzymes in enzyme–antibody immunodiffusion precipitates was primarily intended to allow the identification of an enzyme or group of enzymes in complex mixtures. However, these techniques also may be of use to follow the progressive purification of an enzyme from a crude preparation[22, 23]; to study the purity, homogeneity, and native state of an enzyme preparation; and to study the immunochemical relationship between multiple molecular forms of enzymes having close substrate specificity.[21]

The experimental conditions given below for the identification of indi-

[22] J. Uriel and S. Avrameas, *Biochemistry* **4**, 1740 (1965).
[23] S. Avrameas and J. Uriel, *Biochemistry* **4**, 1750 (1965).

vidual enzymes are those conventionally used in enzymology. However, differences in the optimal conditions of catalytic activity (pH, ionic strength, temperature, and time of incubation) have been found among isodynamic enzymes from different sources. Thus the choice of varying such conditions in a particular case is left to the operator.

Unless otherwise indicated the immunodiffusion plates are washed in saline and dried prior to the identification reactions, and the incubation media are prepared just before use.

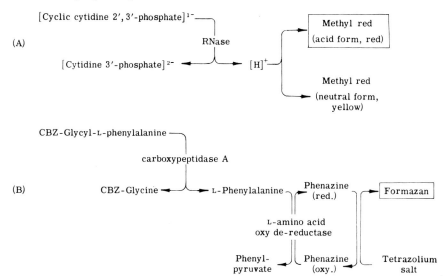

Fig. 3. Models of characterization reactions with nonchromogenic substrates. (A) Demonstration of ribonucleases; (B) demonstration of carboxypeptidase.

In Table I are listed the individual enzymes that have been identified with the aid of the techniques outlined in this section.

ii. Oxidoreductases

A great number of oxidoreductases utilize NAD, NADP, O_2, or H_2O_2 as hydrogen acceptors. This wide group of enzymes may be easily demonstrated by color reactions in gel diffusion media. The electron-transfer reaction is visualized with the aid of appropriate oxidoreduction indicators. Several examples are given below.

(*a*) *NAD or NADP as Acceptors.* Phenazine methosulfate, a redox dye, accepts reversibly electrons from the reduced forms of NAD or NADP. The electron pathway is completed by a tetrazolium salt as final electron acceptor.

(1) *Lactate dehydrogenase (EC 1.1.1.27).*[24]

[24] S. Avrameas and K. Rajewsky, *Nature* **201**, 405 (1963).

Incubation medium. Dissolve in 10 ml of Tris buffer (0.05 M; pH 8.2) 150 mg of sodium lactate, 10 mg of nicotinamide-adenine dinucleotide (NAD), and 50 mg of sodium azide. Add 1 ml ethanol containing 10 mg of MTT* Warm the solution to 45°C and mix with 1.6% melted agar or agarose aqueous solution kept at the same temperature. In the agar–substrate solution dissolve with stirring 1 to 2 mg of phenazine methosulfate. Use at once.

Procedure. Pour over the plates enough agar–substrate solution to obtain a layer of 1 to 2 mm thick and incubate during 60 to 90 minutes at room temperature. Protect the plates from light to avoid the spontaneous reduction of phenazine methosulfate. After incubation, fix the plates during 2 hours in 2% acetic acid. Dry under filter paper.

(2) *Glucose-6-phosphate dehydrogenase (EC 1.1.2.49).*

Incubation medium. Dissolve in 20 ml of 0.05 M Tris buffer (pH 7.5) 40 mg of glucose 6-phosphate, 10 mg of NADP, 50 mg of NaN$_3$, 10 mg of MTT, and 1 mg of Phenazine methosulfate.

Procedure. Dried immunodiffusion plates may be used. Control medium is made by replacing the G-6-P solution with H$_2$O. Pour medium over slides and incubate at room temperature. Development time is variable; several hours may be required. Protect solutions and incubation from light. An example of a G-6-PD reaction is shown in Fig. 1C.

(3) *Glutamate dehydrogenase (EC 1.4.1.2) and alanine dehydrogenase (EC 1.4.1.1)*[†][25]

Incubation media. (a) For glutamate dehydrogenase: Dissolve in 10 ml of 0.05 M Tris buffer (pH 7.5) 100 mg of sodium L-glutamate, 5 mg of NAD, 2 mg of nitro-blue tetrazolium salt (nitro-BT),‡ and 4 mg of phenazine methosulfate. (b) For alanine dehydrogenase: Dissolve in 10 ml of 0.05 M Tris buffer (pH 9.0) 90 mg of L-alanine, 1.2 mg of NAD, 2 mg of nitro-BT, and 4 mg of phenazine methosulfate. Protect the incubation media from light and use at once.

Procedure. Use washed, *but not dried,* immunodiffusion plates. Incubate the plates at 37°C (60 minutes) in substrate (a) and for 90 to 120 minutes in substrate (b). Wash the plates in running water to remove background staining and dry under filter paper. Protect the solutions from light.

(b) *O$_2$ as Acceptor*

(1) *Xanthine oxidase (EC 1.2.3.2).*[26]

* MTT: 3(4,5-dimethyl thiazolyl 1,2)2,5-diphenyl tetrazolium.
† Identifications not tried in this laboratory.
[25] N. Talal, G. M. Tomkins, J. F. Mushinski, and K. L. Yielding, *J. Mol. Biol.* **8,** 46 (1964).
‡ Nitro-BT: 2,2'-di-*p*-nitrophenyl-5,5'-diphenyl-3,3'-(3,3'-dimethoxy-4,4'-biphenylene) ditetrazolium salt.
[26] M. Stanislawski, S. Oisgold, J. Uriel, and S. Avrameas, *Protides Biol. Fluids, Proc. Colloq.* **12,** 228. Elsevier, Amsterdam, 1965.

TABLE I

ENZYMES IDENTIFIED BY THE CATALYTIC PROPERTIES OF THE ENZYME–ANTIBODY
PRECIPITATES OBTAINED IN GEL DIFFUSION MEDIA

EC No.[a]	Enzyme	Substrate	Reference footnote No.	Text page
1.1.1.27	Lactate dehydrogenase	L-Lactate	24	307
1.1.2.49	Glucose-6-phosphate dehydrogenase	Glucose 6-phosphate	19	307
1.2.3.2	Xanthine oxidase	Xanthine or xanthosine	25	308
1.4.1.1	Alanine dehydrogenase	L-Alanine	26	308
1.4.1.2	Glutamate dehydrogenase	L-Glutamate	26	308
1.10.3.2	Ceruloplasmin	p-Phenylenediamine	20	306,310
1.11.1.6	Catalase	H_2O_2	27,42	311
1.11.1.7	Peroxidase	Benzidine	28	311
2.7.7.8	Polynucleotide phosphorylase	Adenosine 5-diphosphate	28a	320
2.7.7.16	Ribonuclease	Cyclic cytidylic acid	29	317
3.1.1	Carboxylic ester hydrolases	2-Naphthyl acetate	30	312
3.1.1	Carboxylic ester hydrolases	1-Naphthyl acetate	31	312
3.1.1	Carboxylic ester hydrolases	Indoxyl acetate	30	312
3.1.1.3	Lipase	2-Naphthyl nonanoate	32	313
3.1.1.7	Acetylcholinesterase	Acetylthiocholine	30	313
3.1.1.8	Cholinesterase	Butyrylthiocholine	30	313
3.1.1.8	Cholinesterase	Carbonaphthoxy choline	30	
3.1.3.1	Alkaline phosphatase	Naphthol AS-MX phosphoric acid	33	313
3.1.3.2	Acid phosphatase	β-Glycerophosphate	34	
3.1.3.2	Acid phosphatase	Naphthol AS-BI phosphoric acid	33	313
3.1.3.9	Glucose-6-phosphatase	Glucose 6-phosphate	19	314
3.2.1.1	α-Amylase	Soluble starch	35	314
3.2.1.2	β-Amylase	β-Amylose	36	314
3.2.1.23	β-Galactosidase	6-Bromo-2-naphthyl-β-D-galactoside	37	315
3.2.1.31	β-Glucuronidase	6-Bromo-2-naphthyl-β-D-glucopyranoside	37	315
3.2.1.30	β-Acetylglucoseaminidase	Naphthol-AS-LC-acetyl-β-D-glucoseaminide	37	
3.4.1.1	Leucine aminopeptidase	Leucyl-4-methoxy-2-naphthylamide	22	315
3.4.2.1	Carboxypeptidase A	Carbonaphthoxy-DL-phenylalanine	4a	315
3.4.2.2	Carboxypeptidase B	Hippuryl-L-arginine	29,38	316
3.4.4.1	Pepsin	Bovine serum albumin	39	319
3.4.4.4	Trypsin	Benzoyl-D,L-arginine-2-naphthylamide	4a	316
3.4.4.4	Trypsin	p-Tosyl-L-arginine methyl ester	29	316
3.4.4.5	Chymotrypsin	Acetyl-D,L-phenylalanine-2-naphthyl ester	4a	317
3.4.4.5	Chymotrypsin	Acetyl-L-tyrosine ethyl ester	29	317
4.1.2.7	Aldolase	D-Fructose diphosphate	40	317
4.2.1.1	Carbonic anhydrase	H_2CO_3	41	318

[a] Code number assigned by the Enzyme Commission (EC) of the International Union of Biochemistry.   (Footnotes 27-41 on page 310.)

Incubation medium. Dissolve 20 mg of xanthosine in 8 ml of 0.05 M phosphate or Tris buffers (pH 7.5). Add 2 ml of ethanol containing 10 mg of MTT tetrazolium salt. Warm the solution to $\approx 45°C$ and mix quickly with 10 ml of a 1.6% aqueous solution of agar or agarose at $\approx 45°C$. Use at once.

Procedure (*see subsection d.ii.(a).*(1)) Incubate the plates at 37°C during 2 to 3 hours. Wash in 2% acetic acid and dry under filter paper.

(2) *Ceruloplasmin* (*EC 1.10.3.2*).[20] Ceruloplasmin, a serum α_2-globulin containing copper, oxidizes p-phenylenediamine and other phenolic compounds. p-Phenylenediamine, on oxidation, yields a quinoid product "Brandrowsky's base," which is brown and insoluble in water (see Fig. 2A).

Incubation medium. Dissolve 21.6 mg of p-phenylenediamine in 100 ml of 0.1 M acetate buffer (pH 5.7) prepared by mixing equal parts of 0.2 M sodium acetate and 0.02 M acetic acid. Warm the solution to 37°C and use immediately.

Procedure. Immerse the plates in the substrate solution during 2 to 3 hours at 37°C. Wash the plates in 2% acetic acid and dry in air. Ceruloplasmin-antibody precipitates stain brown.

Remarks. The enzymatic activity is inhibited by sodium azide. For the control plates, add to the incubation medium 2 ml of a 0.1 M solution of sodium azide.

References for footnotes 27–41 are in Table I.

[27] A. Micheli, F. Peetoom, N. Rose, S. Ruddy, and P. Grabar, *Ann. Inst. Pasteur* **98**, 694 (1960).

[28] N. Rose, F. Peetoom, S. Ruddy, A. Micheli, and P. Grabar, *Ann. Inst. Pasteur* **98**, 51 (1960).

[28a] J. Uriel, M. N. Thang, and J. Berges, *FEBS Letters*, **2**, 321 (1969).

[29] J. Uriel and S. Avrameas, *Anal. Biochem.* **9**, 180 (1964).

[30] J. Uriel, *Ann. Inst. Pasteur* **101**, 104 (1961).

[31] H. Lauffer, *Ann. N.Y. Acad. Sci.* **103**, 1137 (1963).

[32] J. Pascale, S. Avrameas, and J. Uriel, *J. Biol. Chem.* **241**, 3023 (1966).

[33] B. Guilbert and J. Berges, unpublished results (1965).

[34] S. Shulman, L. Mamrod, M. T. Gonder, and W. A. Soanes, *J. Immunol.* **93**, 474 (1964).

[35] J. Uriel and S. Avrameas, *Ann. Inst. Pasteur* **106**, 396 (1964).

[36] P. Grabar and J. Daussant, *Cereal Chem.* **41**, 523 (1964).

[37] V. K. Raunio, *Acta Pathol. Microbiol. Scand. Suppl.* **195**, (1968).

[38] S. Avrameas and J. Uriel, *Compt. Rend.* **261**, 584 (1965).

[39] H. Hirsch-Marie, M. Conte, and P. Burtin, *Rev. Franc. Etudes Clin. Biol.* **9**, 924 (1965).

[40] F. Schapira, G. Schapira, and J. C. Dreylus, *Nature* **200**, 995 (1963).

[41] A. Micheli and C. Buzzi, *Biochim. Biophys. Acta* **84**, 324 (1964).

(c) *H₂O₂ as Acceptor*

(1) *Peroxidases (EC 1.11.1.7)*. Among the reagents employed for the histochemical characterization of peroxidases, Nadi reagent* and benzidine have been employed for the characterization of these enzymes in gelified media. This procedure can be used to detect haptoglobin in serum because of the peroxidase activity of the attached hemoglobin.

The oxidation of Nadi to a colored product, indophenol blue, is accelerated by the peroxide–peroxidase complex and also by other oxidation systems. The use of Nadi has been criticized because of its lack of specificity. However, if certain limits of control are imposed, the test becomes specific for peroxidases.[42]

Incubation media.† (a) Add to 20 ml of fresh H_2O_2-Nadi reagent (see subsection c.iii) 2 ml of 0.1 M sodium azide in 5% acetic acid. (aa) To 20 mg of benzidine in 14 ml of methanol, add 2 ml of acetate buffer (equal parts of 2 M sodium acetate and 2 M acetic acid), 2 ml of 0.1 M sodium azide, and 2 ml of 3% hydrogen peroxide.

Procedure. Immerse the plates for 10 to 15 minutes in substrate (a) or (aa). Wash for 10 minutes in running water, and dry in air.

Remarks. In contrast to benzidine blue, which fades with time, the indophenol blue resulting from Nadi oxidation is a stable-colored product. The sensitivity of the two substrates is approximately the same.

(2) *Catalase (EC 1.11.1.6) by release of oxygen.*[42] The principle of this reaction differs from that of the preceding ones in that it is not the presence of a colored material that is observed at the end of the reaction, but instead the appearance of bubbles of gas within the gel layer. In the case of catalases, the bubbles are molecular oxygen evolved from the substrate hydrogen peroxide through the catalytic action of these enzymes. An example of this reaction is seen in Fig. 1, panel A.

Procedure. Immerse the plates in commercial 3% hydrogen peroxide. Tiny bubbles of oxygen appear immediately on the precipitin lines possessing catalase activity. After a few minutes wash the plates in running water and dry in air.

(3) *Demonstration of catalase by a color reaction.*[43] The incubation medium contains H_2O_2, KI, and soluble starch. H_2O_2 oxidizes the KI to give free iodine which binds starch, resulting in a violet coloration. In the presence of catalase activity, the H_2O_2 is utilized by the enzyme, thus preventing the color reaction.[44]

---

* Equimolar mixture of fresh solutions of α-naphthol and dimethyl-*p*-phenylene-diamine.

. † Either incubation medium (a) or incubation medium (aa) can be used as perferred.

[42] J. Uriel, *Bull. Soc. Chim. Biol.* **40**, 277 (1958).

[43] R. Bartholomew and G. Hermann, personal communication (1965).

[44] L. Beckman, J. G. Scandalios, and J. L. Brewbaker, *Science* **146**, 1174 (1964).

Reagents. (a) Starch–H_2O_2 solution: Equal volumes of 4% soluble starch and 1% H_2O_2 are mixed just prior to use. (b) KI solution: 4% aqueous KI solution acidified, just before use, with a few drops of 2% acetic acid.

Procedure. Immerse the plates (washed, but not dried) for 10 to 15 minutes in the starch–H_2O_2 reagent. Then, wash plates a few seconds in running water and immerse in reagent (b).

Remarks. Catalase–antibody precipitates appear as uncolored arcs on a violet background. The color reaction starts immediately but is not stable.

Peroxidases and amylases can react in the same manner as catalase with this technique. Catalase activity may be distinguished from peroxidase and amylase activities by using two control plates. Replacing the H_2O_2 solution by water in reagent (a) would remove all peroxidase and catalase activity. If NaN_3 (0.01 M final concentration) is included in reagent (a), catalase activity is inhibited.

iii. Hydrolases

(*a*) *Carboxylic Ester Hydrolases.* These enzymes catalyze the hydrolysis of esters of carboxylic acids. They constitute a broad group of enzymes with a large representation in tissues and biological fluids although their specificity is poorly established. Two groups can be distinguished: *short-* and *long*-chained fatty acid esterases. Other classifications have been suggested, some of which have been criticized.[4a]

Panel D in Fig. 1 shows an array of such "nonspecific" esterases in the immunoelectrophoretic pattern of *Neurospora crassa*. They were revealed by the procedure below, which is schematically illustrated in Fig. 2B.

(1) *Carboxylesterases and cholinesterases with 2-naphthyl acetate*[30]

Incubation medium. Dissolve 5 mg of 2-naphthyl acetate in 0.5 ml of acetone or dimethylformamide. Add 25 ml of phosphate buffer solution (pH 7.4, 0.05 M). An opalescent solution results in which 10 mg of diazotized *o*-dianisidine (Diazo Blue B) are dissolved. This solution is filtered and used immediately.

Procedure. Immerse the plates in the incubation medium for 60 minutes at room temperature. Then wash (1 hour) in 2% acetic acid.

Remarks. The choice of the inhibitor(s) of esterase activity is left to the operator. He should start from concentrated solutions that are brought to the desired final dilutions with phosphate buffer (pH 7.4, 0.05 M). The plates are subjected to a preliminary soaking for 30 minutes in these solutions and then immersed in the incubation medium, which also contains the inhibitor at the same final dilution.

Other general substrates of carboxylic ester hydrolases, such as indoxyl acetate[30] and 1-naphthyl acetate,[31] may be employed.

(2) *Acetylcholinesterases (EC 3.1.1.7) and cholinesterases (EC 3.1.1.8), by thiocholine[30] esters*

Incubation medium. Dissolve 5 mg of INT,* nitro-BT,† or MTT‡ in 1 ml of ethyl alcohol. Add 19 ml of barbital buffer (pH 8.2, 0.05 *M*). Dissolve directly in this solution 20 mg of acetylthiocholine or butyrylthiocholine.

Procedure. Warm the above solution to 37° to 40°C and incubate the plates at this temperature for 2 to 4 hours. Wash in 2% acetic acid (1 hour), and dry in air.

Remarks. The time of incubation depends on the rate of esterase activity and on the degree of sensitivity of the tetrazolium salt used. The MTT salt is the most sensitive.

The thiocholine esters, while more specific for the cholinesterases, can be hydrolyzed by other carboxyl ester hydrolases.[30]

(3) *Lipase (EC 3.1.1.3)*[32]

Incubation medium. Dissolve 10 mg of 2-naphthyl nonanoate in 5 ml of diethylformamide to which 20 ml of Veronal buffer (pH 8, 0.05 *M*) is added. Dissolve in this solution 10 mg of tetrazotized *o*-dianisidine (Diazo Blue B) and 100 mg of sodium taurocholate.

Procedure. Immerse the plates for about 2 hours in the substrate solution and wash in 2% acetic acid (1 hour). Dry in air.

Remarks. 2-Napthyl nonanoate seems to be specific for lipases, that is, for the esterases attacking esters of long-chain fatty acids. Esterases of the group that hydrolyzes esters of short-chain fatty acids (carboxylesterases, cholinesterases) do not attack this substrate.

(b) *Phosphoric Monoester Hydrolases (EC 3.1.3)*

(1) *Alkaline (EC 3.1.3.1) and acid (EC 3.1.3.2.) phosphatases*[33]

Reagents. (1a) Substrate solution (for alkaline phosphatase): 5 mg of naphthol AS-MX phosphoric acid in 0.1 ml of dimethyl formamide, 1 ml of 0.25 *M* magnesium chloride, and 19 ml of Tris buffer (0.05 *M*, pH 8.7). (1b) Substrate solution (for acid phosphatase): 5 mg of naphthol AS-BI phosphoric acid in 20 ml of acetate buffer, pH 4.8 (equal volumes of 0.2 *M* solutions of the salt and the acid).(2) Coupling solution: 10 mg of Garnet GBC diazonium salt§ in 10 ml of the same buffer used in (1b).

Procedure. Incubate the plates in the substrate solution, (1a) or (1b), for 2 hours, then in the coupling reagent for 30 minutes. Wash for 1 hour in 2% acetic acid and dry in air.

---

* INT: 2-(*p*-iodophenyl)-3-*p*-nitrophenyl-5-phenyltetrazolium salt.

† Nitro-BT: 2,2'-di-*p*-nitrophenyl-5,5'-diphenyl-3,3'-(3,3'dimethoxy-4,4'-biphenylene) ditetrazolium salt.

‡ MTT: 3(4,5 dimethyl thiazolyl 1,2)2,5-diphenyl tetrazolium.

§ Diazotized *o*-aminoazotoluene.

Antigen–antibody precipitates with nonspecific phosphatase activity stain blue-violet. An example is shown in Fig. 1b.

(2) *Glucose-6-phosphatase (EC 3.1.3.9)*. The identification is carried out using a reaction similar to that serving for the characterization of carboxypeptidase A (see Fig. 3B). D-Glucose 6-phosphate is used as the primary substrate and D-glucose oxidase as the auxiliary enzyme. Phenazine methosulfate and a tetrazolium salt serve as the electron tranfer chain.

Incubation medium. Dissolve in 20 ml of citrate buffer, pH 6.5, the following reagents: 20 mg of glucose 6-phosphate; 50 mg of glucose oxidase (Calbiochem, type II); 10 mg of MTT*; and, just before use, 2 mg of phenazine methosulfate.

Procedure. Incubate the plates at room temperature for 2 to 3 hours. Protect the plates from light. After the incubation wash the plates in 2% acetic acid.

Remarks. The concentration of the auxiliary enzyme, glucose oxidase, depends on the specific activity of the commercial preparation.

(c) *Glycoside Hydrolases (EC 3.2.1)*. (1) *α-Amylases (EC 3.2.1.1) and β-amylases (EC 3.2.1.2)*[35]

Reagents. (1) Agar or agarose solution: 1.6% in Tris-HCl buffer (pH 6.7, 0.05 M) containing calcium chloride at a final concentration of 0.05 M. Melt the powder in the buffer, cool to about 45°, and maintain at this temperature until used. (2) Soluble starch: a 0.1% solution of soluble starch is prepared in the same buffer. Warm the solution to approximately 45° and maintain at this temperature until used. (3) Iodine solution: 0.25% iodine in 1% potassium iodide.

Procedure. Just before use, mix equal parts of reagents (1) and (2). Pour over the plates enough agar–starch solution to obtain a layer 1 to 2 mm thick and incubate for 60 to 90 minutes at room temperature. After incubation, immerse the plates for a few minutes in the iodide solution.

Antigen–antibody precipitates with amylase activity appear as transparent arcs on a blue-black background.

Remarks. A similar technique for the identification of barley and malt amylases in immunodiffusion precipitates has been described.[36] This procedure involves the use of β-amylose (0.25% solution in acetate buffer, pH 4.5) in place of starch. The plates, washed but not dried, are immersed for 2 hours in the amylose solution, then incubated for 1 hour at 37° and dipped for a few minutes in the iodine solution.

Preincubation of the plates for 30 to 60 minutes in a 5×10^{-6} M solution of HgCl$_2$ serves to distinguish α-amylases from β-amylases. Only β-amylase is inhibited by the mercury salt.

* MTT: 3(4,5-dimethyl thiazolyl 1,2)2,5-diphenyl tetrazolium.

(2) *β-Galactosidases (EC 3.2.1.23), and β-glucuronidases (EC 3.2.1.31)*[37]

Incubation media. Dissolve 30 mg of 6-bromo-2-naphthyl-β-galactoside (a) or 6-bromo-2-naphthyl-β-D-glucopyranoside (b) in 4 ml of dimethyl formamide. Add 6 ml of acetate buffer, pH 4.7 (equal parts of 0.4 M sodium acetate and 0.4 M acetic acid). In this solution dissolve 30 mg of Garnet GBC diazonium salt. Warm the solution to about 45° and mix with 10 ml of 1.6% warmed aqueous agar or agarose solution. Maintain at this temperature until time of use.

Procedure. Pour over the plates enough agar–substrate solution to obtain a layer of gel 1 to 2 mm thick. Incubate at 37° for 2 to 3 hours, wash in 2% acetic acid (2 hours), and dry under filter paper.

Remarks. The synthetic substrates (a) and (b) serve for the identification of β-galactosidases and β-glucuronidases, respectively.

Other glycoside hydrolases have been identified in antigen–antibody precipitates using the same principle and appropriate glycoside substrates.

(d) *α-Aminopeptide Amino Acid Hydrolases (EC 3.4.1).* Enzymes of this group hydrolyze peptides, splitting off N-terminal residues with a free α-amino group.

Leucine aminopeptidase (EC 3.4.1.1)[22]

Incubation medium. To 20 mg of L-leucyl-4-methoxy-2-naphthylamide in 3 ml of dimethylformamide add 7 ml of barbital buffer (0.05 M, pH 8.2) containing 10 mg of Diazo Blue B. Prepare the solution just before use. Warm to about 45°, and mix with 10 ml of 1.6% aqueous melted agarose maintained at the same temperature.

Procedure. Pour over the plates enough agar–substrate solution to obtain a layer of gel of 1 to 2 mm thick. Incubate at 37° for 2 to 3 hours, wash in 2% acetic acid (2 hours). and dry under filter paper.

(e) *α-Carboxypeptide Amino Acid Hydrolases (EC 3.4.2).* Enzymes of this group hydrolyze peptides, splitting off the C-terminal amino acid residue.

(1) *Carboxypeptidases A (EC 3.4.2.1)*[4a]. See model reaction in Fig. 3B.

Incubation medium. Dissolve 10 to 20 mg of carbonaphthoxy-DL-phenylalanine in 1 to 2 ml of dimethylformamide, dilute to 10 ml with distilled water, and dissolve 10 mg of Diazo Blue B in this opalescent solution. Warm to about 45° and mix with 10 ml of 1.6% agar solution in Tris or barbital buffer (pH 7.4, 0.05 M). Melt the buffered agar in a boiling water bath and cool to 45° before mixing. Maintain at this temperature until time of use.

Procedure. Pour over the plates enough agar–substrate solution to obtain a layer 1 to 2 mm thick. Incubate at 37° for 2 to 4 hours. Protect the plates from evaporation by placing them in a closed vessel. Wash (2 hours) in 2% aqueous acetic acid. Dry under filter paper. The lines possessing carboxypeptidase A activity are stained red-violet.

(2) *Carboxypeptidases B (EC 3.4.2.2)*[38]. The enzyme–substrate primary pair (carboxypeptidase B–hippuryl-L-arginine) is coupled to an auxiliary enzyme (L-amino acid oxidase) in a manner similar to the model reaction for carboxypeptidase A shown in Fig. 3B.

Incubation medium. Dissolve in 10 ml of barbital buffer (0.05 M, pH 7.4) 30 mg of hippuryl-L-arginine, 5 mg of L-amino acid oxidase (EC 1.4.3.2) from venom of *Crotalus adamanteus* and 5 mg of MTT tetrazolium salt.* Warm the solution at about 45° and mix with 10 ml of 1.6% aqueous solution of melted agarose maintained at 45°. Dissolve with stirring in the agarose–substrate solution at 45° 1 to 2 mg of phenazine methosulfate and use immediately.

Procedure. Pour over the plates enough agarose-substrate solution to obtain a layer 1 to 2 mm thick and incubate during 60 to 90 minutes at room temperature. Protect the plates from light to avoid the spontaneous reduction of phenazine methosulfate. After incubation, fix the plates for 2 hours in 2% acetic acid. Dry under filter paper.

(f) Peptidyl Peptide Hydrolases (EC 3.4.4). (1) *Trypsins (EC 3.4.4.4) with chromogenic substrates*[4a]

Incubation medium. Dissolve 20 mg of *N*-benzoyl-DL-arginine-2-naphthylamide in 2 ml of dimethylformamide. Add 8 ml of distilled water and dissolve 20 mg of Diazo Blue B in this solution. Warm the solution to about 45° and mix with 10 ml of 1.6% agar solution in Tris or barbital buffer (pH 7.4 to 8.2, 0.05 M). Melt the buffered agar in a boiling water and cool to 45° before mixing. Maintain at this temperature until use.

Procedure is same as with complexes with carboxypeptidase-like activity described in preceding section.

(2) *Demonstration of trypsin with nonchromogenic substrates.*[29] The identification reaction is based on the model represented in Fig. 3A. The method consists in demonstrating with an appropriate pH-indicator any enzymatically induced change in the hydrogen ion concentration of the reaction mixture. The reaction takes place in an unbuffered medium, but the reagents, a synthetic ester and a pH indicator, are previously adjusted to a pH presumed to be optimal for the enzyme studied. As the reaction progresses, the pH in the vicinity of the enzyme–antibody precipitate is shifted into the color range of the indicator.

Reagents and procedure. To 20 mg of *p*-tosyl-L-arginine methyl ester (TAME) in 9 ml of 0.2 M NaCl, add 1 ml of neutral red (0.1 gm in 70 ml of ethanol made up to 100 ml with water). Adjust carefully the pH to 8, warm the solution to about 45° and mix with 10 ml of 1.6% melted

---

* MTT: 3(4,5-dimethyl thiazolyl 1,2)2,5-diphenyl tetrazolium.

agarose in neutral water. Pour over the plates enough agarose–substrate to obtain a layer of gel 1 to 2 mm thick.

Remarks. The reaction starts almost immediately. Along the enzyme–antibody precipitates possessing TAMEase activity the color of the indicator changes from yellow to red. Color pictures of the reaction can be taken in the first 10 to 15 minutes. After this time, the activity pattern is progressively blurred by the free diffusion of the reaction products in the gel.

(3) *Chymotrypsins (EC 3.4.4.5)*[4a]

Incubation medium. Dissolve 5 mg of acetyl-DL-phenylalanine-2-naphthyl ester in 2 ml of dimethyl formamide. Add 18 ml of Tris or barbital buffer (pH 7.4, 0.05 M). Dissolve in this solution 10 mg of Diazo Blue B. Filter, if necessary, and use at once.

Procedure. Immerse the plates for 60 minutes in the incubation medium. Wash (30 minutes) in aqueous 2% acetic acid. Dry in air. The precipitates possessing chymotrypsinlike activity are stained red-violet.

Remarks. Acylphenylalanine or tyrosine esters are poorly specific. In addition to chymotrypsin A, other pancreatic peptidohydrolases such as chymotrypsin B, elastase 1, and trypsin hydrolyze these substrates.[29]

Chymotrypsins may be identified with acetyl-L-tyrosine ethyl ester, a nonchromogenic substrate, as described for trypsin in subsection d. iii. (f) (2) above.

iv. Other Enzymes

(a) *Ribonuclease (EC 2.7.7.16).*[29] The identification reaction of this enzyme is based on the model represented in Fig. 3A. The cyclic phosphate, open by the action of the ribonuclease, dissociates, lowering the pH of the reaction milieu. An appropriate hydrogen ion indicator allows one to visualize the catalytic reaction.

Incubation medium. Suspend 20 mg of 2′,3′-cyclic cytidylic phosphate (barium salt) in 9 ml of 0.25 M sodium sulfate, stir gently for a few minutes, and centrifuge (15 minutes at 3000 rpm). To the supernatant, add 1.5 ml of fresh methyl red solution (0.01 gm of the indicator in 1.86 ml of 0.02 M NaOH and 23 ml of water), and adjust the pH of the solution to 6.8 to 7.0, under pH-meter control. The procedure is followed as described for trypsin in subsection d. iii. (f)(2) above.

Remarks. The reaction progressess for about 30 minutes. Ribonuclease–antibody precipitates stain red. Blurring phenomena do not disturb the localization of the activity during 1 to 2 hours.

(b) *Aldolase (EC 4.1.2.7).*[40]* The enzyme–substrate primary pair

---

* Identification not tried in this laboratory.

(aldolase–fructose diphosphate) is coupled to an auxiliary enzyme (glyceraldehyde phosphate dehydrogenase) to visualize the catalytic reaction (model reaction in Fig. 3B).

Incubation medium. Mix aliquot parts (2 ml each) of the following reagents: Tris buffer (0.25 M, pH 7.5), EDTA (10% solution), NAD (6 mg/ml solution), nitro-BT (20 mg/ml solution), D-fructose diphosphate (0.05 M), and sodium arsenate (0.35 M). Add 6 ml of water and 40 μl of a concentrated suspension of D-glyceraldehyde phosphate dehydrogenase (EC *1.2.1.12*).

Quickly dissolve 1 mg of phenazine methosulfate, and use immediately.

Procedure. The author uses washed, but not dried, plates. Immerse the plates in the substrate solution and incubate during 2 to 3 hours at 37°. Wash in 2% acetic acid (1 hour), and dry under filter paper. Aldolase–antibody precipitates stain violet.

(c) *Demonstration of Carbonic Anhydrase (EC 4.2.1.1).*[41]* *Reagents.* (a) Mix 1.0 ml of 0.1 M CoSO$_4$ with 6 ml of 0.05 M H$_2$SO$_4$. (b) Dissolve 1 gm of NaHCO$_3$ in 50 ml of 0.1 M Na$_2$SO$_4$. Just before use add solution (b) to solution (a).

Procedure. The author uses washed, but not dried, plates. Immerse the plates in the substrate solution during 5 minutes. Remove the plates from the solution and allow to stand for 10 minutes in the air. Repeat this operation twice again. The whole incubation takes 45 minutes, after which the plates are dried under filter paper. After drying, remove the filter paper, wash the plates for a few seconds in distilled water and immerse in dilute ammonium sulfide solution.

A black deposit of cobalt sulfide reveals the antigen–antibody complexes possessing carbonic anhydrase activity.

v. *Identification of Enzymes Using Natural Substrates*

(a) *Proteolytic Activity at Alkaline pH.*[4a] This technique is based on the fact that enzymic digestion products of protein are soluble in reagents that precipitate undigested protein molecules. The same principle has been used to detect the proteolytic activity of enzymes after electrophoresis in agar.[45] The modification consists of the use of a second agar plate containing the substrate upon which the "imprint" of the proteolysis will be obtained. This operation is necessary, otherwise the opalescent antigen–antibody precipitates mask their own proteolytic activity.

Incubation medium. (a) Protein substrate solution: Prepare a 1% solution of casein in barbital buffer (0.05 M, pH 8.0 to 8.2). Heat the

---

* Identification not tried in this laboratory.

[45] J. Uriel, *Nature* **188,** 853 (1960).

solution for 15 minutes in a boiling water bath, allow to cool at room temperature, and filter if necessary. (b) Imprint-supporting plate: Prepare a 1% solution of agar in barbital buffer (0.025, pH 8.0 to 8.2). Pour the melted agar on a glass plate in order to obtain a gel layer of 2 to 3 mm thick.

Immerse the agar plate for 20 minutes in the protein–substrate solution. A film of protein forms by diffusion on the surface of the agar plate. Remove the casein solution and soak the plates for 15 minutes in a 2.5% solution of streptomycin in barbital buffer (0.05 M, pH 8.0 to 8.2). The casein precipitates and the protein film becomes opalescent. Remove the plates from the solution and use at once.

Procedure. The immunodiffusion plates are placed over the freshly prepared imprint-supporting plates. The agar film containing the immunoprecipitates must make uniform contact with the surface of the printing plate. Avoid the formation of air bubbles between the two agar surfaces.

After several* hours of incubation at 37°, the two plates are separated. The immunodiffusion plate is washed for about 15 minutes in saline, then it can be reused for other characterization reactions (proteins, lipoproteins, enzymes).

The imprint-supporting plate is fixed for 2 hours in 2% acetic acid, then dried under filter paper, and finally stained with Amido Black as described above in Section E.1.c.i. The "imprint" of the enzyme–antibody precipitates possessing proteolytic activity appears in this plate as uncolored arcs on a colored background.

(b) *Proteolytic Activity at Strongly Acid pH.*[39] The "imprint" technique is not necessary for proteolytic enzymes active at very low pH. At this pH (1 to 2) the solution of the antigen–antibody precipitates allows one to visualize the physicochemical changes in the digested substrate without need of special manipulations.

Incubation medium. A 2% solution of bovine serum albumin (BSA) in glycine–HCl buffer (0.2 M, pH 1.9 to 2.1).

Procedure. The immunodiffusion plates are washed, not in neutral saline as usual, but in saline buffered at pH 5.6. After 16 to 24 hours of washing, the plates are dried under filter paper.

Immerse the plates in the incubation medium for 30 minutes at room temperature. Remove the plates from BSA solution and allow to stand for another 15 to 30 minutes. Place in 80% ethanol containing 5% acetic acid and 1% HgCl$_2$ for 1 hour. Dry in air and stain for proteins with Amido Black as in Section E.1.c.i.

Remarks. Enzyme–antibody precipitates with proteolytic activity

* The time of incubation depends on the degree of activity of the enzymes studied. For long periods of incubation, protect the plates from evaporation.

appear as uncolored arcs in a blue-black background. Pepsin or enzymes with pepsinlike activity may be identified by this technique.

vi. Identification of Nucleotidyl Transferases

The example given below represents a model of characterization reactions that can be applied to the demonstration of a special group of transferases involved in the synthesis of polynucleotides.

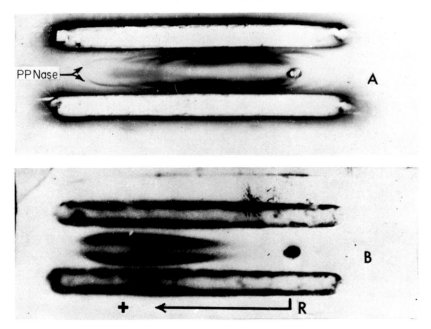

Fig. 4. Immunoelectrophoresis of a soluble extract of *Escherichia coli* B revealed with a rabbit antiserum anti-*E. coli*. (A) Protein. The arrows show the localization of the enzyme polynucleotide phosphorylase (PPNase) on the immunoelectrophoretic pattern. (B) Autoradiography of the same plate. R = starting reservoir. The anode is to the left. From Uriel *et al.*[28a]

The immunoplate containing the enzyme–antibody precipitates is incubated in an appropriate medium which includes a radioactive labeled substrate. The polynucleotide formed remains attached to the enzyme–antibody complex. The plate is then immersed in several baths of a solution of streptomycin; this allows fixation of the polynucleotide as well as washing out of the excess of radiolabeled substrate. Autoradiography of the plate permits localization of the enzyme.

Polynucleotide phosphorylases (CE 2.7.7.8).[28a] This was done using ^{14}C-labeled adenosine 5-diphosphate.

Incubation medium. Prepare a solution of Tris buffer (0.1 M, pH 8) containing 5 mmoles Mg Cl_2 and 0.5 mmole EDTA. Add to this solution a sufficient quantity of radiolabeled nucleotide ADP-^{14}C up to a final activity of 1 μCi per milliliter.

Procedure. Once the immune precipitates are developed, wash the plates in saline for several days in the cold room. Dry under filter paper. Incubate the plates in the medium for about 2 hours at room temperature.

Wash for 4 to 6 hours in several baths of a 1% solution of streptomycin in phosphate buffer, 0.1 M, pH 7. Stain the plates with a protein dye as described above, and remove the excess by washing the plates in a 2% acetic acid solution. Dry in air.

After drying, the plates are covered with a photographic film (Kodirex, Kodak—see Section 14.E.4.b.iii and Appendix I for details) and the film is developed after several days or several weeks, depending on the specific activity of the enzyme–antibody complex. An example of this test is shown in Fig. 4.

Remarks. ADP-^{14}C can be replaced by another labeled nucleotide. The same principle can be applied for the characterization of RNA- or DNA-polymerases.

2. PHOTOGRAPHY OF PRECIPITATES IN GELS*†

a. INTRODUCTION

Because of the transient or changing nature of precipitates in gels, good photographic technique is essential for keeping accurate and complete experimental records. In quantitative studies of diffusion rates, measurements are often made from photographs taken at different times under fixed conditions of enlargement. For publication, fine photographs showing the detail claimed for them should be the goal of all authors and be required by all editors. Although photographs of less technical excellence may serve for notebook records, it is wise to establish high standards of photographic recording from the outset.‡

Unstained antigen–antibody lines in gels can be photographed on

* Section 14.E.2 was contributed by Curtis A. Williams and Merrill W. Chase.

† Acknowledgment is made of helpful advice from Richard F. Carter, Lewis W. Koster, and Henrik Boudakian of The Rockefeller University, Graphic Services.

‡ Alternatives to routine photographic records consist of either sketches and drawings when the precipitate bands are not complex, tracings on paper with the object projected from an enlarger in a darkroom, or preservation of dried gel plates for later photographic copying. For tracings, a fixed magnification should be adopted; also, an auxiliary light which allows retention of dark adaptation will be found useful (20 watt red fluorescent bulb, according to Tobie[1]).

[1] J. E. Tobie, *J. Histochem. Cytochem.* **6**, 271 (1958).

several occasions if necessary, but one must prefocus the projector to allow very rapid handling of the slides to avoid temperature artifacts from heating by the condenser source-light. Further development or spreading of bands can be stopped at any time, based on experience, by placing the slides in a washing bath of saline and Merthiolate 1:10,000, to leach out unreacted proteins. The final dried preparations (14.D.2.e.ii) are stained as described in Section 14.E.1; they give an excellent photographic record. It is advisable to wash out and dry all important gels at the most significant time in their development. For this purpose, a well-planned storage file, index, and recording system should be initiated at the outset.

The choice of photographic method will depend upon the size of plates, the need for color recording as opposed to black-and-white, purpose of the illustration (notebook record or publication), and so on.

If a laboratory is already equipped for photographic work, adaptation for recording precipitates in gels, unstained or stained, is made readily. A darkroom, provided with safelights and sink will be necessary: small rooms can be adapted to darkroom purposes by means of opaque shades that run in light-tight slots.

Because visual observations of antigen–antibody reactions in gels are made by dark field illumination, we consider, first, coupling this type of illumination to recording by a suitable camera. While this method is expensive in equipment and materials (and usually in time), in the hands of experienced photographers the results can surpass all others, particularly for recording faint reactions.

However, since the opaque precipitates are usually formed in clear gels, use of the gels as "negatives" for projection or contact printing is most frequently used (Section 14.E.2.d). In most cases such a procedure is simpler, quite satisfactory, and less expensive.

The special case of radioimmunoelectrophoresis, in which radiolabeled antigen causes registration of its image on film, is discussed separately (Section 14.E.4).

b. Photography by Dark Field Illumination

i. Illuminators

Observations of gel diffusion reactions are made best by dark field: here, the specimen, positioned over a black background, is illuminated by light impinging at an angle. Several types of apparatus are possible. For observation of precipitates arising by double diffusion (Ouchterlony type), the source of light can be a circular fluorescent fixture (such as a 12-inch or an 8-inch circular tube), which offers omnidirectional light.

To examine IEA bands formed by diffusion of reagent from trough(s) cut in a rectangular slide, a light source consisting of two parallel fluorescent tubes is often preferable.

The dark field or angle lighting principle is illustrated in Fig. 1A. The subject is lighted from the side by slanting light while the eye or camera is screened from direct rays of the light source. Bands of precipitate will then be visible against a dark background. For every size and type of subject there is an angle of illumination giving maximum brightness and this angle should be determined for immune precipitates in the gel layers employed. Different gelling materials and different concentrations and thicknesses of gel vary in clarity. Some gels have high light-scattering properties: the strategy in such cases is to maximize contrast between the precipitate and the gel background rather than merely increase the brightness of illumination.

The simplest possible apparatus permitting such adjustments is best described in terms of Fig. 1A. The light source e is a 35-watt 12-inch circular fluorescent fixture, the dark field d is a round piece of black felt, velvet, or dull black construction paper, and the light screen b and subject support c is a piece of cardboard with a hole cut in it, resting on a ring-stand support by which the subject a can be raised or lowered to alter the angle of illumination. With a camera equipped with a "plus" supplementary lens positioned as shown, and Kodak Tri-X-Pan or Panatomic-X film, quite satisfactory pictures of precipitates can be obtained.* Alternatively, a similar device using two parallel fluorescent tubes can be constructed: the circular fluorescent tube offers light which is omni-directional (disadvantageous in examining IEA bands), and which is emitted at varying distances from a rectangular object.

Figures 1B, 1C, and 1D are end-view diagrams of other simple dark field viewers that can be constructed in the laboratory. Figure 1B shows a box enclosing a light-ring, or two parallel fluorescent bulbs, much as in 1A. Figure 1C makes use of an X-ray viewer, tracing stage, or the like; a device of this type provided with a diffuser cover usually of flashed opal glass is feasible only provided there is evenness of illumination (test with an incident-light meter). Figure 1D employs a single fluorescent tube with reflectors on either side of the dark field.

After selection of the light source, the proper height of the object and obliqueness of the light must be determined. An excellent initial test object consists of a 3 × 1-inch slide on which a dilute sodium chloride solution has been allowed to evaporate. This slide can be held at various heights above the source in a dark room, and strips or discs of dull black

---

* Kodak Fine Grain Positive Film is best suited for this purpose. It is currently available only in sheets (4 × 5 inches and larger) or in 35 mm in 100-foot rolls.

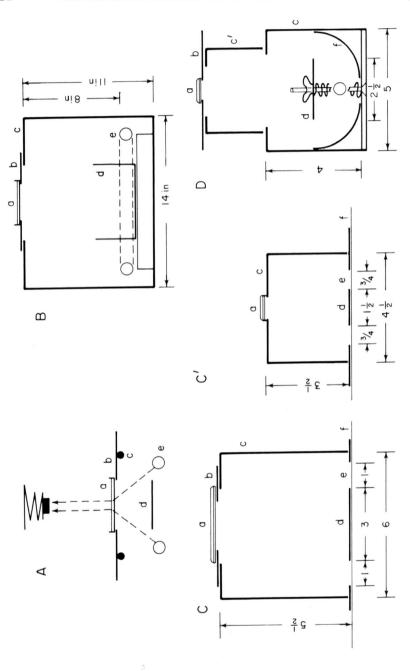

cardboard can be held in various positions over the light source to secure a satisfactory degree of angle lighting and to provide the necessary dark background. Confirmation of this position is made by substituting an actual gel slide. There may be two quite different positions and angles of illumination which can be judged satisfactory—one giving overall brightness and another providing fine delineation. One of us chooses light passing upward at an angle of 70° to 75° from vertical; the other chooses light at an angle of 50° to 60°. Once the dimensions are determined, the construction can be undertaken with confidence. In general, sharper delineation for photographic purposes as constrasted with visual examination will be secured for wet unstained antigen–antibody precipitates by using light which does not pass through a diffuser. Some adjustment of the plate adapter b should be provided: this can be accomplished by shims of dull black cardboard in Figs. 1B and 1C. In Figs. 1C and 1C′, the dark field mask d which is placed on the viewer box is dull black poster board or construction paper. The size and shape of the slits

---

Fig. 1. End-view diagrams of dark field viewers. (A) Schematic diagram of dark-field principle with camera in place: a, subject; b, mask and subject adapter; c, support; d, dark field; e, light source. (B) Fixed-dimension viewer with inbuilt 12-inch circular fluorescent light. The enclosure box is painted dull black inside and serves as the subject support c. The lighting fixture e is mounted permanently in the box. The dark field screen d is one end of a No. 10 (6-inch diameter) food tin, cut off to give 3 inch sides, and painted dull black inside and out—it can be positioned bottom up or bottom down whichever gives the best dark-field view. The dimensions given provide illumination angles between 50° and 60°, but they could be adapted to an 8-inch lighting fixture if a smaller unit is desired. (C and C′) Dark-field viewing system making use of diffused light viewer (e.g., X-ray). A dark-field mask d is cut from black poster cardboard or construction paper with light slits e of indicated width and of any necessary length. The mask is placed on the lighted glass surface f. The enclosure support c for the larger viewer (C) is the lid of a cardboard gift box with a 3-inch wide opening centered in the top and painted dull black inside. Various subject adapters b can be cut from stiff cardboard, or a 5×7 inch photographic glass plate can be used to cover the opening. The subject a shown in (C) represents a large immunoelectrophoresis plate. The smaller version (C′) is used for microimmuno-electrophoresis slides and is shown without an adapter, although with different mask patterns a larger opening and adapters could be useful. The support c is the lid of a $3\frac{1}{4} \times 4$-inch Kodak projection slide package. The dimension given for both (C) and (C′) provide illumination angles between 65° and 75° (compare footnote, page 326). (D) Single lamp reflector viewer with adjustable dark field. The basic unit consists of a sturdy housing c mounted on a bakelite or plastic base. The light source e is a 15-Watt $8 \times \frac{1}{2}$-inch fluorescent tube. The reflectors f are of 2-inch radius quarter-round polished metal. The variable level dark-field plate d is supported by a spring and wing nut on a machine screw at each end through the base. The dimensions given for the basic unit provide illumination angles of 50° to 60° about the center of the opening. If greater angles are desired, the subject a and its adapter b can be raised by elevator supports c′ of whatever height required.

cut in the mask determines the illumination of the object. The dimensions shown provide illumination angles of about 70°. The subject a can be at constant elevation supported by a plate adapter b on an inverted box c serving as a screen. For the large viewer (Fig. 1C), several adapters and masks can be cut for different sizes of plates or for different purposes. The smaller viewer (Fig. 1C′) is for routine work with microslides.* With viewers of this type, equalization of the two parallel light sources can usually be achieved by repositioning the dark field mask so that the light slits are over areas of the diffuser receiving incident light of the same intensity, quality, and angle.

ii. Cameras

Any camera that can be fitted for close-up work can be used, either with a supplementary plus lens or an extension ring between camera body and lens. Through-the-lens focusing is desirable. Some workers choose to record on 36-exposure 35-mm roll film, using high contrast films as described below. The resulting negatives after development are enlarged to the desired size in a second operation. View cameras fitted with sheet film holders (4 × 5-inch size) offer some advantage in individual control in processing; simple contact printing becomes possible for the second operation.

* A simple device for observations of IEA bands on 25 × 75 mm slides, illustrated here, consists of a Thermolyne viewing box, Model LL-6515, and an altered card-

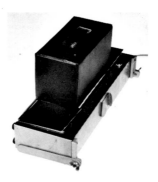

board storage box of the type sold for filing 4 × 6-inch cards (6⅜ × 3¼ × 4¾-inches high). The height is reduced to 90 mm by a complete incision just below the hinged lid; the bottom of the box, inverted, becomes the object carrier by cutting out a central rectangular section 60 × 22 mm in size. All interior and cut surfaces are blackened by one or more coats of Kodak Brushing Lacquer No. 4 Dull Black. In use, a dull black strip of cardboard 37 mm wide is centered over the plastic diffuser to serve as the mask, and the box support is placed over the mask so that equal slits of illumination enter the box. The slide, resting over the rectangular opening, is illuminated by light passing upward from each side at an angle of 70° to 75° from the vertical position. Viewing is done in a partially darkened room.

Polaroid cameras of types accepting only roll film, while they are convenient for notebook records, are not recommended for publication-quality prints. Polaroid roll films are difficult to control for consistent tone qualities in prints. If subjects differ slightly, it may take several exposures each to obtain satisfactory prints. Moreover, it should be noted that simple Polaroid camera set-ups are not the most suitable for recording results of microdiffusion or microimmunoelectrophoresis patterns that will require enlargement for proper examination. Two solutions to this problem are possible. A cut film, Type 55 PN ("positive–negative") ASA50, 4 × 5 inches, is available which yields a positive print and a separate negative of good quality. While this shares the same problems of control found with other Polaroid films, it is possible to compensate somewhat in the enlarging and printing procedures. PN film negatives are not high contrast and they do require additional processing. Thus far, PN films are not available in rolls. Alternatively, although the quality of the print will not be satisfactory for publication purposes, Polaroid positive transparency rolls (3¼ × 4-inch only) can be used to copy (as in rapid preparation of lantern slides) and to make enlargements (film 46 L is used for continuous tone and 146 L for line work only).

iii. Professional Illuminator-Camera Apparatus

To solve the problem mentioned above and to meet the variety of needs in the photographic laboratory, more elaborately planned apparatus is needed. Ideal apparatus should be adaptable to both reflected and transmitted illumination, and dark- and bright-field effects should be obtainable. Individual light sources must be adjustable as to intensity, direction, and distance. In addition it is wise to use a view camera to allow single film exposure and to facilitate controlled results.

The standard MP-3 Polaroid Industrial View Camera can be equipped with a specially designed illumination box (Fig. 2). A 14 × 17-inch hole (dimensions of standard X-ray film) is cut in the hardwood base of the MP-3 and routed to support a clear glass plate or an opal glass diffuser plate and/or with black masking templates. The distance between lights and object, and between object and opaque disc(s) is variable at will. Black masking templates carried on the clear glass plate are used for unstained, wet gels; the opal diffuser and Wratten filters are used for stained, dyed precipitates. The versatility of this illuminator system and the precision of its performance with all types and sizes of subject have fully justified the construction. Few laboratories will have access to such a professional model.

A metal cabinet with inbuilt staging area, illuminator, and camera—accepting Polaroid Type 107 Film Pack or Kodak TX 515 film pack—has been introduced* to allow photography of routine laboratory records

* Cordis Laboratories, Miami, Florida.

at magnifications of 0.9 or 1.9 ×. The higher magnification is judged serviceable for routine photography of antigen–antibody bands for notebook records; micro-Ouchterlony reactions, in contrast, are rather well recorded.

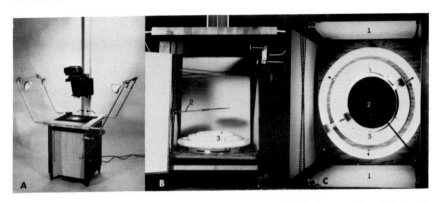

FIG. 2. Professional lighting unit for scientific and medical photography. (A) Front view of MP3 Polaroid Industrial View Camera XL Model with modified baseboard shown attached to specially designed "Illumination Cabinet." (B) Front view of "Illumination Cabinet" with door opened; note the aluminum foil reflecting surfaces appearing as white. (Inside dimensions, 21 × 19 × 24 inches high.) 1, Control handle for adjusting height of lamp unit 3; 2, holder for dark field discs, adjustable vertically; 3, illumination unit containing 3 circular fluorescent lamps and reflector (8½-, 12-, and 16-inch tubes). (C) Top view of Illumination Cabinet, door to the right, showing: 1, opening of 35 × 43-cm (14 × 17-inch) cut in baseboard of MP3 unit; 2, dark-field disc holder, with one of several black discs on disc holder; 3, illumination unit as in (B, 3) immediately above.

The unit was designed by Mr. Henrik Boudakian of The Rockefeller University, Graphic Services Department.

iv. Exposure, Materials, and Processing

(a) *Exposure.* Exposure is determined largely empirically according to the visual effect desired. The amount of oblique light which is refracted by the fine, opaque precipitates is small, hence exposure meters must be highly sensitive even to suggest the range of probable exposures. The final result reflects intensity of the light source and its position in relation to the subject.

Although the light intensity and the time of exposure are equivalent variables, apart from minor adjustments, it is to be noted that in "dark-field" illumination the practice of compensating for increases in one variable by decreases in the other seldom gives equivalent results. For example, twice the light intensity with half the exposure time may lead to a loss of fine detail because of excessive light scattering or "glare" by a dark-field subject. This particularly applies to complex patterns of precipitates in gels and even more so when the gel background is not perfectly clear. It is therefore desirable to have a variable rheostat on tungsten light sources used with black and white films even with the simpler laboratory setups described above. In practice, however, the proper exposure range will soon be determined with precision when a particular apparatus is employed repeatedly for photography.* Light intensity and exposure time should be worked out in the range of aperture settings between f/11 and f/16.

With the modified MP-3 apparatus (Fig. 2), the circular fluorescent fixtures are raised or lowered by a chain mechanism while optical effects on the subject are observed in the ground-glass view screen of the camera. The dark-field disc may also be moved up or down to achieve the best resolution of adjacent bands or spots. The size of the gel plate or subject matter determines the diameter and elevation of the disc used. Most of these or equivalent adjustments can be made with the simpler apparatus shown in Figs. 1C or 1D.†

(b) *Materials.* For rendering fine detail in wet unstained IEA plates, Kodak Fine Grain Positive Film (ASA 10, in tungsten light) has been found most satisfactory; it is available also in 35 mm rolls. Typical exposure times at f/16 would be in the 4- to 10-second range, depending upon the subject brightness. The fact that this film is "color blind" permits development by inspection to bring out desired effects; the film must be developed in full darkness for 3 minutes and can then be inspected at intervals under a Wratten series 2 (dark red) safelight.‡ Typical development time at 20° is 6 to 9 minutes in Kodak D-19 developer.

For photography of stained and dried slides, see Subsections c and d.

(c) *Printing.* The printing of negatives is the point in the process where the most dramatic effects can be achieved. The reason for this, and the reason that producing a photographic negative is a preferred first step of professionals trying to render precipitates in gels, is that the range of tone and the retained detail can be used selectively in printing. In printing on paper, neither detail nor range of contrasts can be increased over that

---

* Best definition is seen when the finished, dry print presents a background just slightly gray rather than fully black. Proper development is not immediately apparent under safelight illumination, where prints appear darker than in the finished state. Accordingly, the temperature of developer and a fixed time of development become important factors in processing exposed paper.

† Only the modified MP-3 apparatus resolved well the bands forming in agar within Cordis plastic immunodiffusion plates, which present multiple reflective surfaces. The circular fluorescent fixture was dropped to the base of the cabinet, the dark-field disc was replaced with a similar disc of polished metal, and the disc was turned empirically to an angle of about 35° from horizontal. The polished metal disc picked up bounce-light from the sides of the box and revealed the bands sharply. (Information by courtesy of Mr. Henrik Boudakian.)

‡ With panchromatic camera films, inspection during development is not possible.

in the negative. But by choosing among the more contrasty papers (grades 4 to 6) and experimenting with exposure and developing times, certain details can be emphasized. When high-contrast negatives are used, the best prints in terms of detail are obtained with printing papers of grades 2 or 3. The exposure and development of prints is described below in Subsection d.

(d) *Retouching.* Where the background is black or very dark on negatives made on high-contrast films, minor dirt spots, scratches, and artifacts can be eliminated by using opaque spotting colors such as Marabu (a water-base suspension which is removable). The transparent spotting colors, such as Spotone, come in many tones and are used for darkening. The latter are not removable, and their use on negatives is risky. Retouching is highly desirable for prints which are to be reproduced for publication or for projection slides. Opaque spotting colors which can be blended to achieve any tone are recommended. Spotting pencils, e.g., Wolff carbon pencils, can be used to darken small areas or spots, but they are used only on matte finishes.

It should be emphasized that retouching is primarily a cosmetic technique and should not be considered an alternative to careful laboratory procedure. Drawings rather than retouched photographs should be submitted with a manuscript when gels are distorted or cracked, when there is excessive background dirt, or when bands of precipitate are distorted by overflow of reagents. Retouching should not be used for intensification or obliteration of precipitate bands. Here also, drawings are preferred, as they are clearly recognized as interpretations and not primary records.

Yet reactions are sometimes faint, and a publishable photograph of the results is required. Contrast may be increased by printing the gel plate as negative on a contrasty film to produce a transparent positive, which in turn is reprinted on contrasty film. This "reprinted" negative may then give on paper a print that would be suitable for reproduction.

c. PHOTOGRAPHY ON FILM BY BRIGHT FIELD ILLUMINATION (STAINED SLIDES)

For delineation of dried, stained slides and plates in black and white photography, different films and processing are required. The same illumination equipment can be employed, however, usually by placing an opal glass or plastic diffuser plate over the light source. (For evenness of bright field, it may be necessary to remove the dark-field disc.) In bright field photography a light meter can be very helpful in determining exposure conditions, particularly when used as an incident-light meter moved over the object area. The most exacting test consists of placing the camera in the intended position over the device, with the light source turned on, and flashing a film (as at $1/500$ sec at f/22). Upon development, such a test film will show, as irregular dense areas of silver grains, any "hot spots" in the illumination. There are several causes of hot spots: poorly positioned lamps as in an X-ray viewing box; insufficient application of the dull black coating inside of the device to assure nonreflective surfaces; reflectors—in the case of parallel lamps—which are unlike either in brightness or in curvature; a box which is too shallow to allow proper diffusion of light rays by the flashed opal glass covering sheet. Faults of this type should become apparent, and repairs can be effected by inserting sections of white cardboard, aluminum foil and the like beneath the bulbs and conforming suitably the curvature of these reflectance materials.

When the subject is a transparent dried gel with stained precipitates entrapped, it is placed directly on the diffuser plate. Peripheral light is excluded by laying masks around the subject. Since the surfaces of dried gels are rough, it is usually wise to wet the surface and superimpose a cover glass before photography. The surface of the slide is wetted; lint which may have been deposited from filter paper during drying is rubbed away with a fingertip; the slide and its intended coverslip (such as No. 1 thickness, 22 × 40 mm or longer), or even another 3 × 1-inch slide, are immersed beneath the surface of water containing a trace of detergent, as Photoflo; the coverslip is brought over the agar film and mated with exclusion of bubbles. The glass–agar–water–glass sandwich is removed, the lower and upper surfaces are carefully dried, and the sandwich is photographed. The procedure has the further advantage of filling the original wells and avoiding reflection images.

Because of the wide range of colored precipitates (see Section 14.E.1), best results will be obtained with panchromatic films coupled with appropriate filters. Suitable films for rendering dark precipitate bands on white background are: Versapan (ASA 125 in tungsten light), or Kodak Panatomic-X (ASA 32 in tungsten light for roll film), or Kodak Plus-X Pan (ASA 125 in tungsten light). Green filters (Wratten 58 or X-2) are used to enhance registration of red dyes, and an orange filter (Wratten No. 22) is employed when blue dye is present. Kodak D-76 is a typical developer for continuous tone photography.

Photography in black and white of dry, stained slides by projection of image upon paper is discussed in Subsection E.2.d.

For color photography, fluorescent bulb illuminators are far from ideal; yet experienced professional operators can usually secure satisfactory results with stained gels. The surest color rendition will occur when light of 3200°K "temperature" is used. Photo-ECT lamps, 120 volts and 500 watts, supplied with 120 volts by passing the current through a Powerstat or Variac (monitored by a voltmeter) represent a stable source of 3200°K light. It is suited to Type B color materials and is adapted to Type A (3400°K) emulsions by interposing an 82A filter.

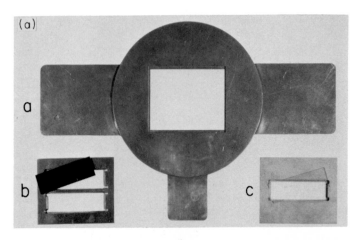

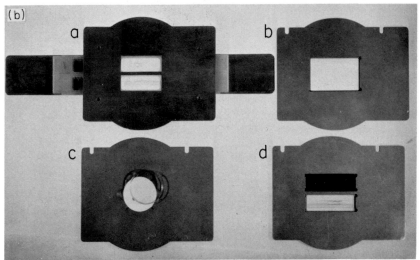

FIG. 3.(a) Adapter for direct projection of gel plates with Omega B8 enlarger. Mask a holds $3\frac{1}{4}$ × 4-inch lantern slide plates or inserts b or c. Insert mask b accepts 1 or 2 slides of 25 × 75 mm, or a black Lucite accessory mask. Insert mask c has a double-depth well with a cemented glass bottom for photography of microscope slides under water. (b) Adapters for direct projection of gel plates with Omega D2 Enlarger, with centering slots for positioning over the condenser. Support mask a is for photographing wet gels by pairs held in 6-slide frames (Gelman); material is $\frac{1}{8}$ inch aluminum, the upper and lower sheets being separated $\frac{5}{16}$ inch by spacer strips which also serve as guides for the slide frame. Mask b is for 3 × 2-inch (75 × 50 mm) glass slides. Mask c is to suspend 50-mm plastic petri dishes by means of the cleats molded on the dish; stock is $\frac{1}{8}$ inch (6.5 mm) aluminum. Mask d is similar to b in Fig. 3A.

d. DIRECT PROTECTION OF GEL PLATES UPON BROMIDE PRINTING PAPER

Excellent prints at ca. 3 × enlargement can be made by direct projection printing from an enlarger upon high-contrast, glossy single weight paper such as Kodabromide No. 5 or Agfa Brovira grade 6, using either unstained or stained antigen–antibody immunodiffusion lines (Ouchterlony or IEA) developed in relatively thin layers (0.8 to 2.5 mm) of clear agar. Immunodiffusion conducted in small plastic petri dishes where agar layers are relatively thick demands especially clear agar; for this purpose, the Allison and Humphrey buffer containing EDTA (see Vol. II, Appendix II.8, Buffer No. 36) is highly recommended. A suitable holder to support the slide or petri dish at the "film plane" of the enlarger is necessary (Figs. 3A and 3B).

The following description dealing with two particular enlargers is representative and may serve as a general guide; each worker must adapt the procedure to the use of other equipment. Further, practical exposures must be arrived at by trial and error until the worker is fully familiar with the equipment and degree of definition. Enlarger size is determined by the ability to photograph, for example, the entirety of a 50 × 75-mm (2 × 3-inch) slide. The darkroom should be provided with suitable safelights such as Kodak series OA (yellow-green) or Dupont S-55X (brownish).

One of the authors uses an Omega D2 enlarger, lamphouse type D of condenser-type lamp source, equipped with a Wollensak Graphic Raptar lens of 5⅜ inches (138 mm) focal length, f/4.5. Timing is done conveniently by a Time-O-Lite Model M-59 control (Industrial Timer Corporation, Parsippany, New Jersey). The object carrier (Fig. 3B) suspends the slide 66.6 cm above the easel of the enlarger, distance from lens to easel being 47 cm when magnification of 2.8 × is desired.* A piece of 5 × 7 single-weight printing paper is placed on the easel upside down, and the specimen is focused in the dark critically, with the enlarger lens stopped down as far as possible. Critical focusing is made conveniently with an enlarger focusing sight ("Magna Sight," Bestwell Optical Instrument Company, 209 Beverly Road, Brooklyn, New York), placed in the path of the projected image. The image is intercepted and brought to focus on the mirror of the sight with the projector lens wide open. The

---

* Corresponding data for the Omega B8 enlarger with 4¾-inch (120 mm) condensers and Wollensak Enlarging Raptar lens of 2½ inches (90 mm) focal length, f/4.5, are as follows for 2.8 × enlargements: object carrier 45 cm above the easel, distance from lens to easel, 33 cm.

lens is then stopped down to the desired aperture and the focusing light is turned off. A sheet of glossy printing paper is placed on the easel, replacing the dummy spacer sheet. A penciled notation of the specimen is written *lightly* on the reverse side of the paper.

For 25 × 75 mm (1 × 3 inch) slides used in immunodiffusion, exposure at f/22 for 9 seconds is usually optimal with unstained slides*; thicker agar in petri dishes requires slightly longer exposure. Exposure is accomplished by the setting of the timing device. Exposed paper may be placed inside a black photo envelope or an empty discarded printing-paper box, if development is to be delayed. Exposed sheets can be held in a paper safe for a week or more before development; obviously it is unsafe to delay development and lose the opportunity of correcting errors unless all exposure conditions are held constant and are well understood.

Stained slides of 3 × 2 inches or 3 × 1 inches are handled in the same way. Surface irregularities of dried agar can present problems, particularly when a condenser type enlarger—the most efficient for fine detail—is used. The problem is minimized, but with loss of some fine detail and sharpness of image, when an enlarger with a diffused light source, e.g., Omegalite B, is used. The surface of the slide is first wetted and all lint is gently removed by rubbing with the finger. A special well in a metal washing frame with cemented glass bottom has been employed (Fig. 3C), sufficiently deep to allow covering the stained slide with water. Or the slide may be immersed under water and a second slide or large coverslip mated to it, the sandwich being wiped dry on top and bottom. Care must be taken lest water fall and dry on the condenser lens.

Depending on the dye used and transparency of the gel, stained slides may require some alteration in exposure from that used with wet, unstained slides.

Different stains give different photographic results depending on the intensity of staining and the particular color imparted. Faint reactions may be almost transparent after slides are dried, and successful registry may depend on the insensitivity of the printing emulsion to the color of the stain. In such cases red (Ponceau R, or Azocarmine) or green (Light Green, or Bromphenol Blue—acid reaction) stains may be a better choice than blue (Amido Black, or Coomasie Blue). Staining procedures are described in Sections 14.E.1 and 14.D.2.c.*viii*. For consistent or comparable results from one experiment to another, it is important that both the staining *and* the destaining of background be rigorously standardized. Some stains dissociate from precipitates during destaining more readily than others, and more readily from some proteins than from others.

* See footnote * on page 329.

e. DIRECT PROJECTION OF MICRO-DOUBLE DIFFUSION (PREER) TUBES

The system developed by Preer (Section 14.C.7) utilizes a 6-mm column of soft agar for development of antigen–antibody bands. Visual examination is made by angled light; yet photography is best carried out by projection from an enlarger on Kodabromide 5 or Agfa grade 6 bromide papers. Owing to the small dimension of the agar column (6 mm × 1.8 mm) within a 4 cm × 3 mm OD tube the photographic enlarger should be arranged for 10× enlargement. For this purpose, an enlarger intended for 35 mm film should be chosen since the angle of emitted light is broader than in the case of standard enlargers. We have used quite successfully a Leitz Focomat 1C enlarger, which has a "condenser-diffuser" light source and a Focotar projection lens 1:4.5, 5 cm. The tubes are laid horizontally on a suitable flat holder, one at a time, and focused critically by means of a "Magna Sight" enlarger focusing sight. Typical exposures with this projector using Kodabromide No. 5 have averaged 15 seconds at f/11 (Fig. 4).

f. LARGE PLATES: REGISTRATION ON FILM AND ON BROMIDE PAPER (Contact Printing)

Object plates greater in size than 3 × 3 inches (75 × 75 mm) present some special problems in recording to the average worker who does not have access to professional photo equipment such as is described in Subsection b.*iii.*

i. Registration on Film Negatives

Cameras that use film larger than 35 mm rolls are recommended. When the subject is a large (macro) IEA plate, it is possible to arrange photography by dark field illumination as in Subsection b—the best record for publication—or bright-field photography as in Subsection c, or contact printing, as described below. For bright-field photography, the plate is placed on the backlighted diffuser plate and peripheral light is excluded by placing masks. For the final photograph made upon full development of the bands, wells and troughs should be filled to brimming with water to prevent refraction or reflection images from the inner surface of the wells. The final photograph of very large subjects, up to the areas of 20 × 17 cm, can be made advantageously under water within a Kodak Duroflex developing tray (8 × 10 inches, 20 × 50 cm) having most of the bottom replaced by a sheet of clear $\frac{1}{16}$-inch Lucite cemented to it. The tray, elevated at the ends by narrow strips of felt that serve to prevent scratching of the Lucite, is placed on a light box proved to emit even illumination. Unused areas of the light box are screened suitably so that stray light does not affect the camera.

The same films are used, namely, Kodak Fine Grain Positive Film, for line drawings and fine antigen–antibody bands, or panchromatic films for stained slides as described in Subsection c.

Fig. 4. Preer double-diffusion tube (6 mm × 1.8 mm agar) photographed at 10 × magnification on Kodabromide No. 5 paper, courtesy of Dr. Huminori Kawata. See text.

ii. *Contact Registration on Sensitized Paper*

Another quite satisfactory method with large plates consists in placing the plate directly on photographic projection paper of grades 5 or 6 in a darkroom and exposing by a suitably weak tungsten light. An enlarger easel can be used as support, and exposure effected by brief exposure from the enlarger light with lens stopped down to f/22. Or if the glass plate is not too thick and there are no nearby reflecting surfaces, a 25 watt unfrosted and unshaded incandescent bulb placed 60 to 80 cm above the plate can be used for the exposure.

The objective is to approach "point source" illumination which makes for more discrete shadows of precipitates and smaller highlights from reflecting surfaces.   If the reagent wells are empty at the time of photography, they should be filled to brimming with water to reduce reflections. When the experiment is to be terminated, photography under water is recommended in order to eliminate surface artifacts. Developing trays of red, yellow, or black plastic can be used, water coming from a standing container; wetted photo paper is slipped under the immersed plates in such manner as not to trap or to produce bubbles. Floating dust and bubbles must be removed from the surface of the water. Fresh tap water contains too much dissolved air and will cause bubbles on the surface.

While the contact method can be used for microdiffusion techniques, e.g., on 25 × 75 mm slides, there is little use in reproducing the small patterns without enlargement.

g. Processing of Photographic Printing Paper

i. Development

Four 8 × 10 trays, for example Kodak Duraflex trays, are arranged as usual in the darkroom, with printing tongs placed by each.   The first tray serves to hold a 6 × 8 inch tray in which developer is poured (the smaller tray is rocked during development); cool water and a few ice cubes are placed in the larger tray. A thermometer is immersed in the developer to check the temperature (20° is desirable). A suitable developer is Kodak Paper Developer D-72,* the same as Dupont 55-D, diluted with 2 parts of water (90 ml of stock developer plus 180 ml of cold water for the 6 × 8 inch tray).

The second tray contains an acetic acid stopbath (Kodak SB-la), made by diluting 34 ml of glacial acetic acid (*caution:* burns skin) or 125 ml of 28% acetic acid to a volume of 1 liter.

The third tray contains the fixing bath (hypo and hardener),† while the fourth tray, placed in the sink, contains wash water kept close to 20° to 25°. (Experts use two successive baths of hypo and hardener;

---

* This is sold commercially as Dektol (Eastman) or Vividol (GAF) or "55D All-Purpose Developer" (Dupont). Store in the refrigerator in glass bottles filled to the neck. Discard when the solution acquires a yellow or brown color.

† Fixing bath with hardener added has a relatively short shelf life. We prefer to store separately 30% sodium thiosulfate ("hypo") and Kodak fixing bath F-6. The two solutions are blended for use (800 ml of 30% hypo and—added slowly with stirring— 200 ml of cool F-6); unused portions of the mixture are stored and are usable as long as precipitate does not form. Used hypo is stored separately; used hypo remaining after paper development must be used only for paper and is stored separately from hypo which has been used for film development. The capacity of this fixative is 60 sheets of 5 × 7-inch paper per quart.

the second bath, fresh for each set of prints, becomes the first bath for the following set of prints.)

The exposed sheets are immersed individually into the developer in the 6 × 8-inch tray, the tray being tilted periodically as the image appears. With correct exposure, the image appears after about 10 seconds and is fully developed by 60 to 75 seconds (fullest tonal scale). Overexposure, indicated by the requirement for using shorter development times, is never advantageous; detail is lost. In a few instances, shorter than normal exposures, requiring longer development than 75 seconds, can be useful for registering fine detail. The sheet is then drained briefly by touching the tray and is transferred upside down into the stopbath. After 15 to 30 seconds, the sheets are lifted, drained, and transferred into the hypo bath. As prints accumulate in the hypo bath, they are "handled" by being moved from top to bottom of the tray. After fixation, which is completed within 20 minutes (according to the type of fixative used), prints are transferred to water and washed thoroughly with several changes of water; a final addition of Kodak Hypo Clearing Agent concentrate (0.5 lb, 225 gm, in 1.9 liters of water) to the rinse water (1:4) is made for a few minutes; the rinse is discarded and the papers are washed for a minimum of 30 minutes before drying.

Prints that exhibit a mottled or streaked background indicate over- or underexposure, not improper development as might be expected (providing, of course, that the paper has been kept *fully immersed* in the developer). Occasionally two gel slides that appear identical to the eye do not record identically on film, probably owing to slight color differences.

ii. Drying

Various dryers for glossy paper are available. The choice will depend on the anticipated volume of output.* Prints are soaked for 5 to 10 minutes in a bath such as Flexogloss Solution (General Aniline and Film Corporation, New York, New York). They are then drained well and laid on the ferrotype plate, glossy surface downward. The single layer of developed prints is covered with large sheets of *photographic* blotting paper (19 × 24 inches) and excess moisture is removed by running a squeegee over the blotting paper. The prints are then dried according to the type of dryer employed.

Dried prints curl away from the ferrotype plate and may retain a slight curl. Severe curl can usually be reduced by drying at a lower temperature. If a print straightening apparatus is used, all prints to be meas-

---

* A dryer suitable for moderate laboratory work loads is the Rexo Print Dryer Model 66 (Burke and James, Inc., Chicago, Illinois).

ured or compared must be passed through the straightener in the same orientation since these devices stretch the prints slightly in one direction.

iii. Mounting

Identification, in the form of *light* pencil marks on the back of the print, will persist during processing and drying. The information is carried to the unexposed margin of the glossy surface by writing with India ink (such as Pelikan, Günther Wagner, Germany) or with a fine-tipped flowbrush using toluol-solvent ink. Sheets of Kodak Dry Mounting Tissue as large as the prints, say 5 × 7 inches, are tacked at two or three points to the backs of the prints by a quick stroke with a tacking iron or the tip of a flatiron. The prints with attached mounting tissue are trimmed on a cutting board before placement on the final support sheet so that the margins of print and mounting tissue coincide. We find $8\frac{1}{2}$ × 11 inch plain white *ledger* paper to be suitable since it is sufficiently stiff to avoid curling when prints are affixed. Final mounting is done by dry heat transmitted through the print to the mounting sheet. For small-scale work, 2 sheets of onion skin paper are placed over the print and 2 sheets below it, and heat is impressed with a flatiron at low setting. Too much heat will discolor the print; with insufficient heat, partial attachment will occur and the print will later separate. The corners should be tested by being bent slightly to determine firmness of adherence. Whenever the facility is available, dry mounting press is recommended.

3. INTERFEROMETRY FOR ANALYSIS
OF ANTIGEN–ANTIBODY REACTIONS IN GELS*

The principle involved in the use of interferometry for the analysis of antigen–antibody reactions in gels is that the accumulation of an antigen–antibody complex is accompanied by a localized increase in optical density, and therefore an increase in the optical path, which can be detected with great sensitivity and measured using an optical interference system of the Fabry–Pérot type.[1]

The method can be used qualitatively for resolving a large number of closely packed precipitin bands, and quantitatively for less complex systems of bands.[2] With the Fabry-Pérot system interference fringes are

---

* Section 14.E.3 was contributed by G. C. Easty.

[1] E. J. Ambrose, *J. Sci. Instr.* **25**, 134 (1948).
[2] G. C. Easty and E. J. Ambrose, *J. Exptl. Biol.* **34**, 60 (1957).

produced where each fringe is a contour line of constant optical path. Where an antigen–antibody reaction takes place an inflexion or peak in the fringes is observed, which is a measure of the quantity of complex present.

a. OPTICAL CELL

The interference system consists of two 6.3 mm (0.25 inch) thick glass plates 52 × 37 mm (2 × 1.5 inches), each ground optically flat on one surface, which is silvered *in vacuo* to give about 10% transmission of white light. The thin silver films are protected by thin coverslips held in contact with the silver films by a thin layer of immersion oil, and sealed around the edges with a cement such as a cold-setting epoxy resin. The two plates, with their silvered surfaces facing each other, are placed horizontally with two sponge rubber spacers about 4 mm thick between them in a rigid metal framework. The framework has four fine-thread vertical screws which can be screwed down on to the four corners of the uppermost plate. This arrangement permits the adjustment of the angle between the plates and controls the spacing between the interference fringes. The plates are adjusted by means of the screws until they are almost parallel. The metal frame carrying the plates is placed on the stage of a low power microscope and illuminated from beneath by a beam of monochromatic light obtained from a low-pressure mercury vapor lamp using a didymium filter. The angle of incidence of the monochromatic light, on which the sharpness of the interference fringes is very dependent, is adjusted by means of a horizontally movable pinhole. The size of the pinhole is important in controlling the sharpness and contrast of the fringes, and it is best made by piercing a thin sheet of copper with a fine tapering needle. The optimum size of the pinhole, which will depend on the dimensions of the optical system, the object and the light intensity, is best found empirically by gradually increasing its size until a suitable compromise between intensity of illumination and sharpness of the fringes is found.

b. DIFFUSION CELL

The gel-diffusions must be carried out in tubes of rectangular cross section of constant dimensions. In practice, quite satisfactory tubes can be made from three microscope slides which are free of gross optical flaws. One slide is split along its length, using a diamond, into halves which are used as spacers, with the other two slides forming upper and lower surfaces. Thus a flat tube, or cell, is formed about 3 to 4 mm wide, 1 mm deep, and 7 cm long. The joints between the slides are sealed by dipping the edges of the cell, held firmly in a bulldog clip, into a dish containing a mixture of soft petrolatum and paraffin wax (1:1). Care must be taken that the wax mixture does not enter the central channel as it is not readily wetted by gelatin or agar gel, and leakage of the reactants along the gel–glass interface may occur with consequent distortion of the pattern of precipitin bands. More permanent cells can be made using epoxy resins as cements.

Molten gelatin or agar is injected into the tube using a hypodermic syringe fitted with an 18-gauge needle, leaving a space at either end for the antigen and antibody solutions. When the gel is set the solutions are introduced into the spaces at either end and sealed with the wax mixture, so that the whole tube is watertight and there is no loss of water by evaporation. Gelatin wets the glass well and forms a good seal, but has other well known disadvantages for gel-diffusion work. Agar undergoes syneresis on setting, and leakage can often occur along one or more of the agar–glass interfaces. The possibility of leakage can be avoided in ordinary gel diffusion work by drying a film of agar gel on the glass before adding the diffusion gel. Unfortunately, in this system this procedure often results in optical inhomogeneities which, although not apparent to the naked eye, are quite conspicuous in the interference system. In practice, the best procedure is to allow the agar to set, then add a little molten gelatin which seals any leaks, removing excess gelatin by draining on to filter papers.

c. ANALYSIS

When the gel-diffusion cell is ready for examination, it is placed between the optically flat plates of the optical cell with a film of immersion oil between the cell and the plates. The interference fringes are produced by adjusting the angle between the plates and the position of the pinhole controlling the angle of incident light, and may be photographed or reproduced with a camera lucida. The region of antigen–antibody reaction appears as a peak in the fringes, which are generally adjusted to run parallel with the length of the diffusion channel. The quantity of complex is directly proportional to the area under the peak and can be calculated from Eq. (1):

$$\frac{\lambda w}{2\alpha} \int_{l_1}^{l_2} n_c \, dl \tag{1}$$

where λ is the wavelength of the light (mercury green), w is the width of the channel in centimeters, α is the specific protein refractive index increment (0.00185 for most proteins), and $\int_{l_1}^{l_2} n_e \, dl$ is the area measured under the peak (Fig. 1) expressed in fringe displacement along the length of the channel. The quantity n_e is the fringe shift relative to the medium on either side of the band, and l_1, l_2 are the extreme edges of the band, in centimeters.

One major difficulty in applying this method is that once a dense precipitate is formed it does not contribute to the refractive index to the

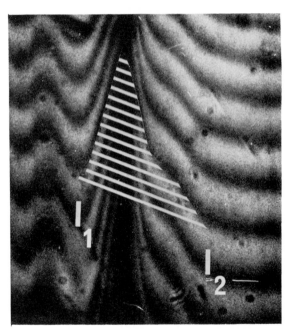

Fig. 1. Interference fringes showing several peaks or inflexions due to the formation of antigen–antibody complexes. The shaded area under one peak, from l_1 to l_2, is proportional to the quantity of complex present.

extent that it would if the same quantity of complex were present in a less densely aggregated form. This difficulty may be overcome by dissolving the precipitate with dilute alkali or reagents such as sodium dodecyl sulfate. As the antigen–antibody complex is dissolved, it slowly diffuses away from its original site, forming a peak which becomes more broad and shallow as diffusion proceeds. The area under the peak can be measured at any stage, but for greatest accuracy it should be measured as soon as a single fringe can be traced through the peak from one side to the other

4. AUTORADIOGRAPHY OF
ANTIGEN–ANTIBODY REACTIONS IN GELS*†

a. INTRODUCTION

A double diffusion reaction concentrates the antigen and antibody in a discrete band in the gel. The gel can be washed free of unreacted material, and dried down to a transparent film on the plate without distorting the pattern of antigen–antibody precipitates. This also further concentrates the reactants (see General Procedures, Section c). If either reactant is isotopically labeled or has a radioactive substance bound to it, the pattern of immune precipitation can be revealed by exposure of a photographic emulsion, film, or plate placed in contact with the dried gel layer (see General Principles, Section b and Appendix I for details).

Autoradiography of immune precipitation patterns in agar gel can be useful in various types of experiments.[1,2] Since autoradiography is usually a more sensitive method than staining procedures for visualization of precipitin bands, faint reactions that would otherwise escape attention can be detected.‡ Thus, purification of labeled antigens or antibodies could be monitored by autoradiography of agar gel patterns often permitting detection of unsuspected impurities.

Another general application may be the study of the nature of the interaction between antigen and antibody in agar gel and the test of the principle of the specific barrier function of immunological precipitation lines. Also, the special binding properties (or carrier functions) of serum or tissue proteins can be demonstrated by the coprecipitation of the protein and isotopically-labeled compounds such as metal ions, hormones, vitamins, or other proteins. When such studies involve mixtures of proteins, autoradiography of immunoelectrophoretic patterns can be of great help

* Section 14.E.4 was contributed by G. J. Thorbecke, G. M. Hochwald, and C. A. Williams.

† Supported by Grants Nos. AI-3076 and NB05024 from the United States Public Health Service. G.J.T. is the recipient of Career Development Award No. 5-K3-GM-15522; G.M.H. was the recipient of Career Development Award No. K3-NB-18,023.
[1] R. Patterson, *J. Lab. Clin. Med.* **57**, 657 (1961).
[2] J. Rejnek and T. Bednarik, *Clin. Chim. Acta* **5**, 250 (1960).
‡ Patterson[1] obtained greater than tenfold increase in sensitivity over ordinary staining procedures, resulting in detection of 0.2 μg of ^{131}I-labeled bovine serum albumin N/milliliter in Ouchterlony plates.

in identifying the impurity in a preparation or in characterizing the binding protein.*

Another major application for radioimmunoelectrophoresis is in the study of protein synthesis. Isotopically labeled macromolecules produced by tissues cultured in the presence of a radioactive precursor can be demonstrated with a high degree of sensitivity. Such studies may help identify tissular origins of certain proteins[5, 6] and specific protein products of subcellular compartments.[7-9] These applications are discussed in Section d.

b. GENERAL PRINCIPLES

   i. Characteristics and Choice of Isotopes[†]

Among the isotopes which have been used for autoradiography of gel precipitate patterns are ^{14}C, ^{32}P, ^{35}S, ^{59}Fe, ^{60}Co, ^{131}I, and [125]I.

Tritium has been used for high-resolution autoradiography of histological sections and for chromatograms.[10][‡] Tritium is a very low energy beat emitter, however, and very high radioactivity would be required for a sufficient number of particles to escape the agar layer and expose the emulsion. The tritium beta particle has a maximum energy of 0.018 Mev, and will penetrate 6 to 7μ in water, but the average particle energy is but 0.006 Mev, so most particles penetrate only 1 μ.[‡][§]

---

* A specialized application of this principle can be found in studies of antigen combining power of immune globulins and their fragments.[3, 4]

[3] H. Miller and G. Owen, *Nature* **188**, 67 (1960).

[4] J. H. Morse, and J. F. Heremans, *J. Lab. Clin. Med.* **59**, 891 (1962).

[5] G. M. Hochwald, G. J. Thorbecke, and R. Asofsky, *J. Exptl. Med.* **114**, 459 (1961).

[6] G. J. Thorbecke, G. M. Hochwald, and E. B. Jacobson, *Ann. N.Y. Acad. Sci.* **101**, 255 (1962).

[7] A. von der Decken, *Biochem. J.* **88**, 385 (1963).

[8] M. C. Ganoza, C. A. Williams, and F. Lipman, *Proc. Natl. Acad. Sci. U.S.* **53**, 619 (1965).

[9] C. A. Williams, M. C. Ganoza, and F. Lipman, *Proc. Natl. Acad. Sci., U.S.* **53**, 622 (1965).

† Chapter 11, (see Sections B.1 and G.2) of Vol. II is devoted to many aspects of radioisotope handling and research, and it should be consulted for theoretical considerations and general practical details. Autoradiography as applied to histological sections is discussed there.

[10] J. Chamberlain, A. Hughes, A. W. Rogers, and G. H. Thomas, *Nature* **201**, 774 (1964).

‡ For chromatograms, sensitivity is expressed in terms of the minimum radioactivity which, when spread over 1 cm² causes recognizable blackening of the emulsion in 1 day's exposure.[10] The minimum sensitivity for this weak beta emitter was estimated at approximately 0.3 μCi/cm²/day. Presumably, such an indication of sensitivity could be devised for precipitation bands, but so far this has not been done.

§ Vol. II, Chap. 11, Section G.2.

The ^{14}C emission, although a beta particle like ^{3}H, has nearly ten times the energy (0.155 Mev maximum). ^{14}C will produce good autoradiographs of precipitates in gel with materials of moderate specific radioactivity.

^{32}P is a very high energy beta emitter (1.7 Mev maximum). Therefore, while there would be no problem obtaining autoradiograms, a number of the higher energy particles will expose the emulsion beyond the confines of a characteristically sharp band of precipitate.

^{131}I has been extensively used as an external label on proteins. Very high specific activities can be obtained, but ^{131}I produces low resolution autoradiograms because of high energy beta particles and a number of high energy levels of γ-rays. The latter emissions are highly penetrating and can be expected to expose an emulsion well beyond the radiation source. ^{125}I emits a very soft (0.035 Mev) γ-ray which is adequate for autoradiography at moderate levels of radioactivity because of the 60-day half-life of the isotope.

ii. Photographic Emulsions

The sensitivity of an autoradiographic system, however, defined for a given isotope, depends in part on the photographic emulsion. Some are more sensitive (faster) than others, and since in general the faster an emulsion the coarser the grain, these also give less resolution.

Various double-coated X-ray sheet films have been used (Kodak Blue Brand, Medical, KK-type industrial No Screen, Ilford Ilfex, Gevaert Osray). These are fast films of comparatively large grain size, but their resolution for precipitation patterns is generally sufficient. Other somewhat less sensitive sheet films such as Kodak Royal Pan or Type A emulsions have slightly better resolution and a lighter background, but a disadvantage is that they have to be handled in complete darkness. These or even slower emulsions, such as Kodak Contrast Process Ortho film, should be used for "ultra micro" methods or where precipitates form very close to one another.

Contrast lantern plates can also be used conveniently, and on special order No Screen and Type A (Kodak) emulsions may be obtained on glass plates 25 × 75 mm (1 × 3 inches) for use with microscope slides. These are especially practical since many gel diffusion analyses are now performed on microscope slides. Film may also be obtained precut to a desired size.

iii. Exposure

Intimate contact between the photographic emulsion and the radiation source is essential for both sensitivity and resolution in autoradiography. Glass is the most frequently used support for gel analyses by double diffusion or by immunoelectrophoresis (see procedures below), and if autoradiography is planned, glass or some other rigid support is essential since the film or photoplate must be pressed tightly against the dried gel layer. A piece of film size similar to the supporting glass is placed with its emulsion against the agar and is "sandwiched" with another glass or rigid support to ensure the close contact. The film and glass are held together with a rubber band (nonsparking). If the emulsion is on a glass plate of the proper size the procedure is even more simple. The exposure preparation is wrapped in aluminum foil or black photo-wrapping paper, and placed in a light-proof box.

Exposure time will vary with type and amount of isotope used. The general rules follow from the discussion above: the optimum exposure time is shortened by higher radioactivity, isotopes with higher energy emissions, faster emulsions, and closer contact between the emulsion and the radiation source. If isotopes with short half-lives are employed it is important to use enough isotope to produce the autoradiogram before the elapse of twice the half-life. Should an emulsion not be sufficiently exposed by three-fourths of the radioactivity available, it is not likely that another eighth will produce the autoradiographs. Among the isotopes mentioned, this consideration would apply principally to ^{32}P ($T = 14\ d$) and ^{131}I ($T = 8\ d$) (see Vol. II, Chap. 11.G.5.)

Among the variables specifically affecting exposure by immune precipitates in dried gels are sharpness of zone or precipitate (i.e., isotope density), thickness of dried gel layer (i.e., emission penetration), and the amount and composition of the precipitate (i.e., self-absorption capacity).

c. GENERAL PROCEDURES

i. Preparation of Precipitation Patterns

Double diffusion or immunoelectrophoresis plates are prepared as described in Sections 14.B.3 and 14.D.2 and in detail in Appendix I. There are certain precautions which should be taken, however, if autoradiographs are to be made of the patterns.

1. Patterns should be washed extensively to remove all traces of unreacted radioactive material. Sometimes material binds to or precipitates nonspecifically in an agar matrix, possibly because of its charge. If this is thought to be a problem, a higher salt concentration (e.g., 3 M, pH 7 to 8) in the wash would help to elute ion-bound material. However, if the experiment concerns a test for nonimmune binding of a radioactive ligand (see Section d.ii), care must be taken not to wash precipitates in a solution which might dissociate the ligand from the antigen.

2. The agar is dried to a thin film on the glass under lint-free filter paper at room temperature or 37°. Any residual dampness will cause the emulsion to swell and possibly stick to the agar, ruining the autoradiograph and often the agar layer as well.

3. For most purposes the pattern can be stained by various dyes either before or after contact with the photographic emulsion. There is no theoretical basis to suspect that such dyes would expose the emulsion in total darkness since their photoactive excited state lasts only a few minutes after their synthesis. However, when in doubt it is best to use unstained preparations. The additional wetting, swelling, and drying may cause surface aberrations which could hinder close contact with the emulsion.

ii. Antigen–Antibody Ratio

The best autoradiographs are obtained from precipitation bands at or near equivalence. Such bands are the sharpest, concentrating the available isotope in the minimum area. It is seen in Fig. 1 that neither antigen excess nor antibody excess reactions can equal a precipitate at equivalence for satisfactory exposure by the same amount of isotope.

In a single setup it may be impossible to achieve ideal ratios for several radioactive components in a mixture of antigens or antibodies. A series of dilutions of one or the other reactant may be required. Perhaps the addition of nonradioactive carrier will be necessary in order to obtain satisfactory precipitates. Carrier is frequently employed in studies of protein synthesis *in vitro* (see Section d.iii below).

iii. Controls

Apart from controlling the form or state of the label, which is a problem more peculiar to the application than to the general procedure, it is important to demonstrate that radioactivity associated with a given precipitate is not due to adsorption to preformed precipitate, coprecipitation by entrapment, or fortuitous cross reaction. Mechanical effects and extraneous chemical exposure must also be controlled.

(a) *Adsorption and Coprecipitation.* The possibility that immunologically noncrossreacting material will cause labeling of a precipitation line which it meets during diffusion on agar can be tested in a number of ways. The radioactive substance may be mixed with an unrelated antigen and diffused against antibody to the latter, or the different reactants may be placed in separate wells so that their diffusion "fields" intersect, as shown in Fig. 2.

(b) *Cross-Reaction.* There are many types of cross-reactions which could interfere with the valid interpretation of autoradiographs of pre-

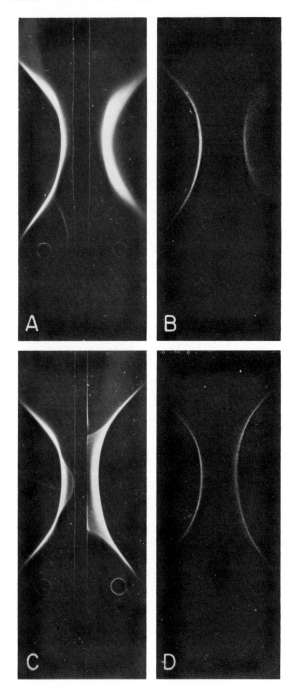

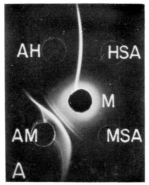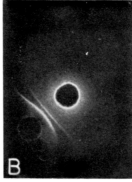

Fig. 2. Control for nonspecific association of radioactive material with an antigen–antibody precipitate. (A) Stained diffusion plate. (B) Autoradiograph. AM, Rabbit anti-mouse serum; MSA, purified unlabeled mouse serum albumin; M, protein products of mouse-liver microsomal incorporation system. The unrelated antigen, human serum albumin, is biologically and physically similar to one of the experimental radioactive antigens—mouse serum albumin from a mouse-liver microsomal incorporation system, M, identified by its "identity" reaction with MSA. This test has the features of controlling for nonspecific coprecipitation over a wide range of relative concentrations of precipitating system to radioactive substance and over a range of state from preformed to nascent precipitate. No detectable radioactivity should associate with the unrelated precipitation band.

cipitation bands in gels. Appropriate absorption of antisera can usually avoid difficulties.

(c) *Mechanical and Chemical Effects.* Photographic emulsion is very sensitive to scratching and other mechanical insults. In fact, after exposure a simple way to mark autoradiographs before development is with a sharp scratching tool, such as a diamond pencil.

Very dense and sharp precipitates will produce a ridge in the dried agar. If such slides are pressed too tightly against the emulsion, a mechanical artifact may result.

Fig. 1. Effect of antigen–antibody ratio on autoradiographic sensitivity. (A) Stained micro-IEA slide of purified ^{14}C-mouse serum albumin (MSA) with 4-times concentrated antibody. Equivalence reaction on left was produced by 24 μg MSA containing about 5 dpm ^{14}C. Antibody-excess reaction on right was produced by 6 μg of MSA with about 1.3 dpm. (B) Corresponding autoradiograph to A. (C) Stained micro IEA slide of ^{14}C-MSA with unconcentrated antibody. Equivalence reaction on left was produced by 6 μg of MSA with 1.3 dpm. Antigen-excess reaction on right was produced by 24 μg of MSA with about 5 dpm ^{14}C. (D) Corresponding autoradiograph to C. Approximately equal amounts of radioactivity (1.3 dpm) are represented in the autoradiographs of the equivalence reaction of D (left) and the antibody-excess reaction B (right). Similarly, equivalence in B (left) can be compared with antigen-excess in D (right) for 5 dpm reactions.

Many laboratory chemicals, particularly reducing agents, will "expose" photographic emulsions. If slides have been properly washed and handled this should not present a problem; but a fingerprint on the emulsion or even on the dried agar slide can ruin an autoradiogram.

It is often advisable to prepare a nonradioactive control slide as nearly as possible like the experimental slide. Duplicate experimental slides are the next best control for these difficulties, and also one can serve to estimate proper exposure time for the other.

iv. Photography

Autoradiographs can be used in a photoenlarger just like stained slides or plates (see Section 14.E.2). It is often useful to prepare negatives when it is necessary to increase contrast for publication. If long autoradiographic exposure times are necessary, the background "fog" from cosmic radiation or diffuse binding of isotope to the agar or incomplete washing may necessitate the preparation of negatives on high contrast plates or film.

d. SPECIFIC APPLICATIONS AND PROCEDURES

i. Demonstration of Serum Antibody Activity

Specific antibody can be detected with great sensitivity by means of labeled antigen in agar gel diffusion reactions. The two principal methods differ only with respect to the time of addition of the labeled antigen. (1) Prior to immunoelectrophoresis the labeled antigen is incubated for a few hours at 37° with the serum containing antibody.[3, 4] (2) The labeled antigen is added to the antiserum used to develop the immunoelectrophoretic pattern of the antibody-containing serum.[11] It can be added to the antibody trough immediately after the antiserum has diffused into the agar; or, alternatively, the labeled antigen can be added to the trough after the pattern has developed and the unreacted material has been washed out of the gel. Specific antibody precipitated by anti-immunoglobulin in the gel will still bind antigen. With both these methods, simple double diffusion in agar can be employed instead of immunoelectrophoresis if a specific antiserum to one of the immunoglobulin classes is used (Appendix I).

The first method is dependent on the formation of soluble complexes in the serum containing the labeled antigen. It is, therefore, most applicable to the study of nonprecipitating antigen–antibody systems, such as insulin.[4, 12] The electrophoretic mobility of the immune globulins may be influenced by interaction with antigen.

[11] Y. Yagi, see Appendix I.
[12] T. J. Merimee, and T. E. Prout, *J. Lab. Clin. Med.* **64**, 412 (1964).

The second method is more easily interpreted when complex antisera are used to develop the immunoelectrophoretic pattern. When the antigen is added immediately after or together with the antiserum, an extra precipitation line may form representing interaction of the labeled antigen with excess antibody in the serum under analysis.[13] This is prevented when the immunoelectrophoretic patterns are developed and washed prior to addition of the labeled antigen to the antiserum trough. Regardless of the procedure used, labeled impurities in the antigen solution may result in nonspecific labeling of precipitation arcs, when they cross-react with serum constituents and, thus, coprecipitate in the corresponding precipitation arcs.[13] It is recommended to use only one labeled antigen per immunoelectrophoresis slide.[14]

When all other conditions are kept constant, the relative intensities of the radioactive lines grossly reflect the relative antibody activities in the different immune globulins. Using approximately 1 μg ($= 1$ μCi) of insulin/milliliter, Yagi et al.[15] were able to detect reactivity in guinea pig sera containing 0.033 μg of antibody-N /milliliter. Similarly, Minden et al.,[14] using 1 μg ($= 1.5$ μCi) ^{131}I BSA/milliliter, detected antibody concentrations in rabbit sera as low as 0.003 μg N anti-BSA/ml.

Besides iodine, other isotopes have been used for the labeling of antigens. ^{32}P-labeled poliovirus[16] and ^{60}Co-labeled vitamin B_{12}-intrinsic factor (see below) have been successfully used for the detection of antibody activity in antisera to these antigens.

ii. Nonimmunological Binding Reactions

Many proteins bind other substances, such as metallic ions, vitamins, hormones, lipids, and other proteins. In many cases these are specific reactions which are interpreted biologically as carrier functions. Some are nonspecific, or at least for the present they are better understood in physicochemical terms. Such binding reactions can be detected and, in some instances, elucidated by using the "binder" protein as an antigen in an immune precipitation system and a radioactive ligand or bound substance.

Autoradiography of diffusion patterns can be performed as with other applications. There may be, however, special technical considerations which depend on the properties of the isotope employed.

[13] H. C. Goodman, E. D. Exum, and J. Robbins, J. Immunol. **92**, 843 (1964).
[14] P. Minden, H. M. Grey, and R. S. Farr, J. Immunol. **99**, 304 (1967).
[15] Y. Yagi, P. Maier, D. Pressman, C. E. Arbesman, R. E. Reisman, and A. R. Lenzer, J. Immunol. **90**, 760 (1963).
[16] E. Ainbender, R. Berger, M. M. Hevizy, H. D. Zepp, and H. L. Hodes, Proc. Soc. Exptl. Biol. Med. **119**, 1166 (1965).

(a) *Metal-Binding Proteins.* The identification of iron-binding proteins in biological fluids, such as transferrin,[17] red protein from milk,[18] and conalbumin from egg white,[19] can be achieved by the use of ^{59}Fe. Precipitation patterns in agar gel, both in immunoelectrophoresis and in Ouchterlony plates, as well as the behavior of iron-binding proteins in starch gel electrophoresis,[20,21] can be studied by means of autoradiography without need for the purified protein.

Labeling of transferrin is easily accomplished by incubation of 1 ml of serum for 1 hour at 37° with 2 μCi FeCl₃. Ferrous salts can also be used, and incubation for 24 hours at 4° is also effective. Subsequent dialysis removes excess unbound iron. Care should be taken that the pH is kept above or at 7 before autoradiography is performed because the complex of Fe with transferrin is not stable below pH 7. Exposure times vary from 1 to 7 days.

(b) *Vitamin- and Hormone-Binding Proteins.* Since vitamin B₁₂ contains a molecule of cobalt, ^{58}Co- or ^{60}Co-labeled B₁₂ can be used to identify proteins in various biological fluids which specifically bind this vitamin. With this method comparisons have been made between gastric juice (intrinsic factor) from normal individuals and from patients with pernicious anemia.[22] Intrinsic factor of normal gastric juice appears to migrate in the β region and may consist of more than one cross-reacting protein. Labeling of the vitamin B₁₂-binding proteins is accomplished by addition of 4 μCi (4 μg) labeled vitamin B₁₂ to 1 ml of a concentrated gastric juice protein solution (40 to 80 mg/ml), followed by incubation for 1 hour at room temperature. Another application of labeled vitamin B₁₂ is in the detection of serum antibody to intrinsic factor.[23]

Insulin, thyroxine, and *pituitary polypeptide hormones* can be labeled with [131]I (see Vol. I, Chap. 4.A.2) in order to study the "carrier function" of serum proteins for these substances. Such studies usually involve methods for the quantitative determination of the degree of binding by serum or serum fractions. Autoradiographs are more often obtained from electrophoretic[24] than from immunoelectrophoretic patterns. However, the most exact qualitative identification of hormone binding proteins is with

---

[17] J. Clausen, R. Rask-Nielsen, H. E. Christensen, and T. Munkner, *Cancer Res.* **20**, 178 (1960).

[18] B. J. Johanson, *Acta Chem. Scand.* **14**, 510 (1960).

[19] J. Williams, *Biochem. J.* **83**, 355 (1962).

[20] E. R. Giblett, C. G. Hickman, and O. Smithies, *Nature* **183**, 1589 (1959).

[21] B. S. Blumberg, and L. Warren, *Biochim. Biophys. Acta* **50**, 90 (1961).

[22] J. Hurlimann, *Helv. Med. Acta* **30**, 126 (1963).

[23] I. M. Samloff, and E. V. Barnett, *J. Clin. Invest.* **44**, 1094 (1965).

[24] W. DiGiulio, Z. Michalak, P. A. Weinhold, J. R. Hamilton, and G. E. Thomas, *J. Lab. Clin. Med.* **64**, 349 (1964).

radioimmunoelectrophoretic patterns. This method has been used for growth hormones[25] and for thyroxine.[26]

Varying amounts of the purified labeled hormone are incubated with serum, and the mixture is analyzed by immunoelectrophoresis with antisera either to the hormone itself or to the serum proteins. For growth hormone 200 μg to 2 mg/milliliter of serum was used, for thyroxine 2 to 16 μg (100 μCi)/milliliter of serum.[24]

(c) *Association of Different Protein Molecules in Solution.* Such studies can be greatly faciliated by the use of ^{131}I-labeling of one of the proteins. Autoradiography of agar gel precipitin patterns was applied to the study of such protein–protein interaction by Lang and Hoeffgen.[27] It was noted by these authors that coprecipitation could be studied systematically by this method in order to elucidate the nonimmunological, physicochemical interference between proteins in a mixture.

This type of "nonspecific" association may cause interpretative difficulties in the use of these methods for the study of protein synthesis. Rigorous controls are required, some of which are discussed below in Section iii.

iii. Demonstration of Protein Synthesis in Vitro

One of the simplest and most reliable methods for the demonstration of sites of synthesis of individual proteins is by autoradiography of immunoelectrophoretic patterns of proteins labeled by the incorporation of radioactive amino acids.

(a) *Preparation of Antigens.* Proteins concentrated from the medium in which tissues or cells have been incubated may be used as antigens.[5, 6, 28–31] This is achieved in a variety of ways: lyophilization, ultrafiltration, salting out, etc. It is important to recognize that only proteins secreted by cells (e.g., serum proteins) can be studied in this fashion. The proteins not normally secreted can be obtained from the tissue itself rather than the medium.

The products of cell-free systems can be examined in a similar fashion.[7–9] If a microsomal system of rat or mouse liver is used, however,

[25] M. M. Grumbach, and S. L. Kaplan, *Ciba Found. Colloq. Endocrinol.* **14**, 63 (1962).

[26] J. Hirschfeld, and U. Soderberg, *Experientia* **16**, 198 (1960).

[27] N. Lang, and B. Hoeffgen, *in* "Protides of the Biological Fluids" (H. Peeters, ed.), Vol. 11, p. 377. Elsevier, Amsterdam, 1963.

[28] R. Asofsky, and G. J. Thorbecke, *J. Exptl. Med.* **114**, 471 (1961).

[29] G. J. Thorbecke, R. Asofsky, G. M. Hochwald, and E. B. Jacobson, *in* "Protides of the Biological Fluids" (H. Peeters, ed.), Vol. 11, p. 125. Elsevier, Amsterdam, 1963.

[30] V. J. Stecher, and G. J. Thorbecke, *J. Immunol.* **99**, 643 (1967).

[31] C. A. Williams, R. Asofsky, and G. J. Thorbecke, *J. Exptl. Med.* **118**, 315 (1963).

export proteins will not be found in the soluble supernatant of the incubation medium, but rather in the microsomal vesicles. They are released most satisfactorily by sonication.[8] The soluble tissue proteins are not bound in the microsomes and may be recovered from the supernatant of the systems.[32] It appears that they are produced on the so-called free ribosomes of the liver cell.

(b) *Incubation Media.* Incubation media used for incorporation by tissues, cells, or subcellular fractions should contain ^{14}C-amino acids of high specific activity (100 to 200 μCi/mmole).

In tissue cultures with 50 to 100 mg of various tissues, 1 μCi of each of two amino acids/milliliter of culture fluid has given satisfactory results[5,28]. The ^{14}C-amino acids that have been used with success are lysine, isoleucine, leucine, and valine. The most suitable amino acids are those which do not contain a free SH group and cannot be converted into ^{14}C-labeled precursors with free SH groups. Algal protein hydrolyzates have been found to cause nonspecific labeling of proteins.[5] Proof that ^{14}C- or ^{35}S-amino acids have been incorporated into an individual protein, and are not simply attached to the surface of the protein molecules, can be obtained by autoradiography of a chromatogram made from the peptide mixture of a trypsin digest of the isolated radioactive protein. Proteins should not become labeled when previously killed cells or tissues are cultured in the presence of ^{14}C-labeled amino acid. The tissue culture medium should contain minimal protein in order to allow sufficient concentration of the ^{14}C-labeled proteins. Good results are obtained using medium with 0.5% ovalbumin or bovine serum albumin. The culture fluids are dialyzed extensively against phosphate-buffered 0.015 M NaCl, pH 7.2; concentration can be accomplished by lyophilization. Adequate labeling of rat serum proteins by cell-free systems is accomplished by a single ^{14}C-amino acid, leucine at 2 μCi/milliliter of medium.[8] It is often found that mixtures of several ^{14}C-labeled amino acids at the same total level of radioactivity will increase the level of incorporated activity significantly, but yeast or algal protein hydrolyzates, as mentioned above, may present a problem due to impurities or to precursors with free SH groups. Ribonuclease inhibitors, e.g., polyvinyl sulfate, are useful to include in mouse-liver cell-free systems.[9]

(c) *Carrier Proteins.* These are required for the formation of sharp precipitation arcs in immunoelectrophoresis. With the micromethod the carrier is added separately to the antigen well prior to 3 or 4 repeated additions of the concentrated culture fluids. When comparisons between different preparations are made, similar carriers and antisera should be

[32] C. A. Williams and M. C. Ganoza, *in* "Plasma Protein Metabolism (M. A. Rothchild ed.). Academic Press, New York, 1970.

used in order to ensure comparable immunoelectrophoretic patterns. The culture fluids, even when concentrated, usually contain so little protein in comparison to the carrier that its effect on the precipitation arcs is negligible.

The technique can also be used for the demonstration of antibody formation *in vitro*.[33,34] In this case the carrier pattern is made from a carrier serum containing enough antibody to give a sharp precipitin arc in the IgG region when developed, after electrophoresis, by the corresponding antigen. If labeled antibody of similar specificity is present in the culture fluid, it will coprecipitate in this line and can thus be detected by autoradiography.

(*d*) *Interpretation of Autoradiographs.* All experiments on the biosynthesis of proteins share a common problem—finding proof that a labeled precursor is incorporated into the protein in question and not merely attached to it. Even the controls illustrated and discussed above (c.iii) can not answer this question conclusively.

It is known that antigen–antibody precipitates, prepared in ^{14}C-labeled tissue culture fluids, bind some labeled tissue products nonspecifically. Similarly, when whole tissue culture fluids are analyzed by means of autoradiography of Ouchterlony plates rather than immunoelectrophoretic patterns, *nonspecific labeling* of lines is often observed in control plates with unrelated precipitin lines.[35–37] Although quantitative differences are usually noted between such nonspecific and specific labeling, autoradiography of Ouchterlony plate patterns is more suitable for the study of partly purified protein products than of whole tissue culture fluids.[38] There are also a few lines in immunoelectrophoretic patterns which seem to bind radioactive substances from culture fluids nonspecifically. They are primarily the α_2-macroglobulin[6,39] and α_2- and α_1-lipoprotein[29] lines. A tentative explanation of this phenomenon can be found in the fact that these α-proteins bind enzymes formed by the tissues.[40,41]

[33] G. J. Thorbecke, and G. M. Hochwald, *in* "Radioisotopes in Medicine: *in Vitro* Studies" (R. L. Hayes, F. A. Goswitz, B. E. Murphy, and E. B. Anderson, eds.), p. 589. U.S. Atomic Energy Commission, Oak Ridge, Tennessee, 1967.

[34] A. M. Silverstein, G. J. Thorbecke, K. L. Kraner, and R. J. Lukes, *J. Immunol.* **91**, 384 (1963).

[35] W. S. Morgan, P. Perlmann, and T. Hultin, *J. Biophys. Biochem. Cytol.* **10**, 411 (1960).

[36] G. J. Thorbecke, unpublished observation (1961).

[37] A. von der Decken, and P. N. Campbell, *Biochem. J.* **84**, 449 (1962).

[38] R. van Furth, and M. Diesselhoff-den Dulk, *J. Immunol.* **96**, 920 (1966).

[39] M. E. Philips, and G. J. Thorbecke, *Nature* **207**, 376 (1965).

[40] S. H. Lawrence, and P. J. Melnick, *Proc. Soc. Exptl. Biol. Med.* **107**, 998 (1961).

[41] J. W. Mehl, W. O'Connell, and J. de Groot, *Science* **145**, 821 (1964).

Until more is known about the specific function of α_2-macroglobulin and about protein–protein interaction between serum proteins, no better explanation can be given.

When two proteins are known to interact, as in the case of haptoglobin and hemoglobin, it is easy to understand why labeling of either component can cause labeling of the line representing the complex. Interpretation in this case is only slightly facilitated by observing whether labeling of the fast or of the slow part of the bimodal precipitin arc predominates, since the 24 hours of diffusion needed to develop the lines can effectively obscure the separation obtained by electrophoresis.

When fluids containing highly labeled albumin or γ-globulin are analyzed on the same slide adjacent to unlabeled fluids, carryover of the label may occur during the immunoelectrophoresis because of lateral diffusion. It may be prudent, therefore, to use only one such radioactive preparation per slide.

Great care should be taken in interpreting the results when an autoradiograph is superimposed on the corresponding immunoelectrophoretic pattern. The sensitivity is such that precipitin arcs are often seen on autoradiographs which cannot be detected with protein staining of the corresponding immunoelectrophoresis slides.

Autoradiography of immunoelectrophoresis of tissue extracts made after culturing of the tissue with ^{14}C-amino acids often reveals the presence of more specific antigens than seen with any other method, and provides a more dynamic impression than ordinary immunoelectrophoresis by showing which proteins are rapidly synthesized.[42, 43] Although this method is essentially qualitative, it can be used for the estimation of *relative synthesizing capacities* of different tissues, when all conditions of incubation, culturing, and immunoelectrophoretic analysis are kept constant and the amount of labeled amino acid present is not rate limiting.[9, 31]

More accurate quantitation of the amount of radioactivity in a single precipitin arc can be done by extraction of a piece of agar cut out around the line.[7] Van Furth et al. estimated the *lower limit* of detectability of formation of immunoglobulins by this method.[44] An amount of 0.002 μg of labeled IgM could still be detected on an immunoelectrophoresis slide. Since this used about one-thirtieth of the preparation, the amount in the total culture could be estimated. When such measurements are made, it should be kept in mind that blackening of the X-ray film is proportional to the radioactivity only at low concentrations of silver grains.

[42] P. Perlmann, and T. Hultin, *Nature* **182**, 1530 (1958).
[43] P. Perlmann, T. Hultin, V. D'Amelio, and W. S. Morgan, *Exptl. Cell Res. Suppl.* **7**, 279 (1959).
[44] R. van Furth, H. R. E. Schuit, and W. Hÿmans, *Immunology* **11**, 1 (1966).

This very sensitive method also lends itself well to a combination with other physicochemical methods of fractionation, such as ultracentrifugation or column chromatography.[30,45] All fractions obtained should, of course, be concentrated to very small volumes before testing. Attempts to combine this technique with the use of other labeled precursors of protein synthesis, such as precursors of the carbohydrate moieties, have not been reported as yet. Autoradiography of immunoelectrophoretic patterns can also be used for the study of serum protein formation *in vivo*.[46]

[45] J. D. Wakefield, G. J. Thorbecke, L. J. Old, and E. A. Boyse, *J. Immunol.* **99**, 308 (1967).
[46] R. Asofsky, Z. Trnka, and G. J. Thorbecke, *Proc. Soc. Exptl. Biol. Med.* **111**, 497 (1962).

F. Preparation of Materials for Diffusion in Gels

1. SELECTION AND PREPARATION OF GELS FOR DIFFUSION*

a. GENERAL CHARACTERISTICS

The purpose of semisolid media used in immunodiffusion tests is to suppress convection current mixing of reactants, at the same time permitting these reactants free diffusion and immunological interaction. Therefore, their properties must be such as to provide antigen and antibody with a suitable physical and chemical environment for their interaction. Since both of these reactants are water-soluble macromolecules of negative charge at the pH range over which they can be used, a supporting medium for immunodiffusion should hold a large volume of water, should be either electroneutral or electronegative, and should have large enough "pores" to permit diffusion of either antibody or antigen and preferably both. Usually such media also should be free of contaminants and of properties that predispose them to interact with antigen or antibody or to interfere with antigen–antibody precipitation. Useful accessory characteristics for these media are transparency, inertness to dyes and other chemical indicators, ease of usage, and dimensional and physical stability.

b. SEMISOLID MEDIA CURRENTLY USED FOR IMMUNODIFFUSION

Numerous media have been tried[1]; of these only four unite enough of the above general desired characteristics to have gained enough acceptance to merit discussion here. In order of present popularity they are: agar and a derivative known as agarose, cellulose acetate membrane, gelatin, and polyacrylamide. Of these, agar, agarose, and polyacrylamide are the

* Section 14.F.1 was contributed by Alfred J. Crowle.
[1] A. J. Crowle, "Immunodiffusion." Academic Press, New York, 1961.

most useful; gelatin and cellulose acetate have disadvantages which give them only accessory status as immunodiffusion support media.

Agar is an acid polysaccharide gum extracted from certain seaweeds. It is soluble in boiling water, and its solutions gel when cooled. A 1% solution of it, prepared by boiling, when cooled to approximately 45°C sets to form a lightly turbid, transparent, slightly elastic, dimensionally stable gel which permits nearly unhampered diffusion and interaction of most antigens with their antibodies. Its chief disadvantages are a strong negative charge and a marked tendency to react with several chemical indicators for polysaccharides as well as with cationic dyes. Similarly, it interacts with positively charged antigens, either impeding or preventing their diffusion, and will precipitate some lipoproteins such as can be found in normal human serum. Since it is a plant product extracted from a crude and heterogeneous source, agar is obtainable in several different grades of variable quality and degree of contamination with organic and inorganic substances. Inorganic impurities found in nearly all grades of agar significantly affect antigen–antibody precipitation, often enhancing it.[1]

Agar is a mixture of agaropectin and agarose.[2] Agaropectin is responsible for some of the unwanted properties of agar, notably its strong negative charge. Therefore, recent development of practical methods for separating agarose from agaropectin[3] have been most welcome in providing, in the former, a nearly ideal gelling medium for immunodiffusion. Agarose still retains agar's disadvantage of reacting with several indicators for polysaccharide, and during its preparation it is not freed of inorganic contaminants which tend to enhance antigen–antibody precipitation.

Polyacrylamide, first used for immunodiffusion tests in 1961,[1] has been employed since then only occassionally for this purpose (e.g., Antoine[4]); it is best known currently as a gel for electrophoresis (see Vol. II, Chap. 6.C.4 and 5). This gel consists of polymerized acrylamide and N,N'-methylenebisacrylamide. It is a stable, sticky, very elastic, water-clear gel with dense enough structural texture to impede diffusion of antigen and antibody somewhat but not too much for immunodiffusion tests. It seems to have nearly all of the properties wanted of an ideal immunodiffusion gel, but because it requires somewhat more rigorous handling than does agar or gelatin, it has yet to gain the popularity it deserves.* Polyacrylamide has two major technical disadvantages which should not be difficult to overcome by making some changes in techniques applied to agar gels: its density makes conventional staining and destaining pro-

[2] S. Hjertén, *Biochim. Biophys. Acta* **53**, 514–517 (1961).
[3] S. Hjertén, *Biochim. Biophys. Acta* **62**, 445–449 (1962).
[4] B. Antoine, *Rev. Franc. Etudes Clin. Biol.* **7**, 612–617 (1962).
* Handling is greatly facilitated by including agarose in a gelling concentration.[4a]
[4a] J. Uriel, personal communication (1970).

cedures much slower than those in agar (cf. Ferris *et al.*[5]), and no convenient way yet is known to dry this gel to a film for permanent storage of original antigen–antibody reactions.

Gelatin is a partially hydrolyzed animal protein soluble, like agar, in hot water and yielding water-clear gels on cooling. In immunoelectrophoresis it shows no electroosmosis.[1] By its chemical constitution it protects labile reactants against denaturation, and it can be mixed with these as a liquid at lower temperatures than is possible with agar. Gelatin gels are clearer than agar gels, especially at refrigerator temperatures; they are not reactive with some polysaccharide indicators which color agar. Gelatin is usable over such a wide range of concentrations (from less than 1% to more than 28%) that it can be employed for selectively blocking diffusion of molecules of different sizes, a procedure useful for determining relative molecular weights.[6] Like agar gels, those of gelatin can be dried for permanent storage of immunodiffusion reactions. Unfortunately, these many advantages largely are offset by three major disadvantages: gelatin gels are weak; they take up protein stains; and they have such low melting points at the usually employed concentrations of from 1% to 5% that they liquefy at room temperature.

Recently, a unique application has been discovered for gelatin gels in immunodiffusion. This is in detecting precipitin reactions between antibody and basic protein antigens.[7] Such reactions could not be observed in gels of agar or agarose because these media complex with and prevent diffusion of these antigens. For this kind of test gelatin can be used at a 2% concentration in pH 6.5, 0.1 M sodium phosphate buffer. Reactant solutions, cooled to 4°C, are applied as droplets to the surface of a thin layer of the gel on a microscope slide, also cooled to 4°C, and reactions are allowed to develop for 24 to 48 hours at this same temperature.

The characteristics and uses of cellulose acetate memebranes in immunodiffusion tests are discussed in Sections 14.B.5 and 14.D.3. Their outstanding advantages of economy, purity, and uniformity are counterbalanced by the considerable disadvantage of opacity. Antigen–antibody precipitation cannot be observed in these membranes until they have been washed and their precipitates stained, after which the membranes can be rendered transparent.

c. Physical and Chemical Conditions Affecting the Use of Semisolid Media

Immunodiffusion media are used with various solvents and solutes. For general purpose single and double diffusion tests they should be

[5] T. G. Ferris, R. E. Easterling, and R. E. Budd, *Am. J. Clin. Pathol.* **38**, 383–387 (1962).
[6] A. C. Allison and J. H. Humphrey, *Nature* **183**, 1590–1592 (1959).
[7] A. J. Crowle and C. C. Hu, *Proc. Soc. Exptl. Biol. Med.*, **126**, 729–731 (1967).

employed with physiological salt solutions buffered to neutral or slightly alkaline pH and protected against contaminating microbial growth either by refrigeration or with added bactericidal or bacteriostatic substances like thimerosal (Merthiolate), sodium azide, phenol, or antibiotics. Refrigeration is preferable to antimicrobial additives, because these can injure immunodiffusion reactants whereas refrigeration tends to preserve the reactants. Moreover, antigen–antibody precipitation usually is more complete in the cold than at room or body temperatures.*

Phosphates and barbitals are the pH buffers most often used in immunodiffusion media. The former are inert; the latter tend to enhance antigen–antibody precipitation, but they also precipitate some serum lipoproteins causing halos of precipitate to form around depots of serum. Other buffers less frequently used include citrate, Tris, borate, acetate, and ethylenediamine. Citrate, ethylenediamine and Tris are chelating agents, which complex with heavy metals contaminating some semisolid media. Because these metals can enhance antigen–antibody precipitation, tests employing chelating buffers are considerably less sensitive than tests using nonchelating buffers. Borate buffers offer the unique convenience of being inherently antimicrobial, but neither borate nor acetate are commonly used because they buffer poorly in the pH 7 to pH 8 range optimal for antigen–antibody precipitation.

Most immunodiffusion buffers approximate physiological strength (i.e., equivalent to 0.15 M NaCl) as well as physiological pH on the justifiable assumption that antibodies should precipitate antigen best when used in an *in vitro* environment closely resembling that *in vivo*. But sometimes stronger or weaker buffers yield better results. For example, fowl antisera may precipitate their antigens better in buffers of 8 to 10 times physiological strength[8] (see Section 13.A.2.c), whereas rabbit antisera to protein-polyamino conjugates have been found to precipitate these antigens best at a very low ionic strength equivalent to one-tenth that of plasma.[9] In electrophoresis performed with buffers of physiological strength, electric current flow would be impractically high, electrophoresis would be very slow, and antigen fractionation poor. Consequently, immunoelectrophoresis buffers usually are about one-third physiological strength. Not only are they of lower ionicity, but also they usually are buffered to higher than physiological pH values between 8 and 9, within which range they seem to yield better electrophoretic fractionation of complex mixtures of antigens like serum. Thus, no one buffered solvent is best for all

---

[8] L. M. Weiner, and M. Goodman, *Federation Proc.* **23**, 141 (1964).

[9] D. J. Buchanan-Davidson, M. A. Stahmann, and E. E. Dellert, *J. Immunol.* **83**, 561–570 (1959).

* Note that examinations must be made at the chosen temperature until the pattern is fully developed (Section 14.A.1).

immunodiffusion tests; to obtain optimal results one may have to depend on preliminary experimentation to select a buffer suited to the antigen–antibody system being studied and to its mode of study.

Additives are used in medium solvents for various purposes.[1] Some media, like polyacrylamide, require special ones to set properly, but often such additives serve important auxiliary functions. For example, various acid dyes have been added to agar gels to improve photography of precipitin bands. Glycine added to agar diminishes this gel's nonspecific precipitation of serum lipoproteins.[10] Both dextrose and glycerin have been added to agar to protect labile antigens from spontaneous denaturation. Antigen–antibody precipitation can sometimes be enhanced by adding cadmium or nickel salts to agar gels in very low concentrations; their effects as natural contaminants of crude agar can be canceled by adding chelators to the buffer. These examples indicate that the composition of solvents in immunodiffusion media is widely flexible and adaptable, and the value of tailoring a medium solvent to an antigen–antibody system in critical experimentation is emphasized.

d. Preparation of Gels

Methods by which support media are prepared will influence results obtained with them. Following are brief descriptions of methods for preparing agar, agarose, gelatin, and polyacrylamide gels suitable for most kinds of immunodiffusion and immunoelectrophoresis tests.

i. Agar and Agarose

Some effects of contaminants persisting through initial preparation of agar have already been mentioned, but there are additional factors. Crude agar will have a stronger negative charge than purified agar, it will be more likely to denature or combine with various reactants, it will yield a weaker gel, it will be less clear, and it will hydrolyze more during heating. The more any agar is heated, the less of it will gel on cooling. This effect, while usually negligible, will be noticed if agar is melted and kept near boiling temperature for more than a few minutes, or if it is melted and gelled repeatedly. This is the most troublesome if critical measurements are being attempted on reactant diffusion rates. This is because hydrolyzed agar that fails to gel increases the viscosity of the gel's fluid phase, and because hydrolysis lowers the concentration of agar capable of gelling. Concentration of gelling agent affects the outcome and interpretation of all immunodiffusion tests. Usually a minimum is selected, one that will yield a gel just strong enough for the type of immunodiffusion test being employed. But sometimes a much higher concen-

[10] S. P. Halbert, L. Swick, and C. Sonn, *J. Exptl. Med.* **101**, 557–576 (1955).

tration is desirable, for example for determining reactant molecular weight by finding the gel density necessary to stop diffusion of a reactant, or for increasing the precipitin band sharpness and resolution.

Agar and agarose gels are prepared in similar manner. Agarose is commercially available, and some workers feel that it should be used in preference to agar whenever possible. Its preparation from agar in the laboratory is described in Section 14.F.2. Grades of agar suitable for gelling bacteriological media are as good as or better than higher priced purified agars for single- and double-diffusion agar gels, but agar employed for immunoelectrophoresis should be more highly purified and preferably with low electroosmotic flow; exceptions are discussed in Section 14.D.2.c.*ii*.

Some degree of agar purification may be desirable as well for other reasons, such as increasing the clarity of the gel, decreasing its viscosity, lowering somewhat the quantity needed to obtain satisfactory gel rigidity, decreasing its electroosmotic effects, decreasing nonspecific interaction with such substances as serum lipids, or studying the effects of individual chemicals added to agar gels on immunodiffusion reactions. Such agars can be purchased, but they also can be prepared easily in several ways from cruder agars.

Agar is clarified somewhat by ridding it of particulate impurities. This is achieved by dissolving it in the solvent and at the pH required for immunodiffusion and then filtering it hot through several layers of lintless cloth, coarse filter paper, or other inert filtering agents like shredded paper, diatomaceous earth, or asbestos. It is freed of dissolved impurities with progressively greater effectiveness by dialyzing its granules or shreds against distilled water, by making it into a gel with distilled water and then cubing the gel and dialyzing or electrodialyzing it in distilled water. In an alternate technique, gelled agar is frozen and then thawed; this breaks the gel, and the resulting shreds of agar are pressed by a plunger in a syringe or within a clean cloth sack to free them of most water and accompanying dissolved impurities. See also Section 14.D.2.b.*v*.

A very pure agar may be obtained by using chemicals that actively sequester most of the impurities. The following method[1] permits ready preparation of a large quantity of agar which is purer as determined by ash residue than most of the specially purified agars marketed.

Mix agar granules with 20 parts by weight of 1% racemic tartaric acid in distilled water, neutralize to pH 7.0 with ammonium hydroxide, and allow to stand with occasional agitation for at least 45 minutes. Pass this suspension through a coarse filter and discard the filtrate. Partially dry the agar granules with several washings of anhydrous methanol. Transfer them to a beaker, stirring them into 20 parts by weight of 1% salicylic acid in 95% ethanol. Again, allow this suspension to stand with occasional shaking for at least 45 minutes and then recover the agar granules on a coarse filter. Rinse these on the filter 4 times with 1% ammonium hydroxide in deionized water and then repeatedly with deionized water alone until the washings are of neutral pH. Such rinsing is facilitated by mixing the agar with the water and then filtering it free of wash water on several layers of gauze. Finally, gather the mass of agar into the center of the gauze filter, twist it closed, and squeeze it free of wash fluid. Dry the agar at 37°C, a process that can be hastened by rinsing the agar with anhydrous acetone. Typically, agar with impurities amounting to 3 to 4% ash on incineration is purified in this manner to an ash residue of only 0.01%, and it is free of calcium and other divalent ions.

Agar and agarose may be used at concentrations below 1% for single and double diffusion tests and up to 2% for immunoelectrophoresis depending on the gelling properties. Dry powder* is weighed out to make slightly more solution than will be required for a particular experiment. In a suitable container the agar granules are suspended gently in the buffer to wet them, and then the tube or flask is placed in a boiling water bath (or in a pressure cooker, in high altitude laboratories) and heated for as few minutes as required to obtain complete solution. This solution can be used immediately for pouring immunodiffusion plates, or it can be cooled first to between 45°C and 50C° for mixing with heat-labile reactant and then poured. If necessary, it can be kept liquid at this lower temperature for several hours without material deterioration. The gel that forms as the solution cools is ready for use unless maximum or constant gel stability is required, in which case it should be left to stand overnight at 4°C.

Poured agar and agarose gels on immunodiffusion plates or in tubes remain stable and useful indefinitely if not dried or contaminated; but gel remaining from the first melt and not used should be discarded rather than remelt. If more agar gel is needed it should be made up anew from the dried powder.

ii. Gelatin

Gelatin for use in bacteriological media is suitable also for immuno-diffusion and immunoelectrophoresis gel media. It is employed at 2 to 4%, and its gels are prepared in the same manner as agar gels, except that they must be refrigerated to set.

iii. Acrylamides (see Vol. II, Sections 6.C.4 and 5)

Polyacrylamide gels are made by polymerizing acrylamides. This can be done in several ways. The following method is easy and reli-

---

* "Dry" agar can contain from 15% to 30% of water. A dry weight basis is described in Section 14.D.2.b.v.

able and provides gels useful for single and double diffusion as well as for immunoelectrophoresis.

Dissolve Cyanogum 41* in barbital or phosphate buffer to make a 5% solution; if necessary, clarify this solution by paper filtration. Add 10% β-dimethylpropionitrile and 10% ammonium persulfate to final concentrations of 0.04% of each; these chemicals catalyze polymerization under anaerobic conditions. Place some clean microscope slides in the bottom of a shallow, level-bottomed vessel, and pour enough Cyanogum solution into this vessel to cover the slides to a depth of 1 mm. Pour over this a layer 2 mm thick of mineral oil or of heptane to exclude atmospheric oxygen. Steam the vessel over a boiling water bath, and within 3 to 5 minutes polymerization will have occurred. This can be verified by dropping the tip of an applicator stick through the heptane or mineral oil onto the Cyanogum: The stick will bounce if the gel has formed.

The resulting gel can be stored indefinitely under its mineral oil cover to prevent dehydration; its own residual toxicity prevents microbial contamination. When a slide is needed, it is cut from the surrounding gel and removed from the original vessel. If mineral oil has been used to cover the Cyanogum solution during polymerization and storage, it can be washed from the gel surface with petroleum ether; if heptane has been used, it will evaporate a few moments after being poured off. Cyanogum gels are sticky. Fingers or implements touching them should be greased to prevent their sticking to the gels. This stickiness is an advantage when some object meant to retain close contact with the gel, such as a template or filter paper impregnated with reactant, is applied to it.

The gels and procedures discussed above have been laboratory tested and their value proved. But the reader should not hesitate to try new kinds of media or improved techniques, since those presently used have been developed empirically and there is considerable room for their further improvement.

---

* A mixture of acrylamide and N,N'-methylenebisacrylamide produced by American Cyanamid Company. This mixture, either as a dry powder or in solution, is toxic until polymerized.

2. THE PREPARATION AND PROPERTIES OF AGAROSE*

a. Some Comparative Properties of Agar and Agarose

The two main components of agar—agarose and agaropectin—are both polysaccharides. Agaropectin contains sulfate and also some carboxyl groups, while agarose is built up from galactose units and is thus

---

* Section 14.F.2 was contributed by Stellan Hjertén.

devoid of charged groups[1, 2] (Fig. 1). The neutral character of agarose often makes it superior to agar for electrophoretic,[2-6] chromatographic[7, 8] and immunological experiments.[9] Agarose exhibits little or no anticomplementary[10] and virus inhibitory effects.[11] Basic substances, which are strongly adsorbed by agar, can often be studied in agarose gels without difficulty. Agarose gels also have the advantage of giving a relatively low electroendosmosis. Agarose has a higher gel strength than agar and gives more transparent gels. The proteins present in commercial agar and

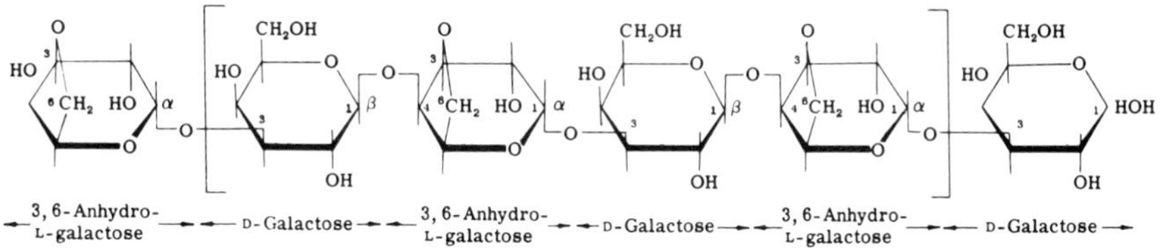

FIG. 1. The structure of agarose, according to Araki.[1] Reproduced from Hjertén[2] with permission of the publisher.

absent from agarose, give a more or less pronounced background in staining procedures.

b. PREPARATION

The method described here for the preparation of agarose is a much simplified version of a procedure published earlier.[12]* Centrifugation in warm rotors has been replaced by filtrations in an oven. The details are as follows.

[1] C. Araki, *Bull. Chem. Soc. Japan* **29**, 543 (1956).
[2] S. Hjertén, *Biochim. Biophys. Acta* **53**, 514 (1961).
[3] S. Hjertén, *J. Chromatog.* **12**, 510 (1963).
[4] V. Gheţie and D. Moţet-Grigoraş, *Studii Cercetări Biochim.* **3**, 409 (1962).
[5] D. Moţet and V. Gheţie, *Rev. Roumaine Biochim.* **1**, 175 (1964).
[6] B. Russell, J. Levitt, and A. Polson, *Biochim. Biophys. Acta* **79**, 622 (1964).
[7] S. Hjertén, *Arch. Biochem. Biophys.* **99**, 466 (1962).
[8] S. Hjertén, *Biochim. Biophys. Acta* **79**, 393 (1964).
[9] S. Brishammar, S. Hjertén, and B. von Hofsten, *Biochim. Biophys. Acta* **53**, 518 (1961).
[10] J. Bernovská, J. Kostka, and J. Sterzl, *Folia Microbiol. (Prague)* **8**, 376 (1963).
[11] B. Russell, T. H. Mead, and A. Polson, *Biochim. Biophys. Acta* **86**, 169 (1964).
[12] S. Hjertén, *Biochim. Biophys. Acta* **62**, 445 (1962).
* This procedure has been modified also by Uriel *et al.*[13] However, their technique has the practical disadvantage of requiring a centrifugation at elevated temperature. Other methods for the preparation of agarose have been described by Hjertén[2] and Russell *et al.*[11]
[13] J. Uriel, S. Avrameas, and P. Grabar, *in* "Protides of the Biological Fluids" (H. Peeters, ed.), Vol. 11, p. 355. Elsevier, Amsterdam, 1964.

Agar (32 gm, Difco Bacto Agar from Difco Laboratories, Michigan) and cetylpyridinium chloride (16 gm) are dissolved by boiling in 800 and 450 ml of water, respectively. (Cetylpyridinium bromide can also be used.) The warm cetylpyridinium chloride solution is with stirring *slowly* added to the agar solution. A precipitate forms from the complex of agaropectin with cetylpyridinium ions. The precipitate is allowed to settle overnight in an open beaker, placed in an oven at 65°. The evaporation increases the agarose concentration; this makes the subsequent precipitation with ethanol more efficient. The supernatant (agarose solution with excess of cetylpyridinium chloride) is separated from the precipitate by suction filtration in the oven on a Büchner funnel (the rubber tubing from the water pump can be introduced into the oven through its ventilation holes). To keep the filtration rate as high as possible, it is important not to stir up the settled precipitate. For this filtration the suction flask, the Büchner funnel, and two moistened filter papers are preheated in the drying oven. About 25 gm of dry fuller's earth* is added to the warm filtrate with stirring. The excess cetylpyridinium ions are efficiently adsorbed to the fuller's earth after about 1 hour at 65° with occasional stirring. Sodium chloride is added to a final concentration of about 7.0% and is dissolved by stirring. This increase in ionic strength is required to break cetylpyridinium complexes and to aggregate the smallest fuller's earth particles so that these will not pass the pores of a filter paper. After 4 hours the fuller's earth is removed by filtration inside the oven in the same way as described above for removal of precipitated agaropectin. Excessive foaming may be prevented by the addition of a few drops of *n*-octanol to the Büchner funnel and the suction flask (if necessary, octanol can be used also in the preceding filtration). The Büchner funnel should have a large diameter (about 20 cm) so that the filtration proceeds as rapidly as possible (within 10 minutes). Otherwise there is a risk that the temperature drop during the suction filtration will become so pronounced that gelling occurs in the filter papers and reduces the flow. In that case the filter papers should be changed.

The agarose is precipitated by 3 to 4 volumes of ethanol. If the agarose has partly gelled in the suction flask during the filtration, it must be dissolved by boiling before this precipitation. Cetylpyridinium salts are soluble in ethanol. Therefore this procedure is efficient also for removal of these salts, in case insufficient fuller's earth has been added. Furthermore, the concentration of sodium chloride in the agarose is also reduced to a minimum by this precipitation with ethanol.

---

* A fuller's earth available from The British Drug Houses Ltd., Poole, England, has been used. No pretreatment or washing of this product (Lloyd's reagent "for adsorption purposes") is necessary.

After some hours a firm precipitate is formed on the bottom of the container. Most of the supernatant is decanted, and the remainder is sucked off on a Büchner funnel. The small amounts of sodium chloride in the agarose can be removed by washing with 70% ethanol. The agarose is washed with ether and then air-dried at room temperature. The final product is completely white; the yield is about 20 gm.*

* The author is much indebted to Professor Arne Tiselius for stimulating interest in this work. He also wishes to thank Mrs. Irja Blomqvist for valuable technical assistance. The investigation has been supported by Research Grant G-18702 from the National Science Foundation and the Swedish Natural Science Research Council.

G. Special Techniques with Diffusion in Gels

1. SINGLE ANTIGEN–ANTIBODY SYSTEMS PREPARED FROM MIXED REACTIONS IN GELATIN*

A specially designed diffusion cell allows gel diffusion of mixed antigens and mixed antibodies to occur over a large cross-sectional area.[1] Appreciable quantities of individual antigen–antibody complexes form as parallel planes in the gel, and these zones are separated by freezing the gel and then cutting sections of it with a freezing microtome.

a. DIFFUSION CELL

The Lucite cell is made in three parts (two ends and a center piece) held together by five brass bolts with wing nuts to form an easily dismantled unit (Fig. 1). The gel (12.7 mm wide; cross-sectional area 38 × 38 mm) is in a space (A) enclosed between two parallel stainless steel gauzes (B) held in frames set in recesses in the ends of the cell. The frames stop leakage along the bottom and sides of the gel. Between the gauzes and the end of the cell are narrow spaces [(C); width 1 mm, approximate capacity 1.5 ml] for the reagents; the volume of these spaces can be varied by placing in them stainless steel plates (D) of various thicknesses (0.92, 0.76, and 0.18 mm). At the bottom corners of these spaces are two small air-access holes (E) which are usually closed with modeling clay.

b. GEL

A solution of gelatin 1.5% in warm (60° to 70°) phosphate-buffered saline, pH 7.3 (NaCl, 4.25 gm; Na_2HPO_4, 8.096 gm; KH_2PO_4, 2.438 gm/liter) containing sodium azide 0.1%, is filtered through Millipore. At 0° to 5° this solution forms a solid gel which liquefies at room temper-

* Section 14.G.1 was contributed by Harry Smith.

[1] H. Smith, B. T. Tozer, R. C. Gallop, and F. C. Scanes, *Biochem. J.* **84**, 74 (1962).

ature. The gel-forming ability of batches of gelatin differ, and the concentration used must be varied slightly from batch to batch.

Warm gelatin solution is poured into the space between the gauzes of the diffusion cell after the reagent spaces have been filled completely by inserting the thickest stainless steel plates. The gel is allowed to set at

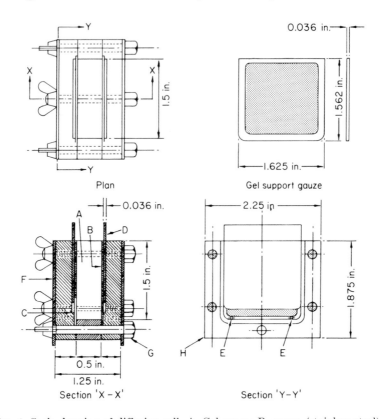

FIG. 1. Scale drawing of diffusion cell. A, Gel space; B, gauze (stainless steel); C, reagent space for antigens or antibodies; D, spacing plate (stainless steel); E, air-access holes; F, clamping plate (brass); G, bolts and wing nuts (brass); H, cell body (Lucite).

0° to 5° for 16 hours. The modeling clay in the air-access holes is pierced and, while the gauzes are held firmly in position, the steel plates are withdrawn to free the spaces for the immunological reagents. If the air-access holes are not opened and the gauzes are not held firm, the gel tends to pull away from the sides of the cell, and this leads to subsequent leakage of reagents. The air-access holes are replugged before the cell is used.

c. Serological Precipitation in the Diffusion Cell

One end of the cell is marked "antigen" and the other "antibody," and the requisite quantities of antigen and antibody solutions (usually 0.75 to 1.5 ml; the antibody is best used as a γ-globulin concentrate, see Vol. I, Chap. 3, Section A.2) are introduced into the reagent spaces. Thin stainless steel plates are then inserted either fully or partially into the spaces until the reagent solution completely fills the available space and can diffuse through the whole area of the gel. To prevent evaporation and cracking of the gel, the cells are placed in a sealed container at 0° to 5° and left until the zones of precipitation appear maximal (1.5 to 3 weeks). Separation of the zones must be more than 1.5 mm apart to allow the individual precipitates to be removed cleanly by the microtome. This is arranged by varying the concentrations of the serological reactants and sometimes by allowing either the antigen or the antibodies to diffuse some days before the other reactant is added. Preliminary experiments in a small cell (12.5 × 12.5 mm) are advisable.

d. Use of a Freezing Microtome to Remove Individual Antigen–Antibody Precipitates

The gel is frozen with solid CO_2 and then the cell is dismantled. The frozen gel is set squarely on the stage of a freezing microtome (An MSE Base Sledge microtome with 90-mm in diameter stage and wedge-shaped 240-mm knife is suitable) and fixed by freezing water around the base. Sections (120 μ thick) from the block are collected with a hairbrush individually and consecutively into 0.9% NaCl (0.1 ml) contained in wells of a Lucite hemagglutination tray at room temperature. The gel melts and the limits of the zones of precipitation are easily seen in the wells of the tray separated by 10 to 20 wells containing little or no precipitate (see Fig. 2 of Smith et al.[2]). The contents of the wells corresponding to the zones of precipitation are removed and combined.

e. Removal of the Gel

A number (10 to 30) of diffusion cells should be used for each experiment. After sectioning, the contents of all the wells containing the same antigen–antibody precipitate are combined (1 volume) and diluted with phosphate-buffered saline (see preparation of gel: 1 volume) and are left at room temperature overnight. The precipitate is removed by centrifugation (1200 g for 0.5 hour at room temperature) and washed six times with phosphate-buffered saline (40, 40, 40, 40, 5, and 5 ml).

[2] H. Smith, R. C. Gallop, and B. T. Tozer, Immunology 7, 111 (1964).

By using a number of cells, 10 to 20 mg of individual precipitates were prepared from several mixtures of two antigens and their corresponding rabbit antibodies; contamination with the extraneous complex was less than 5%.[1, 2]

The potential uses of monospecific antibodies are manifold. Relatively large quantities of these antibodies can be prepared by injecting into rabbits small quantities of the individual complexes separated from mixed antigens and antibodies as described here.[2]

2. PARTICULATE ANTIGENS FOR REACTIONS IN AGAR GEL*

Gel diffusion techniques are usually employed for studies on precipitation reactions involving soluble antigens and their corresponding antibodies; however, they have also been used successfully to examine reactions of particulate antigens of mammalian tissues with their corresponding antibodies.[1,2,3] Most of these studies have dealt with erythrocyte stromata. In addition, investigation was performed on interaction in agar gel between erythrocyte stromata and hemagglutinating viruses in order to obtain reaction lines that would be a counterpart of viral hemagglutination in test tubes.[4]

It is necessary to use a low concentration of agar (0.5%) and to disrupt the antigen into minute particles by sonication.

a. RECOMMENDED PROCEDURES

i. Erythrocyte Stromata

Blood specimens are collected in acid citrate dextrose solution and preserved for not more than 7 days at 4°. Erythrocytes are washed 4 times with 0.15 M NaCl and hemolyzed with distilled water. At least 9 volumes of water are added to 1 volume of packed erythrocytes; however, the most satisfactory preparations are obtained by adding 30 to 50 volumes of water to 1 volume of erythrocyte sediment. The preparation is left at 4° for 8 to 24 hours. The stromata are then washed 4 to 6 times in distilled water and 2 to 4 times in saline solution. After the last washing, the stromata are suspended in saline, using 1 to 4 volumes of saline for 1 volume of the stroma sediment. The preparation is exposed to supersonic vibration at 20,000 cps. We have used the MSE Mullard ultrasonic disintegra-

* Section 14.G.2 was contributed by Felix Milgrom.

[1] F. Milgrom, and U. Loza, J. Immunol. 98, 102–109 (1967).
[2] A. L. Barron, A. Friedman, and F. Milgrom, J. Immunol. 99, 778–784 (1967).
[3] F. Milgrom, and U. Loza, Vox Sanguinis 16, 470–477 (1969).
[4] F. Milgrom, A. L. Barron, and U. Loza, Virology 33, 145–149 (1967).

tor. During sonication the preparation should be submerged in an ice–water mixture. The duration of sonication should be at least 20 seconds, but in those instances in which this treatment does not affect the antigen under investigation, sonication may be extended up to 10 minutes.

For experiments on the interaction of stromata with viruses, no further concentration of stromata is necessary. For experiments with antisera, stromata are concentrated by centrifugation at 60,000 g for 20 minutes and the pellet is resuspended in 1 to 2 volumes of saline. In all cases where the resuspended stromata fail to form a homogeneous suspension, resonication for 5 to 10 seconds should be employed.

Experiments on the reaction of erythrocyte stromata with Rh antibodies requires pretreatment of whole erythrocytes with trypsin. The sediment of washed erythrocytes is suspended in an equal volume of 5% solution of trypsin in a buffer containing, in 100 ml, 800 mg of NaCl, 40 mg of KCl, 6 mg of Na_2HPO_4, 6 mg of KH_2PO_4, and 24.7 mg of $NaHCO_3$. The mixture is incubated for 20 minutes at 37° and the trypsinized cells are washed 5 to 6 times with chilled saline (4°). The erythrocytes are lysed by suspending them in 50 volumes of distilled water for 2 hours at 4°. Following 6 washings in water the stromata are resuspended in 50 volumes of saline and left for 16 hours at 4°. Thereafter the preparation is washed in saline, sonicated for 20 seconds and concentrated as described above.

ii. Myxoviruses

Newcastle disease virus or influenza virus are prepared from infected allantoic fluids of chick embryos.[4] The pooled allantoic fluid is centrifuged at 2000 rpm for 20 minutes in order to remove coarse debris and red blood cells. The supernatant is centrifuged at 78,000 g, and thereafter the pellet is resuspended in plain saline solution or Earle's saline using a volume 200 times less than the original volume of the virus-infected allantoic fluid.

iii. Double Diffusion in Gel

Ionagar No. 2 (Consolidated Laboratories, Inc., Chicago Heights, Illinois) or agarose (Bausch & Lomb, Inc., Rochester, New York) are used as the media for gel diffusion tests. Ionagar is dissolved in an autoclave at 121° and agarose in a waterbath at 100° to give 0.5% solutions in saline and are poured into plastic Petri dishes (Falcon Plastics, Culver City, California) to form layers 2 mm thick. Circular wells 4 to 6 mm in diameter are cut in the solidified gel by means of brass rings. The diffusion distance between wells is 2 to 3 mm. After the wells are filled with reagents, the Petri dishes are closed with lids and incubated at room temperature for 24 hours and at 4° for 2 to 4 days. For some experiments, sonicated erythrocyte stromata should be allowed to diffuse for 24 hours before other wells are filled with antisera or virus preparations.

b. APPLICATIONS

The reactions between erythrocyte stromata and their corresponding antisera usually appear in the form of a heavy line very close to the stromata well [Fig. 1 (1)]. The convexity of the reaction arc is directed toward the antiserum well. The antigen participating in these reactions is composed of particles which may conveniently be seen by phase contrast microscopy [Fig. 1 (2)].

The procedure can be used also as an analytical tool in instances in which an antiserum containing more than one type of antibody is tested against two different antigenic preparations, as exemplified in Fig. 1 parts (3), (4), and (5).

In the experiment, the results of which are presented in Fig. 1 (3), stromata of erythrocytes of CDe/Ce and Cde/ce Rh genotypes were tested against Rh serum containing antibodies to D and G antigens (G antigen is present in erythrocytes containing either C or D or both). It may be seen that the line formed by CD stromata extended in the form of a spur over the line formed by C stromata. Apparently G anti-G line does not constitute a barrier for anti-D antibodies which cross this line to combine with the D antigen.

Infectious mononucleosis serum was tested simultaneously against sheep and bovine erythrocyte stromata [Fig. 1 (4)]. The spur formation demonstrates that the infectious mononucleosis serum recognizes more antigens on bovine than on sheep erythrocyte stromata.

Infectious mononucleosis serum was tested against bovine erythrocyte stromata and Newcastle disease virus [Fig. 1 (5)]. Complete crossing of reaction lines reveals that unrelated antibodies are responsible for the activity of this serum against these two antigens.

In contrast, when two antisera containing different antibody spectra are tested against one stroma preparation, the procedure usually fails as an analytical tool. This is exemplified in Fig. 1 (6a). Unabsorbed anti-M and anti-N sera give an identity reaction with stromata of blood group M erythrocytes. Both these antisera combine with the human species specific antigen but anti-M serum combines in addition, with the blood group M antigen on these stromata. Still, no spur is formed. Apparently the species-specific and the blood-group M antigens reside on the same particles; these therefore cannot cross the line formed in reaction with antibodies directed against one of the antigens. It may be noted in Fig. 1 (6a) that unabsorbed anti-M serum and absorbed anti-M also give identity reaction with stromata of blood group M erythrocytes. Here, the

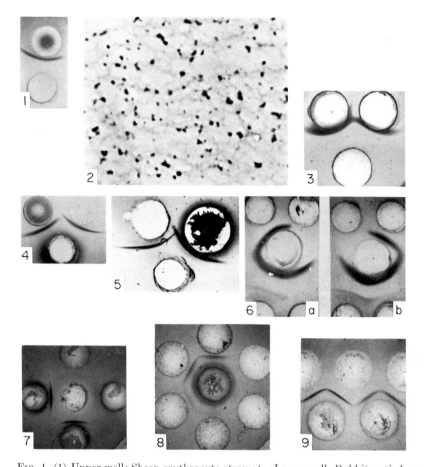

Fig. 1. (1) Upper well: Sheep erythrocyte stromata. Lower well: Rabbit anti-sheep erythrocyte serum. (2) Particles of stromata within a line formed in the reaction of sheep erythrocyte stromata with rabbit anti-sheep erythrocyte serum. Phase contrast microscopy, 3800. The picture was kindly prepared by Dr. O. Haferkamp of the University of Bonn, Germany. (3) Upper left well: Stromata of human erythrocytes, Rh type CDe/Ce. Upper right well: Stromata of human erythrocytes, Rh type Cde/ce. Lower well: Anti-Rh serum with anti-D and anti-G antibodies. (4) Upper left well: Sheep erythrocyte stromata. Upper right well: Bovine erythrocyte stromata. Lower well: Infectious mononucleosis serum. (5) Upper left well: Bovine erythrocyte stromata. Upper right well: Newcastle disease virus, strain VIC. Lower well: Infectious mononucleosis serum. (6) Central well in (a): Human blood group M erythrocyte stromata. Central well in (b): Human blood group N erythrocyte stromata. Lower wells in both figures contain unabsorbed antisera; anti-M on the left, anti-N on the right. Upper wells in both figures: contain absorbed antisera: anti-M serum absorbed with N erythrocyte stromata on the left; anti-N serum absorbed with M erythrocyte stromata on the right. (7) Central well: Human erythrocyte stromata. Top well: PR8 virus, unheated. Right, bottom, and left wells: PR8 virus heated at 56° for 3, 10, and 20 minutes, respectively. (8) Central well: PR8 virus. Top well: Untreated human erythrocyte stromata. Remaining wells, clockwise: Human erythrocyte stromata treated with receptor destroying enzyme (RDE) at dilutions of 1:10, 1:40, 1:160 1:640, and 1:2560. (9) Upper wells: Human erythrocyte stromata. Lower wells: Influenza A; left, PR8 virus; right, Jap/170/62 virus.

unabsorbed antiserum is richer since it contains also species-specific anti-bodies whereas the absorbed serum contains only group-specific anti-bodies. However, no spur is formed because of the above discussed locali-zation of the species-specific and the blood group-specific antigens on the same particle. The result of the experiment with blood group N erythro-cytes [Fig. 1 (6b)] may be explained in an analogous way.

The reactions between erythrocyte stromata and hemagglutinating myxoviruses require prediffusion of stromata for 24 hours. The viruses are heated at 56° in order to destroy viral neuraminidase, which affects stro-mata and prevents their reaction with viral hemagglutinin [Fig. 1 (7)]. The receptor site on the erythrocyte stromata can be destroyed by treatment with RDE as exemplified in Fig. 1 (8). In studying human erythrocyte stromata against various strains of influenza viruses, identity reactions are observed Fig. 1 (9).

Simple analytical studies of insoluble antigens and their antibodies can be made. Many insoluble cell membrane antigens including histo-compatibility antigens can perhaps be investigated. Similarly, studies are possible on the nature of viral hemagglutinin and on the corresponding receptor in various tissues.

CHAPTER 15

Hapten Reactions and Kinetics of Interaction with Antibodies

A. Equilibrium and Kinetic Studies of Antibody–Hapten Reactions*†

Because of the demonstrated divalency of antibodies of the IgG type, and of the polyvalency of antibodies of the IgM type, combination of antibodies with polyvalent, polydeterminant antigens results in the formation of large antibody–antigen aggregates, $(Ab)_x(Ag)_y$, of varying size, complexity, and solubility. Some of these complexes may give rise to heterogeneous systems consisting of precipitates or unstable suspensions. Consequently, antibody–antigen interactions cannot be studied meaningfully by standard physicochemical procedures, used for the determination of the extent and speed of ordinary reactions, unless they can be investigated over a sufficiently low concentration range where phase transitions do not obtain.

On the other hand, with univalent haptens (H), only soluble bimolecular or termolecular products can be formed with divalent antibodies, i.e., complexes of the types AbH or AbH_2, and the interactions involved in these systems may be represented by the elementary and reversible, homogeneous reactions

$$Ab + H \rightleftarrows AbH \tag{1}$$
$$AbH + H \rightleftarrows AbH_2 \tag{2}$$

If the antibody combining sites are considered equal and independent of each other, the first relation suffices to describe the system and the term Ab may then be taken as the concentration of antibody sites, i.e., n times the concentration of antibody molecules where n is the valency of the antibody molecules.

Let us now denote by the letters b and f the molecular species in the bound and free forms, respectively, and by the subscript t the total

* Section 15.A was contributed by A. H. Sehon.

† The research program in the author's laboratory, related to this study, has been supported by grants from the National Institute of Allergy and Infectious Diseases (AI02085), National Institutes of Health, Bethesda, Maryland, and the National and Medical Research Councils of Canada, Ottawa, Ontario.

number of antibody sites or hapten molecules. One can then write on the basis of the law of conservation of mass the following stoichiometric relations:

$$Ab_t = Ab_b + Ab_f$$
$$H_t = H_b + H_f$$
$$AbH = Ab_b = H_b = b$$

Two additional terms, c and r, have been used to denote the concentration of free hapten and the fraction of antibody sites occupied, i.e., $c = H_f$ and $r = b/Ab_t$.

According to the law of mass action and from relation (1), it follows that the equilibrium constant, K, is given by the equation

$$K = \frac{[AbH]}{[Ab][H]} = \frac{[H_b]}{[Ab_f][H_f]} = \frac{b}{[Ab_t - b]c} \tag{3}$$

Furthermore, by making the appropriate substitutions, for a system of antibodies possessing n independent binding sites the mass law equation may be represented by the expression

$$\frac{r}{c} = Kn - Kr \tag{4}$$

Equation (4) has been used widely for representing antibody–hapten binding data on a plot of r/c vs. r, from which the value n can be readily obtained by extrapolation of the experimental curve to the abscissa.[1, 2] If all antibody sites had the same binding affinity for the hapten, one would expect this plot to be linear and K to be equal to the slope of the line, multiplied by -1. However, practically all the systems studied so far exhibit deviation from linearity, which has been interpreted as representing a measure of the heterogeneity of the population of antibody combining sites with respect to their affinities for the hapten molecules.[2–4]

As pointed out in succeeding sections, the distribution of the equilibrium constants and the corresponding spread of free energies has been considered to be Gaussian and each antibody system was characterized by an average equilibrium constant and an appropriate index of heterogeneity. It has been suggested[2] that this heterogeneity is a property unique to the immune response, since it has not been detected in other biopolymer–ligand systems, such as in the formation of enzyme–substrate complexes. Thus, the variability of the strength of the antibody–hapten

---

[1] F. Karush and S. S. Karush, this volume, Section 15.B.
[2] F. Karush, *Advan. Immunol.* **2**, 1 (1962).
[3] J. Cebra, this volume, Section 15.E.
[4] D. Pressman, *Methods Med. Res.* **10**, 122 (1964).

bond for a population of antibody molecules might be regarded as a reflection of subtle conformational differences in and about the combining sites, imparted by the specific mechanism underlying the biosynthesis of antibodies.[2] This hypothesis may not account completely for this unique feature of antibody–hapten interactions, since even in cases where the hapten is attached to only one type of amino acid of a carrier protein, the resulting antigens are likely to be structurally heterogeneous with respect to the conformation of the hapten residue,[5] i.e., depending on the hydrophobic or hydrophilic nature of the amino acids in the environment of the particular amino acid to which the hapten is coupled; accordingly, the heterogeneity of binding constants of antihapten antibodies would reflect also the structural heterogeneity of antigenic determinants. However, further strong support for the heterogeneity of antibodies was provided by the results of an elegant study[6] in which anti-dinitrophenyl(DNP) antibodies, elicited in rabbits by immunization with bovine pancreatic ribonuclease to which one DNP group had been coupled per protein molecule (at the lysine residue in position 41 of RNase), were just as heterogeneous in their binding of ϵ-DNP-L-lysine as most of the antibodies induced by immunization with DNP conjugates of bovine γ-globulin, in which the microenvironments about individual DNP-lysyl residues would be expected to be diverse. Similar conclusions were recently derived from a study in which the univalent hapten–protein conjugate, monodinitrophenylpapain, was used as antigen.[6a] In contrast to these results, however, one may cite the surprising evidence[7] for the singularity of the association constant of "monospecific" antitobacco mosaic virus antibodies, irrespective of whether isolated from serum of single rabbits or from a pool of antisera. Moreover, recently monoclonal myeloma proteins have been isolated possessing anti-DNP activity and properties of homogeneous monodisperse immuhoglobulins.[7a]

For a reversible system represented by relation (1′)

$$Ab + H \underset{k_{21}}{\overset{k_{12}}{\rightleftarrows}} AbH \tag{1′}$$

where k_{12} and k_{21} are the rate constants of the bimolecular association and unimolecular dissociation steps, respectively, the rates of the forward

---

[5] S. J. Singer, *Immunochemistry* **1**, 15 (1964).

[6] H. N. Eisen and G. W. Siskind, *Biochemistry* **3**, 996 (1964).

[6a] L. Brenneman, and S. J. Singer, *Proc. Natl. Acad. Sci.* **16**, 258 (1968).

[7] M. D. Mamet-Bratley, *Immunochemistry* **3**, 155 (1966).

[7a] H. N. Eisen, J. R. Little, C. K. Osterland, and E. S. Simms, *Cold Spring Harbor Symp. Quant. Biol.* **XXXII**, 75 (1967).

and reverse reactions are given by the expressions

$$\text{rate}_{\text{assoc}} = k_{12}[\text{Ab}_f][\text{H}_f]$$
$$\text{rate}_{\text{dissoc}} = k_{21}[\text{AbH}]$$

At equilibrium, the rates of these two reactions are obviously equal and it follows that

$$\frac{k_{12}}{k_{21}} = \frac{[\text{AbH}]}{[\text{Ab}_f][\text{H}_f]} = K \tag{5}$$

This treatment is valid only for reversible reactions, and the reversibility of antibody–hapten reactions has been adequately demonstrated in a number of investigations.[8] As for all ordinary reactions, the determination of equilibrium or rate constants reduces itself inevitably to a determination of the concentrations (or of the change of concentrations as a function of time) of the reactants and/or products. In general, in computing the values of equilibrium and rate constants, all activity coefficients are taken as equal to unity on the assumption that, since the reactions are studies at concentrations below 10^{-5} M, the laws of ideal solutions might be applicable.

Most of the equilibrium constants have been derived from equilibrium dialysis experiments,[1, 2] which provide an absolute basis for measuring the binding between hapten molecules (or any low molecular weight ligands) and antibodies (or any macromolecular species). As described in Section 15.B, this is a general, simple, and direct procedure for the determination of the concentrations of the hapten in the bound and free forms and leaves little latitude for interpretation of the results. By contrast, other procedures, which involve the determination of antibody–hapten association constants in terms of differences in some physical property of the hapten (such as the polarographic reduction potential[8] or extinction coefficient[9]) or of the antibody molecule (such as fluorescence quenching[10] and fluorescence polarization[11]) in the free and bound forms, must be regarded as indirect methods and must be calibrated with reference to data obtained by equilibrium dialysis.

Thus, although in spectrophotometric measurements of antibody–hapten interactions one is forced, for practical reasons, to assume a singularity of the extinction coefficient of the bound form of the hapten, it has

---

[8] H. Schneider and A. H. Sehon, *Trans. N.Y. Acad. Sci.* [2] **24**, 15 (1961).
[9] H. Schneider, S. G. Goldwater, and A. H. Sehon, unpublished data (1969).
[10] H. N. Eisen and J. E. McGuigan, this volume, Section 15.C.
[11] W. Dandliker, this volume Section 15.F.

been inferred recently[9] that the extinction coefficient of the bound form of the hapten is in fact an average value, ϵ_b, defined by Eq. (6)

$$\epsilon_b = \frac{\displaystyle\sum_{i=1}^{i=i} c_i \cdot \epsilon_{b,i}}{\displaystyle\sum_{i=1}^{i=i} c_i} \tag{6}$$

where $\epsilon_{b,i}$ is the extinction coefficient of a hapten at a concentration c_i, bound to an antibody molecule of a particular affinity (i). Moreover, since spectral changes of the hapten are the result of an alteration in molecular environment upon binding and since the extent of antibody–hapten associations would depend on the nature of the forces responsible for these interactions (i.e., ionic, hydrophobic, van der Waals', and hydrogen bonds), which would differ depending on the microheterogeneity of antibody combining sites, one would not expect to find a direct relation between the strength of antibody–hapten interactions and the magnitude of the spectral change induced on binding. In line with these observations, it is to be noted that with certain antibody preparations a variation had been detected in the efficiency of fluorescence quenching as a function of the concentration of bound hapten; this effect may be attributed also to the heterogeneity of the interactions observed.

The change in standard free energy (ΔF°), enthalpy (ΔH°), and entropy (ΔS°), representing the fundamental thermodynamic constants for any system, can be calculated by the use of the classic relations* (7), (8), and (9).

$$\Delta F^\circ = -RT \ln K \tag{7}$$

$$\frac{d \ln K}{d (1/T)} = -\frac{\Delta H^\circ}{R} \tag{8}$$

$$\Delta F^\circ = \Delta H^\circ - \Delta S^\circ \tag{9}$$

The characteristic feature of antibody–hapten reactions is that they occur spontaneously and exceedingly rapidly, i.e., within times shorter than necessary to mix the reagents. The association constants determined for a large number of antibody–hapten systems[2] are in the range of 5×10^4 to 2×10^8 liters/mole, and the corresponding thermodynamic values are of the order of $\Delta F^\circ = -9$ to -14 kcal/mole, $\Delta H^\circ = -7$ to -10 kcal/mole, and $\Delta S^\circ = 9$ to 30 (with one case having an entropy of

* For derivation of these equations, the reader is referred to textbooks of thermodynamics; the application of these equations to immunochemical systems is discussed in detail by Karush.[2]

about -0.8) cal/deg/mole. The relatively small values of $\Delta F°$ for anti-body–antigen reactions indicate that, in spite of their specificity, the bind-ing between antibody and antigen molecules is rather weak, as would be expected for the formation of noncovalent bonds. An unusual feature of antibody–hapten interaction is the positive change in entropy of these reactions. Since antibody–hapten reactions are association processes, it would be expected that these reactions would be associated with losses in rotational and vibrational degrees of freedom, which would be mani-fested by a decrease, rather than an increase, in entropy. To explain this apparent anomaly, it has been suggested that these reactions are accompanied by liberation of some of the water of hydration from the binding sites, which results in an increase in the degrees of freedom of the water molecules released; this effect would thus compensate for any loss in entropy due to the association of the reaction partners, and the net result would be a positive entropy change.

Although it has become a general practice to utilize the methods of chemical kinetics for the elucidation of the mechanisms of most chemical reactions, only very few kinetic studies of antibody–hapten interactions have been made so far, primarily because of the difficulty in determining the rates of these extremely fast reactions even by the use of modern, highly sophisticated instrumentation. In all the kinetic procedures for measuring the speed of antibody–hapten interactions, the rates were determined as a function of a physical property of a system (such as a change, as a function of time, in the absorption spectrum of a dye-hapten or in the quenching efficiency of the tryptophan fluorescence of the anti-body molecule by the specific hapten), which was considered to represent appropriately the change studied.* In general, the rate constant, k, of any time-dependent process may be expressed[12, 13] by the classic Arrhenius equation $k = Ae^{-E/RT}$, where A is the "preexponential term," E = experi-mental activation energy in cal/mole determined from the temperature coefficient of the rate constant k, R = universal gas constant = 1.987 cal/deg/mole, and T = absolute temperature. Hence, for the associa-tion and dissociation steps represented by relation $(1')$, one may write the expressions

$$k_{12} = A_{12}e^{-E_{12}/RT}$$
$$k_{21} = A_{21}e^{-E_{21}/RT}$$

---

* For a discussion of the advantages and limitations of physical methods used for following the kinetics of a reaction, see Chapter 3 of Frost and Pearson.[12]

[12] A. A. Frost and R. G. Pearson, "Kinetics and Mechanism." Wiley, New York, 1953.

[13] S. Glasstone, K. J. Laidler, and H. Eyring, "Theory of Rate Processes." McGraw-Hill, New York, 1941.

From the theory of chemical kinetics of reversible reactions, it can be readily shown[13] that the change in enthalpy, ΔH, in going from the initial to the final state, may be represented by the relation

$$\Delta H = E_{12} - E_{21}$$

Moreover, according to the more rigorous theory of absolute reaction rates,[13] the rate constant for a bimolecular reaction is given by the expression

$$k_{12} = e \frac{\bar{k}T}{h} \cdot e^{-E/RT} \cdot e^{\Delta S^*/R}$$

where e = base of natural logarithms = 2.718, $\bar{k}$ = Boltzmann constant = 1.38×10^{-16} erg/deg, h = Planck's constant = 6.625×10^{-27} erg sec, ΔS^* (in units of cal/deg/mole) = change in standard entropy in going from the initial to the transition state, and E, R, and T as defined previously. In general ΔS^* would be expected to be a positive value if the reorganization of the bonds of the molecules in the transition complex results in the formation of a "looser" structure than that of the reactants. Conversely, if the activated complex were associated with a decrease in the degree of randomness, there would be a decrease in ΔS^*. More complex relations, including the contributions from electrostatic interactions, have been derived for reactions of charged species,[14] which would be more appropriate for the present discussion considering that antibody molecules are polyelectrolytes and that the hapten molecules usually possess charged groups. However, in view of the lack of data on the effect of charge on the kinetics of antibody–hapten reactions, this topic will not be dealt with in this brief survey.

One may calculate the maximum, theoretically limiting rate constant, for an antibody–hapten association reaction, by neglecting any repulsive or attractive electrostatic effects and assuming that every collision between an antibody site and a homologous hapten molecule is "effective." This is equivalent to saying that this reaction would require no activation energy other than that necessary for overcoming the effects of viscosity in a liquid medium and that, consequently, the speed of the reaction would be determined by the rate of diffusion of the reactants, i.e., the reaction would be "diffusion-controlled."

In terms of these assumptions, the rate constant for the diffusion-controlled reaction may be expressed by the equation

$$k_{12} = \frac{2\pi N}{1000} \cdot R_{1,2} D_{1,2}$$

[14] I. Amdur and G. Hammes, "Chemical Kinetics." McGraw-Hill, New York, 1966.

382 HAPTENHAPTEN REACTIONS 15.A]15.A]

where N represents Avogadro's number, $R_{1,2}$ the reaction radius, and $D_{1,2}$ the sum of the diffusion coefficients of the interacting molecules. Using this equation with the reasonable values of 4×10^{-8} cm for the reaction radius and 5×10^{-6} and 4×10^{-7} cm^{-2} sec^{-1} for the diffusion coefficients of the hapten and antibody molecules, respectively, the maximum rate constant for k_{12} would be of the order of 2×10^9 M^{-1} sec^{-1}. Because of steric limitations and electrostatic repulsions arising from the fact that at normal pH the antibody and (also usually) the hapten molecules are negatively charged, it would be expected that the actual values for k_{12} would be smaller than this maximum value by a factor of at least 10. As reviewed in Section 15.D,[15] the values of k_{12} derived from kinetic studies of antibody–hapten systems by the temperature-jump relaxation method were in the range of 2×10^7 and 2×10^8 M^{-1} sec^{-1}. In agreement with these results are the values of the order of 10^8 M^{-1} sec^{-1}, derived for the combination of anti-DNP antibodies with DNP-lysine and DNP-aminocaproate by the use of a stopped flow apparatus* equipped for measurement of fluorescence quenching.[17] It is worth pointing out that fluorescence quenching is a highly sensitive analytical procedure requiring only a small amount of antibodies at concentrations as low as 10^{-7} M. Thus, it would appear that the stopped-flow technique adapted for fluorimetry is capable of yielding precise kinetic data for antibody–hapten reactions and that it might prove to be more generally suited for these studies than the more complex temperature-jump procedure.

The only energies of activation calculated for antibody-hapten association reactions were derived from the above-mentioned studies[17] for the anti-DNP system, the actual values being 4.1 ± 1.0 and 4.4 ± 1.0 kcal/mole with DNP-lysine and DNP-aminocaproate, respectively. These values are comparable to those expected for the energy of activation of viscous flow in liquid media and it would thus appear that antibody–hapten reactions are indeed diffusion controlled. Moreover, in view of the heterogeneity of association constants of an antibody preparation, it would be expected that there should be also some statistical distribution of the rate constants k_{12} and k_{21}, which determine the equilibrium constants [see relation (5)]. Indeed, some suggestive evidence for the heterogeneity of k_{12} values was obtained with the anti-DNP system.[17]

In conclusion, in spite of the scarcity of kinetic data, it is of interest to note that although the intrinsic association constants for the five

---

[15] A. Froese and A. H. Sehon, this volume, Section 15.D.
* For details of stopped-flow techniques, see Roughton and Chance.[16]
[16] F. J. W. Roughton and B. Chance, *Tech. Org. Chem.* **8** (Part 2), 704 (1963).
[17] L. A. Day, J. M. Sturtevant, and S. J. Singer, *Ann. N.Y. Accd. Sci.* **103**, 611 (1963).

different antibody–hapten systems studied differed by almost three orders of magnitude (from 5×10^5 to 10^8 M^{-1}), the values for k_{12} differed within one order of magnitude, i.e., 2×10^7 to 2×10^8 $M^{-1} \sec^{-1}$. Consequently, one would be inclined to infer that the activation energy for the association step (E_{12}) is always negligible and that the strength of an antibody–hapten association would be determined primarily by the activation energy for dissociation (E_{21}), the rate of dissociation thus reflecting the particular forces involved in the interaction between the hapten and the antibody combining site. It is conceivable, therefore, that more information concerning the mechanism of antibody–hapten reactions at molecular level could be obtained by studying the dissociation reactions rather than the association processes.

B. Equilibrium Dialysis*

1. PRINCIPLE OF THE METHOD

Equilibrium dialysis provides a theoretically sound and unambiguous experimental method for the thermodynamic and stoichiometric characterization of antibody–hapten interactions. It is based on the reversibility of this interaction and permits the measurement of the distribution of the hapten between the bound and free forms. The feasibility of the method arises from the impermeability of a dialysis membrane (cellulose) to the antibody molecule and the ready diffusion of haptens through the membrane.

The dialysis unit usually consists of two chambers separated by a membrane. Into one chamber a measured volume of antibody solution is placed and into the other a measured volume of the hapten in the same solvent. Alternatively the antibody and hapten may be placed in the same chamber and solvent in the other. After equilibration, the hapten concentration in the protein-free chamber is measured. This value, except for a possible Donnan correction, represents the concentration of free hapten in equilibrium with the antibody-bound hapten. With the knowledge of the quantities of total hapten and antibody in the dialysis unit, one can calculate the average number (r) of hapten molecules bound per antibody molecule at the corresponding free hapten concentration (c). If a series of such pairs of values is obtained for an appropriate range of c, then the data may be plotted to give a binding curve. As will be described below, alternative methods of graphical representation of binding data have been employed.

* Sections 15.B.1–4 were contributed by Fred Karush† and Sally S. Karush.

† Recipient of a Public Health Service Research Career Award (5-K6-AI-14,012) from the National Institute of Allergy and Infectious Diseases.

Since the antibody molecule constitutes a nondiffusible charged species the distribution of diffusible ionic species between the chambers is subject to the Donnan effect. In practice this effect is reduced to a negligible value for charged haptens by including a sufficient concentration of inorganic ions in the solvent. An ionic strength of 0.1 is generally adequate to render the Donnan effect insignificant.

2. PROCEDURES

a. Dialysis Cells and Membranes

Although equilibrium dialysis can be carried out with dialysis bags prepared with cellulose sausage casing,* the most accurate results, when working with small volumes, e.g., 1 ml, are obtained with the use of the two-section dialysis unit. Several varieties of such dialysis cells have been employed in different laboratories.[1] Our description here, however, will be limited to the type of dialysis cell which has proved satisfactory in our laboratory and which is commercially available.†

The items which comprise the dialysis cell and the brass frame‡ in which it is mounted are shown in Fig. 1. Each section of the cell includes a glass chamber with a ground flange at one end and screw threads at the other end. The outside diameter of the flange is 23 mm and the cellulose membrane which is held between the flanges is of the same diameter. The membranes are cut from sausage casing (20/32, Visking Co., Chicago, Illinois) with a $^{15}/_{16}$-inch cork borer (Arthur H. Thomas, Catalog No. 4073-F). To minimize breakage of the chambers in the assembly of the dialysis cell rubber O-rings (Parker Seal Co., No. 2-112) are placed between the beveled side of the brass plate and the chamber. The chambers are closed with tinfoil-lined screw caps (size No. 15).

The assembly of the dialysis cell with a sufficient but not excessive pressure between the glass flanges is greatly facilitated by the use of a torque nut driver specially designed for this application.‡ The assembled dialysis unit should also be checked for leakage before it is filled with hapten and antibody solutions. A convenient procedure is to connect one side of the dialysis cell to a three-foot glass tube filled with water and look for leakage either through the membrane or between the flanges. This hydrostatic pressure head will reveal almost any leak which is likely to yield an erroneous distribution of the hapten between the two chambers.

* See Vol. II, Chapter 8, Section C.1, for description of such an analytical dialysis cell.
[1] M. E. Carsten and H. N. Eisen, *J. Am. Chem. Soc.* **77**, 1273 (1955).
† Bellco Glass Co., Vineland, New Jersey.
‡ Available from Drummond Scientific Co., 500 Parkway S., Broomall, Pennsylvania.

Before assembly of the cell, new glass chambers are siliconed once prior to use. The membranes are soaked to remove soluble components. If the analytical determination of the free hapten involves the measurement of optical density in the visible spectrum or an assay for radioactivity, then treatment with several changes of distilled water over a period of 1 to 2 hours is adequate. If spectrophotometric measurement in the ultraviolet region is required, then more elaborate extraction procedures may be needed.[2] After appropriate treatment of the membrane it is freed of water with absorbent lens tissue, and while still damp it is placed in

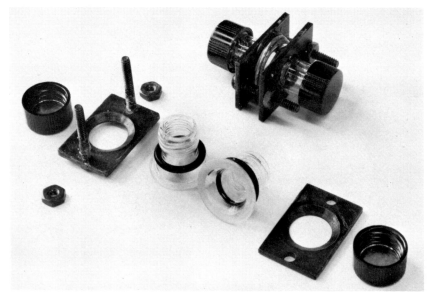

Fig. 1. The assembled dialysis cell and its parts.

position between the flanges. The membrane should be carefully examined for tears or other imperfections and mounted perfectly flat to avoid folds or creases. The care exercised at this stage of the procedure will determine the frequency with which results must be discarded because of leakage of antibody through the membrane. The assembly of the dialysis cell is continued to the point where the cell is firmly secured in the brass frame. Before the chambers are filled with solutions, the membrane is allowed to dry for about 1 hour to avoid significant dilution. More extended drying, such as overnight at room temperature, is not apparently deleterious to the membrane. In addition, before filling, a coat of wax is

2 T. R. Hughes and I. M. Klotz, *Methods Biochem. Anal.* **3**, 265 (1956).

placed along the edge of the flanges to prevent the flow of liquid between the water bath and the cell.

b. MANIPULATIONS AND AUXILIARY EQUIPMENT

The chambers described here were designed to accommodate a volume of 1 ml of solution and provide an air space of about 0.5 ml. The air space serves to facilitate mixing within each chamber during the rocking or rotation of the cell. After the necessary number of cells, which may conveniently range from 12 to 20, are assembled and supported on a test tube rack, they are filled, usually with several different hapten concentrations with duplicate cells for each concentration. For this operation accurate 1-ml volumetric pipets are used. Immediately after the hapten solution is placed in the cell, the caps are screwed on. After all the cells have received their hapten solution they are carefully examined for any evidence of leakage of the hapten solution through the membrane. This is followed by the addition to each cell of 1 ml of antibody solution of which the concentration has been previously accurately determined.

Since precise temperature control and the use of more than one temperature are generally desirable, the equilibration of the contents of the cells is done by rocking or rotating in a constant temperature water bath. A rotating device designed to hold 36 cells mounted in the brass frames is shown in Fig. 2. The shape of this device allows it to be placed in the refrigerated constant-temperature bath (Forma Scientific Inc., Marietta, Ohio) also shown in Fig. 2. With such a bath, the maximum range of temperature control is conveniently available. It is also worthwhile to use two or more fixed thermoregulators (e.g., H. B. Instrument Co., Philadelphia, cat. No. 7530) so that the temperature of the bath can be altered easily and reproducibly. The cells are rotated at a frequency of 5 rpm, which is sufficient to ensure adequate mixing. The period required for equilibration ranges from about 16 hours to less than 48 hours, depending on the temperature and the fractional net transport of hapten across the membrane. If colored haptens are used, it is advisable to avoid exposure of the dialysis cell to fluorescent light and daylight.

After equilibration, the cells are removed from the rotator, drained for a few moments and placed on a test-tube rack with the protein-free solution on top. After a thermal equilibration period of 30 to 60 minutes, the hapten solutions are removed for analysis. If a measurement of optical density is to be made, the hapten solution can be transferred directly to the absorption cell with a Pasteur pipet fitted with a rubber bulb. The 1-ml absorption cells available for use with the Beckman and Zeiss spectrophotometers are satisfactory. The volume of 0.7 to 0.8 ml of solution which can be removed from the chamber provides a sufficient height of liquid in these cells. In removing the screw cap from the dialysis chamber, care should be taken to avoid the liquid trapped in the threads from running into the chamber. This possibility may be virtually eliminated by sealing the screw cap to the chamber with wax. The transferred hapten solutions in the absorption cells should be examined for turbidity which occasionally develops from bacterial growth or inadequate cleanliness. The use of duplicate samples for each hapten concentration is

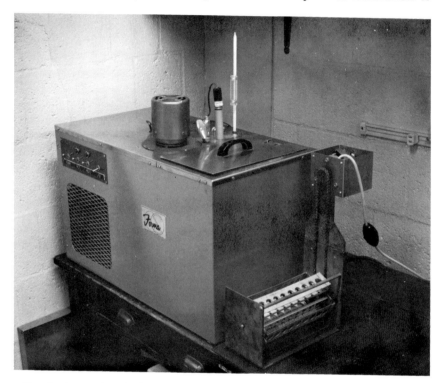

Fig. 2. A rotating device for equilibrium dialysis and the refrigerated constant temperature bath in which the device is immersed.

invaluable since the not infrequent leakage or breakage of a dialysis cell can be readily recognized from the failure to find agreement between duplicate cells. With adequate precautions and the use of accurate volumetric pipets, optical density readings from duplicate cells will generally agree to within 2%.

c. Experimental Conditions and Controls

The method of equilibrium dialysis is based on the assumption that the free hapten concentration in the chamber containing antibody is equal to that in the protein-free chamber. The time required for the practical attainment of this state of equilibrium, the equilibration period, varies with such factors as temperature, the nature of the hapten, and the distribution of the hapten between the bound and free forms. A minimum value of the equilibration period can be ascertained by dialyzing the hapten solution against solvent and measuring the hapten concentration on both sides of the membrane. However, a longer equilibration period is required if the antibody binds a substantial fraction of the total hapten in the system. It is generally advisable to ensure the adequacy of the period of dialysis by the demonstration that the same free hapten concentration is obtained regardless of the initial location of the hapten. This need only be done, at a particular temperature, for that set of conditions which leads to the maximum fraction of bound hapten.

One of the undesirable features of the dialysis method is the fact that frequently the commonly used haptens, particularly azo dyes, are adsorbed to the cellulose membrane. The amount of hapten adsorbed is often a significant quantity compared to that bound to antibody, and correction for this nonspecific binding must then be made. Since in general the amount of hapten adsorbed on the casing is a function of the free hapten concentration, it is necesssary to establish a casing correction curve at each temperature over the appropriate range of free hapten concentrations. This is done by filling both sides of pairs of dialysis cells with a series of hapten solutions and allowing them to dialyze under the usual test conditions. It is advisable then to measure the free hapten concentrations on both sides of the membranes and average the values. The quantity of adsorbed dye is calculated for each of the free measured hapten concentrations, and a correction curve is plotted from which the amount of adsorbed dye can be read off for any concentration of free hapten. The numbers in column 4 of Table I were obtained from such a plot.

For maximum accuracy of the binding results, the antibody concentration selected should be sufficient for the binding of not less than one-half of the total hapten. This condition is desirable because, as will be illustrated below, the bound hapten is calculated as the difference between total hapten and free hapten. The fractional error in the measurement of these quantities will be amplified in the bound hapten if the latter is relatively small. Another advantage gained by the condition that most of the hapten is bound is the reduction in the casing adsorption correction. Since this correction is rather variable from cell to cell, a substantial improvement in accuracy is gained by maintaining the casing correction small relative to the quantity of hapten bound.

In principle the need for a casing adsorption correction can be avoided by measurement of the hapten concentrations in both chambers. Aside from the difficulty introduced by spectral changes associated with hapten binding, the concentration measured in the antibody-containing chamber will be the sum of the free and bound hapten. If this value is to be used for calculation of bound hapten, the protein concentration must be redetermined after dialysis since a substantial volume change may have occurred. Since there are technical difficulties in making the appropriate concentration measurements with the equilibrated antibody solution, it is generally preferable to measure only the free hapten and include a casing adsorption correction in the calculation. Under some circumstances, however, particularly when the fraction of hapten bound is small, it is useful to measure the hapten concentration on both sides of the membrane and to ascertain the change in antibody concentration.

The equilibrium dialysis method can be extended to the measurement of the association constants of weakly bound haptens. Such haptens are encountered, for example, in the study of the energetic contribution of portions of the homologous hapten. For haptens whose association constant (K_A) does not exceed about 10^4 liters/mole it is not feasible to carry out direct binding measurements. In such cases binding is evaluated indirectly by the inhibition of the interaction of the homologous hapten or a related ligand with high association constant. In designing inhibition experiments, one must choose the concentrations of the inhibitor and the control hapten so that the binding of the control hapten is reduced to a value falling in the range of approximately half-saturation of the antibody.

3. CALCULATIONS

The analysis and interpretation of the binding data obtained by the method of equilibrium dialysis proceeds from the recognition that the antibody and hapten interact reversibly to form a soluble complex of molar ratio, r. If all the antibody combining sites possess the same intrinsic association constant for the hapten the relation between r and the free hapten concentration, c, can be described by the adsorption isotherm, as follows:

$$r = \frac{nK_A c}{1 + K_A c} \tag{1}$$

where n is the valence of the antibody molecule. A more useful form of the equation is

$$r/c = nK_A - rK_A \tag{2}$$

since the assumption of energetic homogeneity leads to a linear relationship between r/c and r. When the experimental results are plotted in this way, it is found almost invariably that they do not fall on a straight line. Such deviation from linearity constitutes a demonstration that the antibody population is heterogeneous with respect to its affinity for the hapten under study. For the quantitative description of this heterogeneity the assumption is usually made that the distribution of affinities may be described by a Gauss error function or by the closely related Sips distribution function.[3] In this way, as will be seen shortly, a heterogeneity index can be assigned to each preparation of antibody with respect to a particular hapten.

Given a sufficient range of data a plot of r/c vs. r, regardless of nonlinearity, allows for the determination of n and an average value of the association constant K_0, corresponding to the maximum value in the above distribution functions. The value of n is given by extrapolation of the experimental curve to the abscissa and the value of K_0 by the value of r/c on this curve which corresponds to half-saturation, i.e., $r = n/2$.

Binding data are sometimes represented in the form of a plot of $1/r$ vs. $1/c$ in accordance with the following linear equation, which can be derived from Eq. (1):

$$1/r = 1/nK_A c + 1/n \tag{3}$$

Such a plot also serves to reveal heterogeneity of affinity but the extrapolation of the experimental curve to the ordinate to obtain n is less reliable than in the plot of r/c vs. r.

An illustration of the calculations which are required for a plot of r/c vs. r is shown in Table I for the binding of the azo dye p-(p-dimethylaminobenzene azo)phenyl-β-lactoside (*lac* dye) by rabbit anti-*lac* antibody.[4] It will be noted that the computations are independent of volume changes during dialysis since the only concentration term involved is that for the free hapten. The casing adsorption correction shown in column 4 was obtained from a casing adsorption curve set up as described above.

The results of these calculations are shown in Fig. 3 for two temperatures.[4] It is apparent that the experimental points can be extrapolated to the abscissa to yield a value of 2.0 for the valence of anti-*lac* antibody with an uncertainty of about 5%. The average association constants are then found from the binding curves to be 1.57×10^5 liters/mole at 25.0° and 4.48×10^5 liters/mole at 7.1°. The average standard free energy $(\Delta F°)$ is calculated in the usual way from the relation

$$\Delta F° = -RT \ln K_0 \tag{4}$$

[3] F. Karush, *Advan. Immunol.* **2**, 1 (1962).
[4] F. Karush, *J. Am. Chem. Soc.* **79**, 3380 (1957).

TABLE I

CALCULATION OF BINDING CURVE FOR THE INTERACTION OF LAC DYE WITH PURIFIED RABBIT ANTI-LAC ANTIBODY

Initial moles $\times 10^8$	Free dye conc. (c) ($M \times 10^5$)	Moles of free dye $\times 10^8$	Moles of dye adsorbed on casing $\times 10^8$	Moles of bound dye $\times 10^8$	r^a	r/c $\times 10^{-4}$
2.99	0.399	0.798	0.15	2.04	0.800	20.0
3.79	0.571	1.142	0.20	2.45	0.961	16.84
4.76	0.815	1.630	0.27	2.86	1.121	13.76
5.75	1.148	2.296	0.35	3.10	1.216	10.59
7.70	1.828	3.656	0.50	3.54	1.388	7.60
9.48	2.48	4.96	0.60	3.92	1.537	6.20

[a] Initial concentration of antibody was 2.55×10^{-5} M based on a molecular weight of 156,000.

and the unitary free energy,[3] ΔF_u, is obtained from the equation

$$\Delta F_u = \Delta F^\circ - 7.98T \qquad (5)$$

where R is the gas constant and T is the absolute temperature.

In Fig. 3 the curves are theoretical and were derived on the assumption that the distribution of affinities could be described by an error function (w) in the free energy of complex formation as follows:

$$w(\Delta F) = \frac{1}{\sigma \sqrt{\pi}} e^{-(\Delta F_0 - \Delta F)^2/(RT\sigma)^2} \qquad (6)$$

where ΔF_0 is the average free energy corresponding to K_0 and σ is the heterogeneity index. Expressed in terms of association constants, the distribution function assumes the following form:

$$w(K) = \frac{1}{\sigma \sqrt{\pi}} e^{-[\ln (K/K_0)]^2/\sigma^2} \qquad (7)$$

It can be shown[5] that Eq. (7) leads to the following relation between the fraction of antibody sites occupied and the concentration of free hapten:

$$r/n = 1 - \frac{1}{\sqrt{\pi}} \int_{-\infty}^{\infty} \frac{e^{-\alpha^2}}{1 + K_0 c e^{\alpha\sigma}} d\alpha \qquad (8)$$

where α is $\ln (K/K_0)/\sigma$. The determination of σ for any particular system involves numerical integration over an appropriate range of c with

[5] F. Karush and M. Sonenberg, J. Am. Chem. Soc. 71, 1369 (1949).

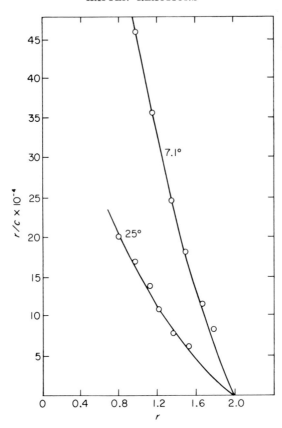

FIG. 3. Binding results at 25° and 7.1° for *lac* dye and purified anti-*lac* antibody. The points are experimental, and the curves are theoretical. [F. Karush, *J. Am. Chem. Soc.* **79**, 3380 (1957).]

selected values of σ and the matching of the experimental result with the theoretical curves thus obtained (for details, see Karush[6]). For the results shown in Fig. 3, a value of 1.5 for σ was found in this way.

The Sips distribution function[7] is more convenient, and probably equally satisfactory, since it leads to the following relatively simple relation:

$$r/n = \frac{(K_0c)^a}{1 + (K_0c)^a} \tag{9}$$

in which a, the heterogeneity index, may range from 0 to 1. For $a = 1$, Eq. (9) reduces to the simple case of noninteracting identical sites

[6] F. Karush, *J. Am. Chem. Soc.* **78**, 5519 (1956).
[7] R. Sips, *J. Chem. Phys.* **16**, 490 (1948).

[Eq. (1)]. For the analysis of binding data, Eq. (9) is expressed in the following form:

$$\log [r/(n - r)] = a \log c + a \log K_0 \tag{10}$$

The adequacy of the Sips distribution function is tested by plotting the experimental data in the form of $\log [r/(n - r)]$ vs. $\log c$ over a sufficient range of c. If the plot is linear, then the values of a and K_0 can be ascertained directly. The relation between the two heterogeneity indices may be expressed as follows:

$$\sigma = 2 \sqrt{\pi} \cot \left(\frac{\pi a}{2}\right) \tag{11}$$

4. LIMITATIONS

Because it relies on the impermeability of the membrane to antibody, the equilibrium dialysis method is limited to haptens that are small enough to diffuse readily through the membrane. This limitation generally precludes the study of the interaction of protein antigens with antibody. Conversely, the study of active fragments derived from antibody is also subject to a lower size limit. In addition the dialysis method, in contrast, for example, to the method of fluorescence quenching, is unable to exploit the extreme rapidity with which antibody and hapten interact. It requires equilibration times of the order of hours in spite of the fact that the interaction is practically instantaneous.

5. MICROTECHNIQUE*

Equilibrium dialysis with scarce or precious materials may be carried out in a microdialysis chamber† such as that described in Fig. 1.[1]

Pieces of dialysis membrane (32/32) are placed in distilled water which is brought to boiling. The membranes are allowed to soak in the hot water for 30 to 60 min after which they are repeatedly soaked in several changes of water at room temperature. After blotting the washed membrane nearly dry on filter paper, discs of 1.5 cm diameter are cut from them, e.g., by punching with a cork borer. The nearly dry discs are then laid tautly over the well in one-half of the chamber. The other half is slipped over the screws and clamped tightly. The two halves of the chamber are then loaded with the appropriate protein and ligand solutions, the access hole screws placed in position and tightened firmly, and chambers are placed at the desired temperature for equilibration. Each

---

* Section 15.B.5. was contributed by Herman N. Eisen.

† If facilities for machining the chambers are not available, they may be purchased from Gateway Serum Co., Box 1735, Cahokia, Illinois 62206.

[1] E. W. Voss, Jr., and H. N. Eisen, *Federation Proc.* **27**, 684 (1968).

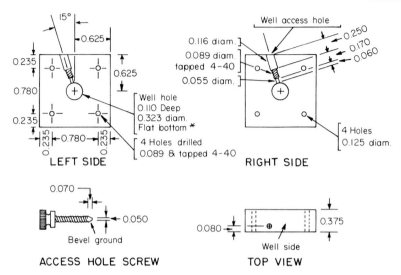

LEFT SIDE   RIGHT SIDE

ACCESS HOLE SCREW   TOP VIEW

Fig. 4. Microdialysis chamber. The bodies of the chamber are machined from ⅜ inch Plexiglas stock. All screws and nuts are stainless steel. The wells should be polished smooth to facilitate adequate cleaning. Note that in this drawing the interfaces of the two halves are shown and that when assembled the two access holes make an angle of 30 degrees with respect to each other for greater ease in filling and sampling. The halves are assembled using 4-40 × 1 inch stainless steel bolts. The screw portions are threaded through the tapped holes in the left half until the heads are flush with the outer surface and may remain there permanently. The right half is then bolted to the left using hexagonal nuts and a screwdriver-type wrench to tighten them. The well access hole screw can be fabricated by cutting the head off of a 4-40 × 1 inch stainless bolt, threading one end into a knurled nut, and peening this end to tighten it; the other end should be beveled as shown. There is one detail which is not adequately shown in the drawing. The portion of the access hole which enters the well must have a minimum diameter of 0.050 inch without impinging on the bottom surface of the chamber. Mr. Richard MacDonald, Dept. of Microbiology, Washington Univ. School of Medicine, St. Louis, provided the diagram and fabricated the chambers for the work on which this Section is based.

side of the membrane can accommodate 100 μl, but 50 μl in each half chamber is satisfactory and is frequently used. Equilibration is usually carried out readily without agitation since the liquid layers are relatively thin. Filling is easily accomplished using serological pipets to which a Luer adapter has been sealed and fitted with 22-gauge stainless needle with a blunt tip. Sampling is performed usually with calibrated capillary pipettes* in conjunction with a pipette filler.† When 50 μl is used per half chamber, one 25 μl sample is readily withdrawn. With 100 μl per half chamber, replicate samples (e.g., 25 μl each) can be taken.

* Such as those supplied by Drummond Scientific Co., Broomall, Pennsylvania.
† Such as one available from the Manostat Corporation, 20 N. Moore St., New York, New York, as their "Accropet-Size A."

C. Quenching of Antibody Fluorescence by Haptens and Antigens: A Method for Determining Antibody–Ligand Affinity*

Fluorescence quenching has been used to study the specific binding of heme, flavins, and pyridine nucleotides by globins and certain enzymes (e.g., Weber and Teale[1] and Velick[2]), as well as the specific reactions of antibodies with haptens and antigens.[3] As a method for measuring the affinity (intrinsic association constant) of an antibody–ligand pair, fluorescence quenching has some attractive advantages over equilibrium dialysis, but also some severe limitations.

1. PRINCIPLES

A molecule is said to fluoresce when it absorbs light of one wavelength and then loses part of the absorbed energy by an almost instantaneous emission of light of a longer wavelength. (The time-lapse between absorption and emission is of the order of 10^{-9} second.) The light emitted by antibody molecules irradiated at 295 mμ has maximum intensity at about 345 mμ, and intensity is greatest when the exciting incident light is at 295 mμ (Fig. 1). Since these maxima are characteristic of tryptophan, the 345 mμ fluorescence of antibody (excited at 295 mμ) is due almost entirely to its tryptophan residues. The other aromatic amino acid residues (phenylalanine and tyrosine) can also fluoresce, but their absorption and emission maxima are at lower wavelengths and are much less intense.

When certain ligands (haptens or antigens) are specifically bound by antibodies, the energy emitted by excited tryptophan residues is transferred intramolecularly by a radiationless process to the bound ligand, which disposes of its absorbed energy by various means, e.g., exchange of vibrational energy with neighboring solvent molecules, or fluorescence at some still longer wavelength (> 350 mμ). (The latter phenomenon is called sensitized or enhanced fluorescence.) In any event, the end result

* Sections 15.C.1–5† were contributed by Herman N. Eisen and James E. McGuigan.

† Supported in part by a Public Health research grant (AI-03231) and a training grant (5T1-AI-257), both from the National Institute of Allergy and Infectious Diseases, and a contract with the Research and Development Command, Department of the Army, recommended by the Commission on Immunization of the Armed Forces Epidermiological Board (DA-49-193-MD-2330).

[1] G. Weber and F. W. J. Teale, in "The Proteins" (H. Neurath, ed.), Vol. 3, p. 445. Adademic Press, New York, 1965.

[2] S. F. Velick, in "Light and Life" (W. D. McElroy and B. Glass, eds.), p. 108. Johns Hopkins Press, Baltimore, Maryland, 1961.

[3] S. F. Velick, C. W. Parker, and H. N. Eisen, Proc. Natl. Acad. Sci. U.S. **46**, 1470 (1960).

of the transfer of excitation energy to bound ligand is damping or quenching of the antibody molecule's tryptophan fluorescence.

Excitation energy can be transferred over intramolecular distances as
large as the molecular dimensions of an Fab fragment of a γG molecule,
e.g., about 50 Å.[4] The efficiency of transfer depends on (1) the orientation

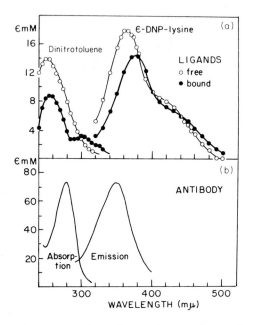

Fig. 1. (a) Absorption spectra of 2,4-dinitrotoluene and ϵ-2,4-dinitrophenyllysine,
unbound (free) or bound specifically by anti-DNP antibody. Both ligands quench the
antibody's fluorescence to nearly the same extent. From H. N. Eisen and G. W.
Siskind, *Biochemistry* **3**, 966 (1964).

(b) Absorption and emission spectra of purified rabbit antibody (anti-DNP).
The maximum emission band is arbitrarily drawn to the same height as the maxi-
mum absorption band. Based on S. F. Velick, C. W. Parker, and H. N. Eisen, *Proc.
Natl. Acad. Sci. U.S.* **46**, 1470 (1960).

of excited tryptophan residues relative to the bound ligand (the probability of transfer is maximal with parallel donor and acceptor groups, and
zero when the groups are at right angles; see Weber and Teale[1]; and (2)
the overlap between the antibody's emission spectrum and the ligand's
absorption spectrum; the latter is often altered when the ligand is bound
(Fig. 1), and, of course, it is the spectrum of the bound ligand which is
relevant. Effective transfer can occur even when the spectral overlap

[4] L. Stryer and R. P. Haugland, *Proc. Natl. Acad. Sci. U.S.* **58**, 719 (1967).

appears trivial; e.g., antibodies to the 2,4-dinitrophenyl (DNP) group are quenched almost as well by 2,4-dinitrotoluene, which absorbs very little in the region of maximal antibody emission (330–350 mμ) as by ϵ-DNP-lysine, which absorbs strongly in this region (Fig. 1).

Ligands with NO_2 groups are particularly effective as quenchers because excited nitro groups return to the ground state via a relatively long-lived "triplet" state, with a correspondingly large probability for deactivation through interactions with solvent molecules.[5] Many other ligands are also effective quenchers, e.g., an azobenzene arsonate[3] and a penicillenate derivative of p-mercuribenzoate.[5a] Most of the commonly used haptens with an aromatic ring can probably quench. Simple sugars would not be expected to quench, but conjugated to benzenoid moieties—such as nitrobenzenes—they might conceivably cause specific quenching of antisugar antibodies.

Fluorescence quenching can be used only with antibody–ligand pairs that form soluble complexes, e.g., those that involve univalent haptens or univalent antibody fragments.[3] Certain univalent antigens have also been studied with the corresponding bivalent antibodies, e.g., IgG anti-DNP molecules with mono-DNP-ribonuclease[6] and with mono-DNP-insulin.[7] The latter antigens not only are univalent, by virtue of having one DNP group per molecule, but also lack tryptophan; hence their fluorescence at 345 mμ is negligible compared to that of the antibody.

Fluorescence quenching is carried out as a titration by adding increasing amounts of ligand to a solution of antibody, and recording the fluorescence after each addition. The antibody must be purified; in whole serum or a globulin fraction of serum, the nonspecific proteins provide too much of a background of unquenchable fluorescence.

Once it is established by preliminary studies how much of the antibody's fluorescence is quenched when its ligand-binding sites are saturated (Q_{max}) it is possible to determine for each level of total ligand the average number of ligand molecules bound per antibody molecule (r), the concentration of free, i.e., unbound, ligand (c), and the proportion of the antibody's sites occupied, r/n, where n, the total number of ligand-binding sites per antibody molecule, is best derived from independent studies, e.g., by equilibrium dialysis. (All the IgG antibodies so far studied are bivalent, i.e., $n = 2$.) Given n and several pairs of r and c, one can

[5] E. J. Bowen and F. Wokes, "Fluorescence in Solutions." Longmans, Green, New York, 1953.

[5a] C. W. Parker, personal communication.

[6] H. N. Eisen, E. S. Simms, J. R. Little, and L. A. Steiner, *Federation Proc.* **23**, 559 (1964).

[7] R. B. Counts and J. R. Little, *Federation Proc.* **25**, 677 (1966).

calculate two values of interest with the logarithmic form of the Sips distribution function[8]

$$\log \frac{r}{n - r} = a \log K + a \log c \qquad (1)$$

(i) the average intrinsic association constant for the reversible binding of the ligand by the antibody; this constant, K_0, is also referred to as average affinity, or as *affinity;* (ii) the heterogeneity of the antibody with respect to affinity, i.e., the dispersion (a) of association constants K about the average value, K_0.

2. PROCEDURE

With a commercially available spectrophotofluorometer, such as the Aminco-Bowman, samples are irradiated with incident light at 295 mμ, and the intensity of emitted light is recorded at 345 mμ. An accurately measured volume of about 1.0 ml, containing a known quantity of antibody, usually about 40 μg, is added to a clean, dry cuvette. Fluorescence is recorded initially, and then again after each addition of ligand in increments of 0.01 to 0.03 ml to a total of 0.2 ml. After each addition the solution is mixed *gently* with a glass rod; vigorous stirring should be avoided. A blank, deducted from each of the fluorescence values, is simply the fluorescence of the solvent alone (e.g., phosphate-buffered saline); it is usually less than 5% of the initial protein fluorescence. Each fluorescence value is also corrected for volume change; e.g., if the initial and final volumes are 1.0 and 1.2 ml, respectively, the final blank-corrected fluorescence value is multiplied by 1.2.

Antibody fluorescence decreases with increasing temperature, and it is necessary to allow the antibody solution to reach a constant temperature (and fluorescence value) before commencing the titration. Ten minutes is usually sufficient. The solution is shielded from exciting light by a shutter, except when fluorescence readings are made. Hollow cuvette holders* can be connected to a constant temperature water bath with circulating pump for thermostatic control (e.g., $\pm 0.1°$ over the range 5° to 60°). In the nonthermostatted cuvette holder, the temperature of the antibody solution usually stabilizes at about 31° ($\pm 1°$).

3. CALCULATIONS AND PLOTTING

Some representative titrations and calculations are shown in Tables I and II, and are plotted in Fig. 2. These calculations were made on the

[8] F. Karush, *Advan. Immunol.* **2,** 1 (1962).
* Made by Mr. Oliver Tretter, Department of Chemistry, Washington University, St. Louis, Missouri, or obtainable from American Instrument Co., Silver Spring, Maryland.

basis of $Q_{\max} = 75$. Automatic digital computing facilities are extremely helpful and a program† is given in Section 15.C.6. For each titration $\log r/n - r$ is plotted vs. $\log c$ [see Eq. (1)]; a, the heterogeneity index, is obtained as the slope, and K_0, the average intrinsic association constant or affinity, from the value of c at $r = n - r$ (i.e., K_0 is the reciprocal of c,

TABLE I

REPRESENTATIVE FLUOROMETRIC TITRATION OF LOW-AFFINITY ANTIBODY[a]

Hapten added (ml)	Fluorescence (arbitrary units)	Quench	Hapten bound (mμmoles)	Free hapten conc. (c) $(M \times 10^6)$	Ratio: moles hapten bound/mole antibody (r)	Ratio $r/n - r$
0	89.2	—	—	—	—	—
0.010	83.6	5.6	0.034	0.043	0.148	0.080
0.020	78.2	11.0	0.067	0.086	0.294	0.172
0.040	70.6	18.4	0.113	0.191	0.492	0.326
0.060	65.6	23.0	0.141	0.308	0.614	0.443
0.080	60.4	28.1	0.172	0.417	0.749	0.599
0.100	57.0	31.1	0.191	0.534	0.829	0.708
0.120	53.8	34.0	0.208	0.648	0.907	0.829
0.150	50.8	36.2	0.222	0.822	0.966	0.934
0.180	48.0	38.4	0.236	0.988	1.024	1.049
0.200	46.0	40.1	0.246	1.093	1.070	1.151

[a] Antibody: 0.23 mμmole in 1.0 ml of 0.15 M NaCl–0.01 M phosphate, pH 7.4, based on A_{278}, $E_{1cm}^{1\%} = 15.5$, and assumed mol. wt. 160,000. Hapten: ϵ-DNP-L-lysine, 7.8 mμmoles per ml, based on A_{360}, molar absorbance 17,530 in the same buffer. Temp. 30°; K_0, 1.2 $\times$ 10^6 M^{-1}; a 0.8 (titration No. 815-1).

the free ligand concentration, when one-half of the total antibody sites are occupied).

The concentration of the free ligand (c) is determined from the difference between the concentrations of total ligand added (L_i) and bound ligand (L_b) (see Tables I and II); and

$$L_b = n\mathrm{Ab}\frac{Q_i}{Q_{\max}}$$

where Q_i is the observed quenching after L_i is added, Ab is antibody concentration in moles liter^{-1}, and n refers to the number of binding sites

† Developed by Mr. Richard Dammkoehler and Mr. Tom Gallagher, of the Washington University Computing Facilities.

per antibody molecule. Thus, the value of Q_{max} is critical, and values are different with different antibodies. With the two systems in which fluorescence quenching has been used most extensively (anti-2,4-dinitrophenyl and anti-2,4,6-trinitrophenyl), it appears that the Q_{max} value is fixed for antibody of a given specificity, regardless of the ligand used to

TABLE II

REPRESENTATIVE FLUOROMETRIC TITRATION OF HIGH-AFFINITY ANTIBODY[a]

Hapten added (ml)	Fluorescence (arbitrary units)	Quench	Hapten bound (mμmoles)	Free hapten conc. (c) ($M \times 10^6$)	Ratio: moles hapten bound/mole antibody (r)	Ratio $r/n - r$
0	75.0	—	—	—	—	—
0.010	60.5	15.6	(0.088)[b]	—	—	—
0.020	51.5	27.9	(0.157)[b]	—	—	—
0.040	38.4	45.9	0.258	0.014	1.225	1.579
0.060	31.2	55.8	0.314	0.090	1.488	2.903
0.080	28.3	59.4	0.334	0.196	1.585	3.815
0.100	27.0	60.7	0.342	0.309	1.619	4.250
0.120	26.0	61.6	0.347	0.421	1.643	4.597
0.150	24.6	62.9	0.354	0.582	1.677	5.184
0.180	24.0	62.9	0.354	0.740	1.678	5.206
0.200	23.5	63.1	0.355	0.841	1.684	5.325

[a] Antibody: 0.22 mμmole in 1.0 ml of 0.15 M NaCl–0.01 M phosphate, pH 7.4, based on A_{278}, $E_{1cm}^{1\%} = 15.5$, and assumed mol. wt. 160,000. Hapten: 2,4-dinitroaniline, 6.8 mμmoles per ml, based on A_{345}, molar absorbance 14,000 in the same buffer. Temp. 30°; K_0, 3.9 $\times$ 10^8 M^{-1}; a 0.3 (titration No. 662-2).

[b] For the first two additions of ligand (0.010 and 0.020 ml) the amount of ligand bound, by calculation, is greater than the amount added. This obvious inconsistency probably arises from heterogeneity in fluorescence and in extent of fluorescence quenching for anti-DNP molecules. This heterogeneity is especially pronounced in high-affinity antibodies (see Fig. 3). For purposes of calculation of K_0 and a, these first two data points are omitted. See Section 15.C.6 and reference 12, this Section.

establish that value. For example, IgG rabbit anti-DNP has the same Q_{max} (about 75) with ε-DNP-L-lysine, 2,4-dinitroaniline, or ε-TNP-L-lysine; similarly, IgG rabbit anti-TNP has $Q_{max} = 50$ to 60, regardless of whether this value is obtained with a DNP- or TNP-ligand.[9, 10]

[9] J. R. Little and H. N. Eisen, *Biochemistry* **5**, 3385 (1966).
[10] J. R. Little and H. N. Eisen, *Biochemistry* **7**, 711 (1968).

Evaluation of Q_{max}. Two approaches have been used.

1. A highly concentrated solution of ligand is added to the antibody solution, and quenching is measured. Correction is made for nonspecific attenuation of incident and emitted light by adding the *same* highly concentrated solution of ligand to a solution of tryptophan or nonspecific γ-globulin. The concentration of hapten is chosen to be large enough to

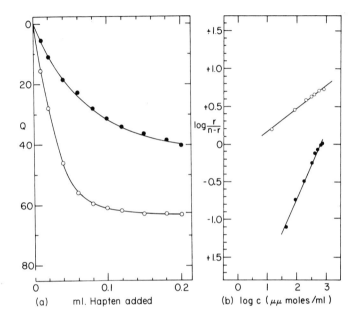

(a)   ml. Hapten added   (b) log c ($\mu\mu$ moles/ml)

FIG. 2. (a) Fluorescence quenching (Q) of a low affinity (●) and a high affinity (○) anti-DNP antibody by DNP-ligands. (b) Data of the left-hand figure plotted according to the logarithmic form of the Sips equation (see text). For the high affinity antibody (○) K_0 is 4×10^8 M^{-1} and a, the heterogeneity index, is 0.3. For the low affinity antibody (●), $K_0 = 1 \times 10^6$ M^{-1} and a is 0.8.

saturate the antibody combining sites, but not so large as to reduce (through light absorption by unbound ligand) the fluorescence of tryptophan or nonspecific γ-globulin by more than about 75%. Because of the latter limitation, this method is useful only with antibodies (e.g., anti-DNP) of affinity $\geq 5 \times 10^5$ M^{-1}. *Sample calculation:* 0.2 ml of 4×10^{-4} M ϵ-DNP-aminocaproate was added to 1.0 ml each of anti-DNP antibody and nonspecific γ-globulin or tryptophan (control). After subtraction of solvent blank fluorescence, correction for dilution, and normalizing for the initial fluorescence (i.e., dividing corrected final fluorescence by the corrected initial value), the corrected fluorescence values dropped from

100 to 8 for the antibody and from 100 to 28 for the control, respectively. The Q_{max} value was thus 71 [i.e., $100 - 100 \ (8/28)$]. A more refined procedure, which is similar in principle and yields the same value for a given antibody is described by Day.[11]

2. In the second method for establishing Q_{max}, equilibrium dialysis and fluorescence quenching titration are both carried out with a given antiboby and ligand. It is thus possible to determine for particular concentrations of total ligand and antibody (a) the concentrations of free and

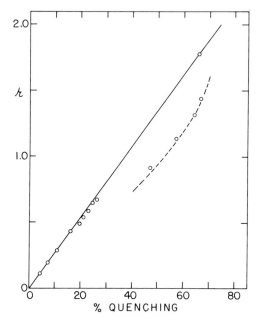

FIG. 3. Fluorescence quenching as a function of the number of ligand binding sites occupied per antibody molecule (r). For the low affinity antibody ($\bigcirc—\bigcirc$), $K_0 = 5 \times 10^5 \ M^{-1}$, quenching is linear with r, and Q_{max} is 75 ($r = 2$). For the high affinity antibody ($\bigcirc\cdots\bigcirc$), $K_0 \geq 10^8 \ M^{-1}$, quenching is *not* linear with r, and Q_{max} cannot be determined by extrapolation. From J. E. McGuigan and H. N. Eisen, *Biochemistry* **7**, 1919 (1968).

bound ligand and the average number of occupied and vacant binding sites per antibody molecule and (b) fluorescence quenching.[12] As Fig. 3 shows, extrapolation to saturation of an IgG antibody ($r = 2$) gives a limiting value for quenching, Q_{max}. This method is not feasible with highly heterogeneous antibodies, whose quenching vs. r plots are non-

[11] L. J. Day, Thesis, Yale University (1962).
[12] J. E. McGuigan and H. N. Eisen, *Biochemistry* **7**, 1919 (1968).

linear. Thus, with rabbit IgG antibodies to the 2,4-dinitrophenyl (DNP) group, high affinity preparations, whose Q_{max} is easily measured by the first procedure (see above), are usually too heterogeneous for measurement of Q_{max} by this second procedure. Conversely, with low-affinity anti-DNP antibodies, which tend to be more homogeneous, Q_{max} is readily measured by this second procedure but not by the first (Fig. 3) (see McGuigan and Eisen[12]).

Earlier studies of rabbit anti-DNP antibodies[13, 14] used $Q_{max} = 72.5$, but currently we use a value of 75 (Fig. 3). The effect of this difference on computed affinity and heterogeneity index is negligible with antibodies of low or moderate affinity ($K_0 = 10^5$ to 10^6 M^{-1}), but may be significant with antibodies of high affinity ($K_0 > 10^7$ M^{-1}) (see Table IV).

4. PRECISION, ACCURACY, AND RANGE

Fluorescence quenching has so far been used most widely with anti-DNP antibodies and DNP-ligands. In replicate titrations with this

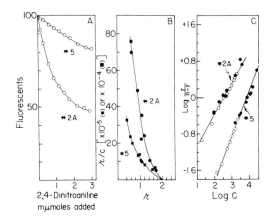

FIG. 4. Agreement between fluorescence quenching and equilibrium dialysis. The binding of 2,4-dinitroaniline-^{14}C by two antibodies, one of low (#5) and the other of high affinity (#2A), were studied by fluorescence quenching (○), in the left panel, and by equilibrium dialysis (●), in the middle panel. Both sets of data are in agreement when plotted together by the Sips equation in the right-hand panel. From H. N. Eisen and G. W. Siskind, *Biochemistry* **3**, 996 (1964).

system, the average deviation of K_0 values from their mean is $\pm 50\%$ when K_0 lies in the optimum range for the method, between about

[13] H. N. Eisen and G. W. Siskind, *Biochemistry* **3**, 996 (1964).
[14] H. N. Eisen, *Methods Med. Res.* **10**, 115 (1964).

5×10^5 M^{-1} and 5×10^7 M^{-1}; at the measurable extremes, about 5×10^4 M^{-1} and 5×10^8 M^{-1}, replicate K_0 values usually agree within factors of 2 or 3.

The accuracy of the method is assessed by determining the extent to which it provides values for K_0 that agree with those obtained by equilibrium dialysis (Section 15.B). Agreement has been satisfactory over a wide range in association constants (5×10^4 to 5×10^7 M^{-1}), as is shown in the representative data of Fig. 4.

5. COMPARISON WITH EQUILIBRIUM DIALYSIS

As a method for measuring affinity, fluorescence quenching offers the following advantages over equilibrium dialysis.

1. Less antibody is necessary. For a single fluorescence titration 40 μg purified antibody is required. To obtain comparable information by ordinary equilibrium dialysis techniques one needs about 5 to 10 mg of low-affinity antibody (about 10^5 M^{-1}) and about 1 mg of high-affinity antibody (10^7 M^{-1} or higher).*

2. Wider range of conditions can be tolerated. Many hours are required to reach equilibrium in dialysis experiments (e.g., 5 to 48, depending on volumes, temperature, etc.), whereas a fluorescence titration can be completed within 15 minutes. Hence when antibodies are subject to denaturation, e.g., at elevated temperature, at low or high pH, or merely by long standing at low concentration, fluorescence quenching may be used whereas equilibrium dialysis may not.

3. Ligands need not be dialyzable. Antigens are nearly always non-dialyzable. Their interactions with antibody cannot, therefore, be studied by equilibrium dialysis, but they can be studied by fluorescence quenching, provided that insoluble aggregates are not formed. Thus, K_0 values for the reaction of some anti-DNP molecules with the immunogen that induced their formation has been determined with mono-DNP-RNase[6] and ϵ-DNP-insulin.[7]

However, fluorescence quenching suffers from the disadvantage that it is less accurate than equilibrium dialysis; i.e., there is less certainty that the values measured are "true" values. The uncertainties arise for the following reasons.

---

* Equilibrium dialysis chambers have recently been adapted to a micro scale; e.g., to the use of 50 μl of protein solution per chamber. A wide range of r and c values can thus be obtained in equilibrium dialysis with as little as 40 μg antibody if affinity is high (about 10^7 M^{-1}), or 500 μg if affinity is low (about 10^5 M^{-1}). Blueprints for construction of the small dialysis chambers may be obtained from the Department of Microbiology, Washington University School of Medicine, St. Louis, Missouri. For procedure, see Section 15.B.5.

1. Fluorescence quenching depends on excitation energy transfer. When two antibody preparations differ in the K_0 values determined by fluorescence quenching it is conceivable that they differ in the efficiency with which excitation energy is transferred (e.g., in Q_{max}), rather than in affinity for the ligand. It is thus necessary with a novel set of reagents or conditions to check the results with a less ambiguous method, such as equilibrium dialysis or ultracentrifugation.[15] Although we have not so far observed serious discrepancies between affinity values measured by

TABLE III

DEPENDENCE OF CALCULATED VALUE OF AFFINITY ON ASSIGNED MOLECULAR
WEIGHT OF ANTIBODY

Titra-tion number	Anti-body	Hapten	Assigned molecular weight			
			180,000		150,000	
			K_0 $(M^{-1} \times 10^{-6})$	a^a	K_0 $(M^{-1} \times 10^{-6})$	a^a
220	1	2,4-Dinitroaniline	2.8	0.7	3.9	0.6
221	1	ϵ-DNP-L-lysine	27	0.8	160	0.6
225	2	2,4-Dinitroaniline	0.14	0.98	0.14	0.97
226	2	ϵ-DNP-L-lysine	0.46	0.8	0.47	0.8
420-3	3	2,4-Dinitrotoluene	160	0.4	1200	0.3
423-2	4	2,4-Dinitrotoluene	12	0.3	22	0.2
428-2	5	2,4-Dinitrotoluene	2.6	0.5	3.2	0.4
435-2	6	2,4-Dinitrotoluene	0.13	0.7	0.13	0.7

^{a} a is heterogeneity index; see Eq. (1) in text. Rabbit IgG anti-DNP antibodies, $Q_{max} = 75$.

the latter methods and fluorescence quenching, it is necessary to remain cautious since experience is still limited.

2. Uncertainties in concentration of free ligand. In equilibrium dialysis the concentration of free ligand is measured *directly* (in the protein-free compartment). Measurements can thus be made with precision, although with high affinity antibodies it is necessary to use highly sensitive assays, and radioactively labeled ligands of high specific activity are a virtual necessity. Fluorescence quenching circumvents this restriction; but in doing so it suffers from another severe limitation, because the concen-

[15] H. K. Schachman, L. Gropper, S. Hanlon, and F. Putney, *Arhc. Biochem. Biophys.* **99**, 175 (1962).

tration of free ligand in this method is estimated *indirectly* from the difference between total ligand added and ligand bound (L_b) (see above). The latter, in turn, depends upon accurate knowledge of the molar concentration of antibody sites (i.e., antibody concentration in weight units, molecular weight of the antibody, number of binding sites per antibody molecule), and upon the Q_{max} value chosen (see above). For example, as Tables III and IV show, the computed K_0 values depend on the choice of molecular weight of antibody and Q_{max}; and the dependence is especially pronounced with high-affinity antibodies.

Experience with the DNP-specific system leads us to conclude that for

TABLE IV

DEPENCENCE OF CALCULATED VALUE OF AFFINITY ON ASSIGNED VALUE OF Q_{max}[a]

Titration number	Antibody preparation	Q'	Q_{max}	K_0 $(M^{-1} \times 10^{-6})$	a
636-1	7	34	50	3.3	0.7
			55	2.2	0.6
			60	1.6	0.6
			65	1.2	0.6
			70	0.96	0.6
			75	0.74	0.6
647-2	8	45	50	570	0.4
			55	40	0.6
			60	20	0.5
			65	9.6	0.6
			70	6.3	0.7
			75	4.5	0.7

[a] For definition of K_0 and a see Eq. 1 in text. Q' is the quenching observed at the end of titration, corrected for volume and blank, and normalized to initial fluorescence value; i.e., Q' of 34 means that the corrected final fluorescence, after addition of 0.2 ml of hapten solution, was 66% of the initial fluorescence ($Q' = 100 - 66$).

many purposes the method of fluorescence quenching is highly satisfactory; it is flexible, simple to perform, requires small amounts of antibody, and for well-characterized systems it provides dependable values for association constants over a 1000-fold, or possibly a 10,000-fold, range. However, this method must be used with caution, and critical results should be checked whenever possible by an unambiguous method, such as equilibrium dialysis. Put in another way, we feel that the method of fluorescence quenching is too good to give up, but not good enough to rely upon as an exclusive method for measuring affinity.

6. COMPUTER PROGRAM FOR ANALYSIS OF FLUORESCENCE QUENCHING OF ANTIBODIES BY LIGANDS*

```
C*****************************************************************
C     DEFINITION OF INPUT VARIABLES
C          MARK = * (11-4-8 PUNCHES)
C          NAME(I) = ANY 9 CHARACTER ALPHAMERIC IDENTIFICATION
C          NSITE = NUMBER OF SITES PER ANTIBODY MOLECULE
C          CONAB = CONCENTRATION OF ANTIBODY
C                  (MILLI-MICRO MOLES/ML)
C          CONL = CONCENTRATION OF LIGAND
C                 (MILLI-MICRO MOLES/ML)
C          BVOL = BEGINNING VOLUME (ML)
C          STFL = STABLE FLUORESCENCE (WITH ANTIBODY PRESENT)
C          SOLBK = SOLVENT BLANK (FLUORESCENCE VALUE WITH NO
C                  ANTIBODY PRESENT)
C          QMAX(I) = EXTENT OF QUENCHING WHEN ALL SITES ON THE
C                    ANTIBODY ARE OCCUPIED BY LIGAND
C                    MOLECULES
C          ADDL(I) = AMOUNT OF LIGAND ADDED (ML)
C          AMTFL(I) = AMOUNT OF FLOURESCENCE
C          NOP = NUMBER OF PAIRED VALUES OF AMTFL(I) AND
C                ADDL(I)
C          NOQ = NUMBER OF DIFFERENT VALUES OF QMAX(I)
C*****************************************************************
      DIMENSION    NAME(2),   QMAX(25), ADDL(25), AMTFL(25),
     1 TLIG(25), TFL(25),   R(25),    X(25),     Y(25),
     2 C(25),    YLG(25),  CLG(25),  Q(25),    BO(25),
     3 R2(25),   CHSAT(25),AFFIN(25),DO(25),   D1(25),
     4 R2D(25),  DHSAT(25),DAFIN(25),B1(25),   NM(25)
C*****************************************************************
C          INPUT DATA SECTION
C*****************************************************************
      INTP=1
      IOUT=2
  100 READ(INTP,1000) MARK,(NAME(I),I=1,2),NSITE, CONAB,
 1001  CONL, BVOL, STFL, SOLBK, NOQ, NOP
      IF(XABSF(MARK)-2600000000) 110,112,110
  110 SENSE LIGHT 1
      GO TO 100
  112 IF(SENSE LIGHT 1) 114,116
  114 TYPE 1002,(NAME(I),I=1,2)
  116 READ(INTP, 1004)(QMAX(I), I=1,NOQ)
      READ(INTP, 1004)(ADDL(I), I=1,NOP)
      READ(INTP, 1004)(AMTFL(I), I=1,NOP)
```

* Section 15.C.6 was contributed by Richard A. Dammkoehler and Tom L. Gallagher.

```
C*******************************************************************
C    DEFINITION OF CALCULATED VALUES
C         BFL = INITIAL STABLE FLUORESCENCE MINUS
C               SOLVENT BLANK
C         Q(I) = NORMALIZED QUENCHING
C         R(I) = LIGAND MOLECULES BOUND PER
C                MOLECULE ANTIBODY
C         X(I) = CONCENTRATION OF BOUND LIGAND
C         Y(I) = RATIO OF OCCUPIED TO VACANT SITES
C                ON ANTIBODY
C         YLG(I) = COMMON LOGARITHM OF Y(I)
C         C(I) = CONCENTRATION OF UNBOUND LIGAND
C         CLG(I) = COMMON LOGARITHM OF C(I) TIMES 1000
C                  (MICRO-MICRO MOLES/ML)
C         CHSAT(I) = CONCENTRATION OF UNBOUND LIGAND WHEN
C                    1/2 OF TOTAL ANTIBODY SITES ARE
C                    OCCUPIED (MOLES/LITER)
C         B0(I) = INTERCEPT OF YLG(I) VS CLG(I) REGRESSION
C         B1(I) = SLOPE OF YLG(I) VS CLG(I) REGRESSION
C         R2(I) = CORRELATION COEFFICIENT
C         AFFIN(I) = 1/CHSAT(I)   (LITERS/MOLE)
C         NM(I) = NUMBER OF PAIRS OF Y(I) AND C(I) OF
C                 WHICH NEITHER ARE ZERO OR NEGATIVE
C         DHSAT(I) = SAME AS CHSAT(I) WITH ELIMINATION
C                    OF DATA POINTS WHOSE C(I) IS ZERO
C                    OR NEGATIVE  (REDUCED DATA)
C         D0(I) = SAME AS B0(I) WITH REDUCED DATA
C         D1(I) = SAME AS B1(I) WITH REDUCED DATA
C         R2D(I) = SAME AS R2(I) WITH REDUCED DATA
C         DAFIN(I) = SAME AS AFFIN(I) WITH REDUCED DATA
C*******************************************************************
C              DATA REDUCTION SECTION
C*******************************************************************
       BFL = STFL - SOLBK
       DO 200 I= 1,NOP
       TLIG(I)= CONL*ADDL(I)
       TFL(I) = (AMTFL(I)- SOLBK) * (BVOL + ADDL(I))
   200 Q(I) = 100.*(1.- TFL(I)/BFL)
       DO 399 J= 1,NOQ
       QX = QMAX(J)
       DO 299 I=1,NOP
       R(I) = FLOATF(NSITE)* Q(I)/QX
       X(I) = CONAB* R(I)
       Y(I) = R(I)/(FLOATF(NSITE)-R(I))
       IF(Y(I)) 202,202,204
   202 YLG(I)= 0.0
       GO TO 206
   204 YLG(I) = LOGXF(Y(I))
   206 C(I) =   (TLIG(I) - X(I))/(BVOL + ADDL(I))
       IF(C(I)) 208,208,210
   208 CLG(I) = 0.0
       GO TO 299
```

```
    210 CLG(I) = 3.0 + LOGXF(C(I))
    299 CONTINUE
C***************************************************************
C             INTERMEDIATE OUTPUT SECTION
C***************************************************************
        WRITE(IOUT, 3000)
        WRITE(IOUT, 3001)(NAME(I),I=1,2)
    300 WRITE(IOUT, 3002)   NSITE, CONAB, CONL, BVOL, STFL,
   3001 SOLBK, QX
        WRITE(IOUT,3003)
        DO 302 I= 1, NOP
    302 WRITE(IOUT,3004)  ADDL(I),TLIG(I), AMTFL(I), Q(I),
   3021 X(I), C(I), R(I), Y(I), YLG(I), CLG(I)
        WRITE(IOUT, 3006)(NAME(I),I=1,2)
        NN= NOP
    310 CALL LSQ (J,NOP,NN,CLG,YLG, BO(J), B1(J),R2(J),
   3101 CHSAT(J), AFFIN(J))
        DO 320 I= 1,NOP
        IF(YLG(I)) 320,322,320
    322 CLG(I)= 0.0
    320 CONTINUE
        DO 340 I= 1,NOP
        IF(CLG(I)) 342,342,340
    342 YLG(I)= 0.0
        NN = NN - 1
    340 CONTINUE
        NM(J) = NN
        IF(NOP-NN) 399,399,350
    350 CALL LSQ(J,NOP,NN,CLG,YLG,DO(J),D1(J),R2D(J),
   3501 DHSAT(J), DAFIN(J))
    399 CONTINUE
C***************************************************************
C             FINAL OUTPUT SECTION
C***************************************************************
        WRITE(IOUT, 4000)
        WRITE(IOUT,3001)(NAME(I),I=1,2)
        WRITE(IOUT,4002)
        DO 400 J= 1,NOQ
    400 WRITE(IOUT, 4004) QMAX(J),BO(J), B1(J), R2(J),
   4001 CHSAT(J), AFFIN(J)
        DO 410 J= 1,NOQ
        IF(NM(J)-NOP) 412,410,412
    412 WRITE(IOUT, 4010) NM(J)
    408 WRITE(IOUT, 4004) QMAX(J),DO(J), D1(J), R2D(J),
   4081 DHSAT(J), DAFIN(J)
    410 CONTINUE
        WRITE(IOUT,3006)(NAME(I),I=1,2)
        GO TO 100
C***************************************************************
C             FORMAT SECTION
C***************************************************************
   1000 FORMAT(A1,A4,A5,I5,5F10.0,2I5)
```

```
1002 FORMAT(19H ERROR NEAR SAMPLE  ,A4,A5)
1004 FORMAT(8F10.0)
3000 FORMAT(1H1, 41X, 23HFLUORESCENCE QUENCHING
30001   24HOF ANTIBODIES BY LIGANDS  /
30002   1H0, 49X, 29HDATA AND INTERMEDIATE RESULTS  )
3001 FORMAT(101X, 7HSAMPLE ,A4,A5)
3002 FORMAT(1H0, 44X, 26HNUMBER OF SITES            , I9/
30021         45X, 26HCONCENTRATION OF ANTIBODY       /
30022         45X, 26H (MILLI-MICRO MOLES/ML)    , F11.3/
30023         45X, 26HCONCENTRATION OF LIGAND         /
30024         45X, 26H (MILLI-MICRO MOLES/ML)    , F11.3/
30025         45X, 26HBEGINNING VOLUME (ML)      , F11.3/
30026         45X, 26HSTABLE FLUORESCENCE        , F11.3/
30027         45X, 26HSOLVENT BLANK              , F11.3/
30028       1H-, 53X,   4HQMAX  , F12.2    )
3003 FORMAT(1H0, 25X, 4HADDL, 4X, 4HTLIG, 4X, 5HAMTFL, 6X,
30031   1HQ, 8X, 1HX, 8X, 1HC, 8X, 1HR, 8X, 1HY, 6X,
30032   6HLOG(Y), 4X, 6HLOG(C)  /)
3004 FORMAT(22X, 2F8.3, F8.1, F10.3, 4F9.3, 2F10.4 )
3006 FORMAT( 7(1H-/), 100X, 7HSAMPLE ,A4,A5 )
4000 FORMAT( 1H1,54X,18HSUMMARY OF RESULTS    )
4002 FORMAT( 1H0, 36X, 4HQMAX, 8X, 2HB0, 6X, 5HSLOPE, 4X,
40021   11HCORRELATION, 8X, 5HCHSAT, 12X, 5HAFFIN  /
40022   66X, 11HCOEFFICIENT, 4X, 13H(MOLES/LITER), 4X,
40023   13H(LITERS/MOLE)  /1H  )
4004 FORMAT( 34X, F7.2, F11.4, F10.4, F13.4,  2(1PE17.3))
4010 FORMAT(1H0, 25X, 4HONLY, I3,
40101   37H ITEMS ARE CONSIDERED IN THE AVERAGE   )
     END


C*********************************************************************
C        SIMPLE LINEAR LEAST SQUARES ROUTINE
C*********************************************************************
     SUBROUTINE LSQ(J,NOP,NP,CLG,YLG,A,B,R2,C,D)
     DIMENSION    CLG(1),   YLG(1)
     EN=NP
     SY2 = 0.0
     SX2 = 0.0
     SXY = 0.0
     SX = 0.0
     SY =0.0
     DO 150 I=1,NOP
     SX=SX+ CLG(I)
     SX2=SX2+CLG(I)*CLG(I)
     SXY=SXY+CLG(I)*YLG(I)
     SY=SY+YLG(I)
150  SY2=SY2+YLG(I)*YLG(I)
     BDEN = SX - (EN*SX2/SX)
     BNUM = SY -(EN*SXY/SX)
     B = BNUM/BDEN
     A = (SXY - B*SX2)/SX
     P = (SXY/EN) - (SX/EN)*(SY/EN)
     SIGX = SQRTF((SX2/EN)- (SX/EN)*(SX/EN))
     SIGY = SQRTF((SY2/EN)- (SY/EN)*(SY/EN))
     R2= P/(SIGX * SIGY)
     C = 1.0 E-09 * 10.**(-A/B)
     D=1.0/C
     RETURN
     END
```

```
      10        20         30        40        50        60        70        80
* 761-2      2   0.215    9.94      1.0      75.0      5.0      2   10
  72.5      75.0
  0.01      0.02      0.04      0.06      0.08      0.10      0.12      0.15
  0.18      0.20
  62.5      51.0      38.5      35.5      34.0      33.5      32.5      31.0
  30.5      30.5
```

FIG. 1. Sample input data.

FLUORESCENCE QUENCHING OF ANTIBODIES BY LIGANDS

DATA AND INTERMEDIATE RESULTS, RUN 1

SAMPLE 761-2

NUMBER OF SITES		2
CONCENTRATION OF ANTIBODY (MILLI-MICRO MOLES/ML)		0.215
CONCENTRATION OF LIGAND (MILLI-MICRO MOLES/ML)		9.940
BEGINNING VOLUME (ML)		1.000
STABLE FLUORESCENCE		75.000
SOLVENT BLANK		5.000

QMAX   72.50

ADDL	TLIG	AMTFL	Q	X	C	R	Y	LOG(Y)	LOG(C)
0.010	0.099	62.5	17.036	0.101	-0.002	0.470	0.307	-0.5127	0.0000
0.020	0.199	51.0	32.971	0.196	0.003	0.910	0.834	-0.0788	0.5027
0.040	0.398	38.5	50.229	0.298	0.096	1.386	2.255	0.3532	1.9816
0.060	0.596	35.5	53.814	0.319	0.262	1.485	2.880	0.4594	2.4175
0.080	0.795	34.0	55.257	0.328	0.433	1.524	3.205	0.5058	2.6363
0.100	0.994	33.5	55.214	0.327	0.606	1.523	3.194	0.5044	2.7824
0.120	1.193	32.5	56.000	0.332	0.768	1.545	3.394	0.5307	2.8856
0.150	1.491	31.0	57.286	0.340	1.001	1.580	3.765	0.5758	3.0005
0.180	1.789	30.5	57.014	0.338	1.230	1.573	3.682	0.5661	3.0898
0.200	1.988	30.5	56.286	0.334	1.378	1.553	3.471	0.5405	3.1394

DATA AND INTERMEDIATE RESULTS, RUN 2
PARAMETERS AS IN RUN 1

SAMPLE 761-2

QMAX   75.00

ADDL	TLIG	AMTFL	Q	X	C	R	Y	LOG(Y)	LOG(C)
0.010	0.099	62.5	17.036	0.098	0.002	0.454	0.294	-0.5318	0.2334
0.020	0.199	51.0	32.971	0.189	0.010	0.879	0.785	-0.1054	0.9810
0.040	0.398	38.5	50.229	0.288	0.105	1.339	2.028	0.3070	2.0229
0.060	0.596	35.5	53.814	0.309	0.272	1.435	2.540	0.4049	2.4339
0.080	0.795	34.0	55.257	0.317	0.443	1.474	2.799	0.4470	2.6464
0.100	0.994	33.5	55.214	0.317	0.616	1.472	2.791	0.4457	2.7895
0.120	1.193	32.5	56.000	0.321	0.778	1.493	2.947	0.4694	2.8912
0.150	1.491	31.0	57.286	0.328	1.011	1.528	3.234	0.5097	3.0047
0.180	1.789	30.5	57.014	0.327	1.239	1.520	3.170	0.5011	3.0932
0.200	1.988	30.5	56.286	0.323	1.388	1.501	3.008	0.4782	3.1423

SUMMARY OF RESULTS

SAMPLE 761-2

QMAX	BO	SLOPE	CORRELATION COEFFICIENT	CHSAT (MOLES/LITER)	AFFIN (LITERS/MOLE)
72.50	-0.3592	0.3136	0.9730	1.397E-08	7.156E 07
75.00	-0.4998	0.3410	0.9763	2.923E-08	3.422E 07

ONLY 9 ITEMS ARE CONSIDERED IN THE AVERAGE

72.50	-0.1694	0.2443	0.9869	4.934E-09	2.027E 08

ELAPSED TIME 00.01.41.12

FIG. 2. Sample output data.

D. Determination of the Kinetics of Antibody–Hapten Reactions with the Temperature-Jump Method*

1. INTRODUCTION

As has been shown in the preceding section[1] and in the introduction to this chapter, antibody–hapten reactions are too fast to be studied by conventional techniques of chemical kinetics, unless the concentration of the reactants can be reduced to levels of the order of 10^{-7} to 10^{-11} M.[2-4] At higher concentrations the rate of mixing of the reactants becomes the rate-determining step and the reaction reaches equilibrium before changes in concentration can be measured as a function of time.[5] In general, it is impossible to drop the concentration of the reagents below 10^{-5} to 10^{-6} M, since the available analytical procedures for following the rates of these reactions are not sufficiently sensitive at lower concentrations.

In contrast to standard kinetic techniques, the relaxation methods developed within the last few years by Eigen and his collaborators[6] lend themselves to the determination of the rates of very rapid reactions, including those of diffusion-controlled systems. The equilibrium conditions of such reactions are perturbed almost "instantaneously," i.e., within extremely short time of less than microseconds, and the readjustment of the system to the new state of equilibrium imposed by the perturbation is followed as a function of time, usually on an oscilloscope. Perturbation of the equilibrium can be achieved by a sudden change in a physical parameter, such as temperature,[7] pressure,[8] or electric field strength.[9] It will be shown below that the "relaxation times" determined can be related to the rate constants of the reactions involved by relatively simple mathematical expressions. The term "relaxation" has been coined mainly by physicists to describe the molecular process of self-adjustment of a perturbed molecular system to the equilibrium conditions.[6]

Most reactions are associated with a change of enthalpy and can therefore be readily perturbed by a sudden change in temperature, which

---

* Section 15.D was contributed by A. Froese and A. H. Sehon.

[1] H. N. Eisen and J. E. McGuigan, this volume, Sections 15.C.1–5.

[2] L. A. Day, J. M. Sturtevant, and S. J. Singer, *Ann. N.Y. Acad. Sci.* **103**, 611 (1963).

[3] S. A. Berson and R. S. Yalow, *J. Clin. Invest.* **38**, 1996 (1959).

[4] H. M. Grey, *J. Immunol.* **91**, 90 (1963).

[5] H. Schneider and A. H. Sehon, *Trans. N.Y. Acad. Sci.* [2] **24**, 15 (1961).

[6] M. Eigen and L. DeMaeyer, *Tech. Org. Chem.* **8**, Part 2, 793 (1963).

[7] G. Czerlinski and M. Eigen, *Z. Elektrochem.* **63**, 562 (1954).

[8] H. Strehlow and M. Becker, *Z. Elektrochem.* **63**, 457 (1959).

[9] M. Eigen and J. Schoen, *Z. Elektrochem.* **59**, 483 (1955).

forces new equilibrium conditions onto a preequilibrated system according to the van't Hoff relation

$$\frac{d \ln K}{dT} = \frac{\Delta H}{RT^2} \tag{1}$$

Consequently, the temperature-jump method is the most widely applicable technique among all relaxation procedures for very rapid chemical reactions.[6] Obviously, the reequilibration process can be followed provided that it is slower than the rate of the temperature rise. This is achieved usually within times of less than microseconds by discharging a high voltage condenser (at 30,000 or 100,000 volts) through the electrolyte solution to be studied. The temperature rise occurs in accordance with the relation

$$\Delta T_t = \int_0^t \frac{V_0^2 \exp\left(- \dfrac{2t}{RC}\right)}{C_p R} \, dt \tag{2}$$

where ΔT_t = temperature rise during an interval of time t; R = resistance of the circuit; C = capacitance of the condenser; V_0 = initial voltage of the condenser; C_p = heat capacity of the solution. The total change in temperature is given by

$$\Delta T_\infty \simeq \frac{C V_0^2}{2 C_p} \simeq \frac{C V_0^2}{2 c_p \rho v} \tag{3}$$

where c_p, ρ, and v are the specific heat, the density, and the volume of the solution, respectively. It can be seen that the total temperature change is practically independent of the resistance R and, therefore, of the ionic strength of the solution. The time constant of the temperature rise, on the other hand, which is given by the relation

$$\tau_T = RC/2 \tag{4}$$

depends on the ionic composition of the solution.

If deviations from equilibrium due to the temperature rise are small, the linearized rate equation for a one-step reaction of arbitrary order may be expressed as

$$\tau \frac{d(\Delta C)}{dt} + \Delta C = \Delta \bar{C} \tag{5}$$

where $\Delta \bar{C}$ is the difference between the new equilibrium concentration of a given reactant and a time-independent reference value C_0, ΔC is the difference between the actual concentration at any time t and C_0, and τ

is the relaxation time. Since the rate of disappearance of a small difference is proportional to the difference itself, relation (5) may be represented by Eq. (6)

$$-\frac{d\Delta C'}{dt} = \frac{1}{\tau}\Delta C' \tag{6}$$

which on integration yields the first-order rate expression

$$\Delta C'_t = \Delta C'_\infty \exp\left(-\frac{t}{\tau}\right) \tag{7}$$

For two different intervals of time, t_1 and t_2, the ratio of the terms $\Delta C'_{t_1}/\Delta C'_{t_2}$ can be written as

$$\frac{\Delta C'_{t_1}}{\Delta C'_{t_2}} = \exp\ (t_2 - t_1)/\tau \tag{8}$$

This equation can be also expressed in the logarithmic form

$$\ln \frac{\Delta C'_{t_1}}{\Delta C'_{t_2}} = \frac{t_2 - t_1}{\tau} \tag{9}$$

and it is clear that the relaxation time, τ, is equal to the difference $(t_2 - t_1)$ when the ratio $\Delta C'_{t_1}/\Delta C'_{t_2} = e$. In other words, the relaxation

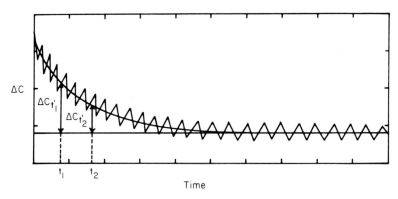

FIG. 1. Relaxation curve recorded on oscilloscope.

time τ is that time after which $1/e$ of the reaction remains to be completed.

In practice the relaxation time for a given reaction is evaluated from photographic recordings of the relaxation curves visualized on an oscilloscope. One fits a curve through the relaxation pattern (Fig. 1) and then the logarithms of the vertical distances, between the points on this curve and the horizontal baseline, are plotted against time. For each simple process the points on the corresponding semilogarithmic plot are expected to lie on a straight line, the slope of this line being equal to the reciprocal of the relaxation time of the process in question, i.e., $1/\tau$. Alternately, the relaxation time may be calculated from the half-lifetime of the reaction, i.e., when

$$\frac{\Delta C'_{t_{1/2}}}{\Delta C'_{\infty}} = \frac{1}{2}$$

From relation (7) it is obvious that

$$\tau = t_{1/2}/0.693 \tag{10}$$

For a reaction consisting of a single reversible process of the type

$$A + B \underset{k_{21}}{\overset{k_{12}}{\rightleftarrows}} C \tag{11}$$

it may be shown[6] that

$$\frac{1}{\tau} = k_{21} + k_{12}[(\bar{A}) + (\bar{B})] \tag{12}$$

where $(\bar{A})$ and $(\bar{B})$ are the free equilibrium concentrations of reactants A and B, corresponding in this specific case to the concentrations of free antibody sites and hapten molecules. It is evident from Eq. (12) that τ depends on the concentrations of both reactants; moreover, as previously alluded to, for each type of reaction mechanism there is a distinct mathematical relationship between τ and the concentrations of the reactants, and appropriate relations have been worked out for different reaction types involving single equilibria.[6] Thus, for example, for a more complex reaction involving two coupled equilibrium steps, such as

$$A + B \underset{k_{21}}{\overset{k_{12}}{\rightleftarrows}} C \tag{13a}$$

$$C + D \underset{k_{32}}{\overset{k_{23}}{\rightleftarrows}} E \tag{13b}$$

two relaxation times will be determined. Mathematical expressions for these two relaxation times can be derived from a set of simultaneous differential equations in terms of the appropriate rate constants and concentrations. These are, however, not identical to the relaxation times that would be calculated for the two individual equilibrium steps, if they occurred independently from each other.

2. APPARATUS

A schematic diagram of the temperature-jump apparatus developed by Eigen and de Maeyer at the Max Planck Institute for Physical Chemistry

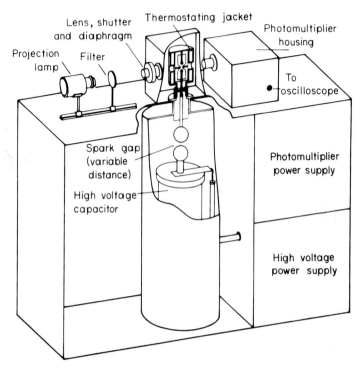

FIG. 2. Schematic diagram of the temperature-jump apparatus. Permission from the publishers to reproduce this illustration from M. Eigen and L. DeMaeyer [*Tech. Org. Chem.* **8**, Part 2, 793 (1963)] is acknowledged with thanks.

in Göttingen is shown in Fig. 2.* For the temperature-jump relaxation technique, concentration changes are best followed using optical techniques, such as light absorption, fluorometric and polarimetric methods. For the study of the kinetics of antibody–hapten reactions, measurements of the changes in concentration of the free hapten were made by absorption spectrophotometry in the visible range.

a. THE REACTION CELL

The reaction cell shown in Figs. 3 and 4 is made of sturdy Plexiglas and has a total volume of about 40 ml; with a special adaptor in the

* The apparatus in the authors' laboratory was also built in the workshops of this Institute. An updated model equipped with an optical system for measurements in the ultraviolet range and with a 1 ml cell can be purchased from Messanlagen Studiengesellschaft mbH., Göttingen, Germany. Other commercial instruments are available from Beckman Instruments Corp., Palo Alto, California; Durrum Instruments Corp., Palo Alto, California; American Instruments Co., Silver Spring, Maryland.

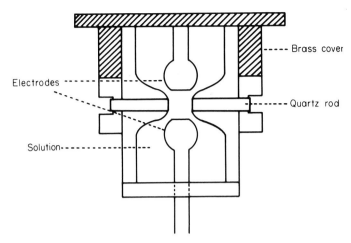

FIG. 3. Schematic diagram of the reaction cell.

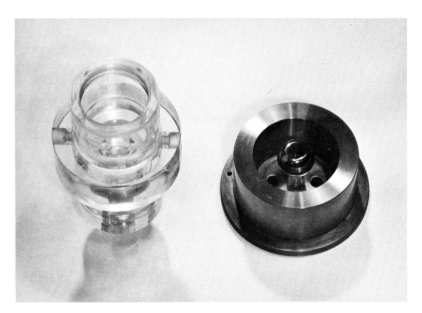

FIG. 4. The reaction cell.

lower half of the cell, as little as 12 ml may be used. The electrodes are designed so as to permit uniform heating in the actual reaction zone (limited to 1–1.3 ml); they are made of brass and are usually platinum or gold plated. Quartz rods are inserted as windows so as to allow visible and ultraviolet radiation to pass the cell. The heavy brass cover of the reaction cell is grounded and is in close contact with a thermostatted jacket, in which the cell rests during the experiment. The temperature within the cell is thus maintained constant.

b. THE HIGH VOLTAGE DISCHARGE SYSTEM

The high voltage condenser (0.1 μF, 30,000 volts) is commercially available from Plastic Capacitors, Inc., Chicago, Illinois. The high voltage power supply may be purchased from Neutronic Associates, Hampstead, New York.

c. THE OPTICAL SYSTEM

It is important that the light source provide high intensity; mercury and xenon high pressure arc lamps satisfy this requirement. Quartz iodide lamps (e.g., Sylvania 6.6A/T2 1/2 Q/CL 45W) with a tungsten filament have been also found useful because of their high surface brightness. Similarly, ordinary tungsten projection lamps may be employed advantageously if the relaxation effects are fairly large. The advantage of tungsten filament lamps is their stability. Mercury and xenon high pressure lamps exhibit arc fluctuations, which at times may make it impossible to measure some slower relaxation effects. The light sources are operated by a direct-current stabilized power supply or a battery, and preferably by a series of batteries. Monochromatic light of the desired wavelength can be obtained by passage of the light beam through an interference filter or by using a monochromator.

To minimize fluctuations in the light source, the beam is split by a half-silvered mirror. One beam passes through the reaction cell and the other through air. The two emerging beams fall onto two RCA 1P28 photomultipliers, operated by a "special" power supply. The signals from the photomultipliers are passed through a cathode follower, are amplified with a differential preamplifier [Tektronix 53/54D] and are then viewed on the screen of a wide-band oscilloscope [Tektronix 545, 531]. Triggering of the horizontal sweep at the instant of discharge of the condenser is achieved by placing an induction coil in the vicinity of the spark gap and connecting one end of this coil to the sweep input of the oscilloscope. The oscilloscope can be equipped with an ordinary 35 mm camera or a Polaroid camera for recording the oscillographic pattern.

3. METHODS

a. CHOICE OF HAPTEN

Since in the temperature-jump technique spectrophotometric methods are used for measuring the concentration changes as a function of time, it is imperative that one of the reactants (e.g., antibody or hapten) undergo a change in absorption properties on combination. This has been achieved by incorporating the haptenic determinant group into an azo dye, which has properties of a pH indicator. The resulting molecule is referred to as a dye-hapten. So far dye-haptens incorporating the 2,4-dinitrophenyl,[10] the *p*-nitrophenyl,[11] and the phenyl arsonate[12] residues

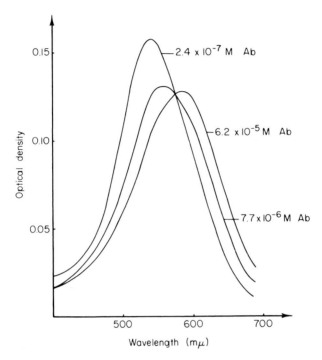

FIG. 5. The effect of rabbit anti-arsanilic antibodies on the absorption spectrum of the dye-hapten 1-naphthol-2-sulfonic acid-4-[4-(4′azobenzene azo)benzene arsonic acid]; the concentration of the dye-hapten was 4.8×10^{-6} *M* in Tris-NaCl buffer (pH 7.5, $\Gamma/2 = 0.1$).

have been used. Spectral changes occurring on combination of the latter dye with homologous antibodies are shown in Fig. 5. It should be pointed out, that not all dye-hapten molecules will undergo sufficiently marked spectral changes on combination with the homologous antibodies to render the system amenable to kinetic studies with the temperature-jump

[10] A. Froese, *Immunochemistry* **5**, 253 (1968).
[11] A. Froese and A. H. Sehon, *Immunochemistry* **2**, 135 (1965).
[12] A. Froese, A. H. Sehon, and M. Eigen, *Can. J. Chem.* **40**, 1786 (1962).

technique. This limitation is primarily due to the temperature-jump being usually of the order of only 6° to 8°, and in consequence the imposed concentration changes are small. It is obvious that the sensitivity for detecting these concentration changes will depend on the extent of the spectral change of the reactant(s), as well as on the enthalpy change of the reaction.

At the present time the choice of the proper dye-hapten depends somewhat on trial and error. It does appear, however, that dye-haptens with good pH indicator properties undergo the largest spectral shifts on combination with antibodies; therefore, one may attribute these shifts, at least in part, to a change in the pK of the dye-hapten.[10,13-15]

Another important factor in choosing the best dye-hapten is its solubility. Most azo dyes, owing to their high content of aromatic rings, are only slightly soluble in aqueous solutions and the formation of micelles may further complicate the systems. Consequently one ought to establish for each dye-hapten the concentration range within which Beer's law is obeyed.

b. PURIFICATION OF ANTIBODIES

The isolation of immune globulins by salt fractionation (e.g., precipitation with sodium or ammonium sulfate) has proved satisfactory. Great care should be taken, however, to eliminate any traces of serum albumin from these preparations of immune globulins, since albumin interacts with a great number of azo dyes causing changes in the absorption properties of the dye molecules. In principle, it may seem profitable to use "pure" antibody preparations isolated with antigenically specific adsorbents or other special procedures. However, in the systems studied so far, normal nonantibody globulins did not appear to affect the spectrum of the dye-haptens and, therefore, the cruder salt fractionation procedures were used for the isolation of antibodies.

c. DETERMINATION OF THE CONCENTRATION OF THE REACTING SPECIES

It was shown in the Introduction that the relaxation time for a given system depends on the concentration of the reacting species. In the temperature-jump apparatus described, concentration changes are measured spectrophotometrically; it is therefore imperative to establish the number and nature of the absorbing species, as well as their concentration. For an ideal case there would be only two absorbing species in the visible

---

[13] H. Metzger, L. Wofsy, and S. J. Singer, *Arch. Biochem. Biophys.* **103**, 206 (1963).
[14] J. M. Sturtevant, L. Wofsy, and S. J. Singer, *Science* **134**, 1434 (1961).
[15] A. Froese and A. Sehon, unpublished results (1964).

spectral range, namely the free and bound forms of the hapten. This will be manifested by a common crossing point (Fig. 5), i.e., one isosbestic point for different absorption curves obtained at different antibody concentrations, the hapten concentration being kept constant. The concentrations of the free and bound forms of the hapten can be then calculated

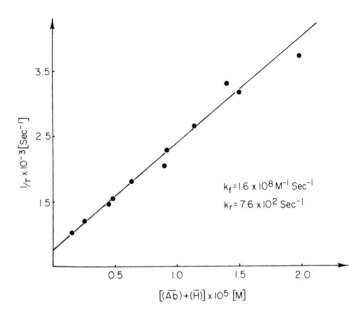

FIG. 6. Concentration dependence of $1/\tau$ for the anti-p-nitrophenyl antibody system.

with the aid of a relationship originally suggested by Klotz[16] for the determination of protein–dye complexes.[12,17]

$$\beta = \frac{\epsilon_f - \epsilon_{app}}{\epsilon_f - \epsilon_b} \tag{14}$$

In the above relationship, β represents the fraction of dye-hapten in the bound form, ϵ_f and ϵ_b represent the molar extinction coefficients for the free and bound forms of the dye-hapten, respectively, and ϵ_{app} is the apparent molar extinction coefficient of a solution containing both forms of the hapten. Since it is desirable to limit the reacting system to only two absorbing species, the experiments are made at a pH (compatible

[16] I. M. Klotz, in "The Proteins" (H. Neurath and K. Bailey, eds.), Vol. 1, Part B, p. 727. Academic Press, New York, 1953.
[17] U. Westphal, B. B. Ashley, and G. L. Selden, J. Am. Chem. Soc. 80, 5735 (1958).

with the stability of the antibody–hapten complex), at which only one of the absorbing species of the dye predominates in the absence of antibody, i.e., at a pH removed far enough from the pK of the chromophoric group of the dye-hapten where mainly the ionized or nonionized form of this group prevails. Thus, any spectral change resulting on addition of antibody can be interpreted in terms of a two-component system. If the absorption maxima of the two forms of the dye hapten are far apart, it is preferable to make spectrophotometric measurements at the two wavelengths, corresponding to the two absorption maxima.[18,19]

The interpretation of spectrophotometric measurements may become rather involved if more than two absorbing species are present. It is advisable to establish the validity of the spectrophotometric method for determining the binding of antibody and hapten with reference to binding data calculated from equilibrium dialysis experiments. It might be visualized that the electronic structure of haptens interacting with antibody sites of varying affinities will be affected to a different extent depending on the degree of steric complementariness, i.e., on the orientation of the hapten within the antibody site, and different molar extinction coefficients would be expected for the different forms of the hapten bound by a heterogeneous antibody population. This complication will obviously render the binding data derived from spectrophotometric measurements somewhat less precise than those obtained by equilibrium dialysis; however, this limitation might be outbalanced by the complication due to absorption of the dye-hapten by the dialysis membrane. Obviously, this limitation is common to all indirect methods in which the concentration of a reacting species is measured in terms of a physical parameter.

The choice of the buffer ions is determined chiefly by the desired pH and the particular antibody–hapten system, since some ions have been found to inhibit the reaction. If a nonbuffering electrolyte is added, it is advisable to avoid halide ions, since these will interact with the electrodes of the temperature-jump cell. Potassium nitrate has so far been found to be the most suitable supporting electrolyte.

4. EXPERIMENTAL PROCEDURE AND RESULTS

Only a general outline of the procedure of a temperature-jump experiment will be given here.

Measurements are made at a wavelength at which the difference in

[18] D. F. Boltz, *in* "Selected Topics in Modern Instrumental Analysis" (D. F. Boltz, ed.), p. 105. Prentice-Hall, Englewood Cliffs, New Jersey, 1952.
[19] C. A. Davies and T. A. Geissman, *J. Am. Chem. Soc.* **76**, 2307 (1954).

extinction coefficients of the bound and free forms of the dye is maximal, provided the sensitivity of the photomultipliers at this wavelength is sufficiently high. The antibody–hapten solution is precooled to the desired temperature in the reaction cell itself. The experiment is then performed at the maximum possible signal–noise ratio, which is a function of the light intensity, the anode load resistance, and photomultiplier sensitivity; care must be taken to work below the saturation of the photo-multipliers. The anode load resistance should always be operated at its highest possible value in order to obtain maximum sensitivity; the greater this resistance, the smaller must be the bandwidth of the transmitted signals.

For any antibody–hapten system, the entire time range of which the instrument is capable should be investigated to detect all relaxation effects. The instrument used by the authors could measure reactions with relaxation times greater than 5 microseconds.

For a solution of a given antibody concentration the temperature is "jumped" several times and the relaxation effect is recorded each time, care being taken to allow the system to return to the temperature of the thermostat, which may require 2 to 3 minutes. If the temperature jump effect is small, it is essential to perform a large number of measurements and average values of the relaxation times are used for appropriate calculations.

Relaxation times greater than 1 second cannot be accurately deter-mined because of convection which sets in after this time. This disturb-ance is brought about by differences in the density of the solutions in the actual reaction volume (bounded by the electrodes and the quartz rods) and the remainder of the cell.

The concentration dependence of the relaxation time must be thor-oughly investigated before one can assign the appropriate mechanism for the reaction and before one can determine the rate expression relating to the rate constants of the individual reaction steps, which participate in the overall reaction. For example as stated previously for the antibody–hapten systems studied so far, the reaction mechanism could be repre-sented by the simple relation*

$$Ab + H \underset{k_{21}}{\overset{k_{12}}{\rightleftharpoons}} AbH \tag{11'}$$

The concentration dependence of τ for such a reaction system is given by Eq. (12). It should be pointed out that if the dye-hapten undergoes a

* However, for other systems the reaction mechanism might be more complex involv-ing additional steps.

change in pK on binding to the antibody combining site, the more detailed mechanism given below may be postulated

$$
\begin{array}{ccc}
\mathrm{I} & & \mathrm{II} \\
& k_{12} & \\
\mathrm{Ab} + \mathrm{DH} & \rightleftarrows & \mathrm{AbDH} \\
& k_{21} & \\
\kappa \updownarrow & & \updownarrow \mathcal{K} \\
& k_{34} & \\
\mathrm{Ab} + \mathrm{D}^- & \rightleftarrows & \mathrm{AbD}^- \\
& k_{43} & \\
\mathrm{III} & & \mathrm{IV}
\end{array}
\qquad (15)
$$

where DH and D^- represent the protonated and ionized forms of the dye-hapten, respectively. If one assumes that equilibration processes between states I and III and between II and IV are fast, it can be shown that*

$$
\frac{1}{\tau} = k_{21}\left(\frac{\mathrm{H}^+}{\mathrm{H}^+ + \mathcal{K}}\right) + k_{43}\left(\frac{\mathcal{K}}{\mathrm{H}^+ + \mathcal{K}}\right)
$$
$$
+ \left[k_{12}\left(\frac{\mathrm{H}^+}{\mathrm{H}^+ + K}\right) + k_{34}\left(\frac{K}{\mathrm{H}^+ + K}\right)\right] [(\overline{\mathrm{Ab}}) + (\overline{\mathrm{D}}_{\mathrm{T}})] \quad (16)
$$

This expression can be further simplified by lumping the concentration dependent and independent parameters into the two terms of Eq. (17), which is formally equivalent to Eq. (12), the two terms $k_{r.app.}$ and $k_{f.app.}$ are the apparent rate constants for the reverse and forward overall reaction steps.

$$
\frac{1}{\tau} = k_{r.app.} + k_{f.app.}\ [(\overline{\mathrm{Ab}}) + (\overline{\mathrm{D}}_{\mathrm{T}})] \qquad (17)
$$

Equations (16) and (17) can be reduced to the simpler expression (12) where the free and bound forms of the hapten are in the same state of ionization. Since Eqs. (17) and (12) have the same concentration dependence, the true values for the rate constants can be determined only if the pH dependence of the reaction is accurately determined.[22] To establish the validity of Eqs. (12) or (17), it is best to vary first one of the reactants keeping the other constant, and then reverse the procedure. In practice, the highest sensitivity of the measurements is limited to a rather small concentration range, usually the concentrations of bound

---

* A similar relationship was derived by Alberty and co-workers[20, 21] for protein–ligand interactions.

[20] D. E. Goldsack, W. S. Eberlein, and R. A. Alberty, *J. Biol. Chem.* **241**, 2653 (1966).

[21] H. B. Dunford and R. A. Alberty, *Biochemistry* **6**, 447 (1967).

[22] A. Froese, S. G. Goldwater, and A. H. Sehon, *Protides Biol. Fluids* (H. Peeters ed.), Vol. 16, p. 167. Pergamon Press, Oxford, 1969.

and free forms of the hapten being almost equal and the total optical density being close to 0.4. The large degree of heterogeneity of some antibody preparations, with respect to the binding constants of the different antibody molecules, may render the interpretation of the effect of concentration changes on τ somewhat ambiguous. Thus, at the lower concentrations of the dye, the contribution of the binding sites with the higher affinities will be more pronounced, and on increasing the concentration of the dye the binding sites having weaker affinities will come into play.

The temperature-jump method has so far been applied to the study of three antibody–hapten systems: (i) antibodies specific to the phenyl arsonate ion; (ii) antibodies to the p-nitrophenyl determinant; and (iii) antibodies to the 2,4-dinitrophenyl determinant. The dye-haptens used in these studies were (i) 1-naphthol-4[4-(4′-azobenzeneazo)benzenearsonic acid] (N-R′); (ii) 4,5-dihydroxy-3-(p-nitrophenylazo)-2,6-naphthalene disulfonic acid (4,5N-2,6S-3pNP); and (iii) 1-hydroxy-4-(2,4-dinitrophenylazo)-2,5-naphthalene disulfonic acid (1N-2,5S-4DNP), respectively. The kinetics of the reactions of antibodies to the 2,4-dinitrophenyl determinant was also studied with the cross-reacting hapten 1-hydroxy-4-(4-nitrophenylazo)-2,5-naphthalene disulfonic acid (1N-2,5S-4pNP). As can be seen from Fig. 6, the kinetic data for system (ii) were represented by the linear relationship (13). From the slope and intercept of this straight line, the rate constants were calculated as $k_{12} = 1.8 \times 10^8 \ M^{-1}$ sec^{-1} and $k_{21} = 750$ sec^{-1}, respectively. This value for the rate constant for the association step in reaction (11′) is lower than the maximum rate constant for a diffusion-controlled reaction by about one order of magnitude and agrees well with the values calculated for the rate constants of other antibody–hapten systems[2, 12] studied so far. These values are compared in Table I. It is evident from these data that the rate constants for the combination of each type of antibody with its homologous hapten do not differ by more than one order of magnitude and approach the value for a diffusion-controlled reaction within a factor of 10 to 100. Thus, antibody–hapten reactions appear to be some of the fastest processes involving biopolymers.

Whereas in the past kinetic experiments have been performed mainly in order to determine the rate constants for the reactions of various antibody–hapten systems, additional information about the mechanisms and nature of such reactions could also be gained.

Since antibody–hapten reactions are reversible, the equilibrium constant for reaction (11′) is given by Eq. (18).

$$K = \frac{k_{12}}{k_{21}} \tag{18}$$

Thus, changes in K could be due to changes in either k_{12}, k_{21}, or both. Equilibrium constants can, therefore, only provide information as to the overall affinity of the antibody for the hapten. When antibodies specific to the 2,4-dinitrophenyl determinant were reacted with cross-reacting haptens incorporating the p-nitrophenyl or the 2,4-dinitrophenyl determinant, it was shown[10] (see also Table I) that appreciable differences were observed only in the rate constant of dissociation (k_{21}). The fact that k_{12} did not exhibit a significant difference for the two dye-haptens would indicate that the activation energy for the two forward reactions was about the same. This would mean that the steric hindrance, if any, in the antibody-combining site for the two dye-haptens was about equal.

TABLE I

VALUES FOR RATE CONSTANTS OF ANTIBODY–HAPTEN SYSTEMS

Antibodies to	Dye-hapten	$k_{12}(M^{-1} \sec^{-1})$	k_{21} (sec^{-1})	Reference
ϕ-A$_s$O$_3$H$^-$	N-R'	2×10^7	50	a
ϕ-NO$_2$	4,5N-2,7S-3pNP	1.8×10^8	760	b
ϕ-(NO$_2$)$_2$	1N-3,6S-2DNP^e	8×10^7	1.4	c
ϕ-(NO$_2$)$_2$	1N-2,5S-4DNP	1.6×10^7	80	d
ϕ-(NO$_2$)$_2$	1N-2,5S-4pNP	1.4×10^7	410	d

^{a} A. Froese, A. H. Sehon, and M. Eigen, *Can. J. Chem.* **40**, 1786 (1962).
^{b} A. Froese and A. H. Sehon, *Immunochemistry* **2**, 135 (1965).
^{c} L. A. Day, J. M. Sturtevant, and S. J. Singer, *Ann. N.Y. Acad. Sci.* **103**, 619 (1963).
^{d} A. Froese, *Immunochemistry* **5**, 253 (1968).
^{e} 1-Hydroxy-2-(2,4-dinitrophenylazo)-3,6-naphthalene disulfonic acid.

Reactions with other cross-reacting haptens of different stereochemical configuration could conceivably exhibit a different kinetic behavior. Kinetic experiments could, therefore, provide additional information about the stereospecificity of antibody–antigen reactions.

Moreover, kinetic experiments with the temperature-jump relaxation technique could in principle be used to detect any conformational change in the antibody molecule itself as a result of combination with hapten, as suggested by Grossberg et al.[23] Additional steps in the antibody–hapten reaction would lead to more than one relaxation effect. Indeed, such a second effect of small amplitude has been observed in some investigations,[10, 22] suggesting that the mechanism for the antibody–hapten may be more complex than that represented by relation (11). In this

[23] A. L. Grossberg, G. Markus, and D. Pressman, *Proc. Natl. Acad. Sci. U.S.* **54**, 942 (1965).

connection it is worth noting that Kirschner *et al.*[24] have demonstrated that the temperature-jump relaxation method can be successfully applied to solve the complex reaction mechanisms of protein–ligand interactions which involve conformation changes in the protein molecule.

It should be pointed out that the use of the temperature-jump relaxation technique could also be extended to the study of antibody–antigen reactions, provided precipitation could be avoided by using univalent antigens or univalent antibody fragments. Such reactions would have to exhibit spectral changes of sufficient magnitude in order to be amenable to present spectrophotometric methods of detection. However, it is conceivable that other detection methods, such as fluorescence quenching or optical rotation, could be used to follow the reaction.

ACKNOWLEDGMENTS

The work done in the authors' laboratory and referred to in this paper has been supported by grants from the National Institute of Allergy and Infectious Diseases, National Institutes of Health, Bethesda, Maryland; the Medical Research Council of Canada and the National Research Council of Canada, Ottawa, Ontario.

[24] K. Kirschner, M. Eigen, R. Bittman, and B. Voigt, *Proc. Natl. Acad. Sci. U.S.* **56**, 1661 (1966).

E. Hapten Inhibition of Reactions of Antibody with Conjugated Haptens*

1. INTRODUCTION

Comprehensive studies of the cross-precipitation or lack of reaction between each of a series of hapten–protein conjugates and antiserum elicited by any one particular hapten attached to a different carrier have helped to define the degree and diversity of antibody specificity. The variable ability of different haptens to cause greater or lesser inhibition of the precipitation of a particular conjugate by its antiserum was also noted in these early studies and, when semiquantitated, permitted examination of the specificities of antibodies.[1] Pauling and his co-workers[2] quantitated hapten inhibition of precipitation, recognized the heterogeneity of anti-hapten antibodies, and established the theoretical basis for the calculation of relative average association constants for a series of haptens reacting with a particular antibody. Even at present, hapten inhibition of precipitation is used to deduce something of the size and

* Section 15.E was contributed by John J. Cebra.

[1] K. Landsteiner, "The Specificity of Serological Reactions," 2nd ed., Harvard Univ. Press, 1945; reprinted by Dover Publications, Inc., New York, 1962.
[2] L. Pauling, D. Pressman, and A. L. Grossberg, *J. Am. Chem. Soc.* **66**, 784 (1944).

heterogeneity of the combining sites of antihapten antibodies.[3] Other sections in this chapter describe elegant methods which permit the direct measurement of hapten–antibody interactions and the calculation of absolute values for reaction parameters.

2. APPLICATIONS

a. COMPARISON OF RELATIVE BINDING OF A SERIES OF HAPTENS

When only relative hapten–antibody association constants are being sought, the hapten inhibition method offers an advantage over many other methods in that antiserum or crude immunoglobulins can be used as a source of antibodies, and hence purified antibodies need not be isolated.

The nature of the haptens may also determine whether the inhibition method should be used. For example, measurement of hapten binding by antibody using the method of equilibrium dialysis requires that molar concentrations of hapten of the same order as those of the antibody $(10^{-4}$ to $10^{-5} M)$ be accurately determined. If a sensitive spectrophotometric or colorimetric method is not available for all members of a series of haptens, or if radiolabeled compounds are not obtainable, then the method of hapten inhibition must be employed to determine relative association constants.[3]

b. DETECTION OF ANTIBODIES SPECIFIC FOR SUPPOSEDLY NONIMMUNOGENIC NATURAL COMPOUNDS

Antibodies specific for certain naturally occurring compounds, such as steroids, nucleic acids, and antibiotics, have been sought after deliberate immunization or have been suspected in certain disease states. If precipitating antibodies are found, their specificity can be established by testing the inhibitory effects of the appropriate natural compounds or fragments thereof. An example might be the inhibition by water-soluble derivatives of steroids of a system containing the supposed immunogen or a conjugate of the natural compound (see Section 1.E.5, Vol. I).

c. TEST FOR SUCCESSFUL AFFINITY LABELING OF ANTIBODY SITE

Wofsy et al.[4] have presented a method for labeling the active site of anti-hapten antibody. Approximately equal concentrations of purified antibody and a chemically reactive hapten (a diazonium fluoroborate derivative) are allowed to react. Specific permanent inhibition of the

[3] V. P. Kreiter and D. Pressman, *Biochemistry* **3**, 274 (1964).
[4] L. Wofsy, H. Metzger, and S. J. Singer, *Biochemistry* **1**, 1031 (1962).

ability of the antibody to precipitate hapten–protein conjugate is taken as one criterion for successful labeling in the region of the antibody site.

3. METHODS FOR QUANTITATIVE INHIBITION STUDIES

a. MATERIALS

The advisability of using an immunoglobulin fraction rather than whole serum as a source of antibody, the recommended procedure for the preparation of the stock solution of immunoglobulin, and the buffers to be used as solvents are all noted in Section 13.B.4 on inhibition of protein–antiprotein precipitation reactions. An amount of immunoglobulin containing a defined quantity (1 to 2 mg) of anti-hapten antibody in a volume of 0.5 ml is used for each reaction tube.

i. Hapten–Protein Conjugate (Test Antigen)

The test antigen is used to define and determine the amount of anti-hapten antibody in the immunoglobulin. Ordinarily it consists of the same hapten employed in the original immunogen, attached instead to a protein carrier that does not cross-react with the carrier in the immunogen. For instance, if the carrier in the immunogen was bovine γ-globulin, test antigen containing ovalbumin would be appropriate. Another combination might be horse ferritin in the immunogen and human serum albumin in the test antigen. Unlike many protein antigens, artificial conjugates are not homogeneous; they usually consist of a population of molecules containing varying numbers of substituent haptens attached to a number of different amino acid residues of the carriers. The test antigen chosen for the inhibition system should be soluble in neutral buffers and should contain sufficient substituent haptenic groups so that all molecules of the test antigen are precipitable by antibody. However, it should have a reasonably narrow distribution of number of haptenic groups about the average number of substituents. Methods for preparation of soluble conjugates are given in Volume I, Chapter 1, Section E. If the substituents are primarily reactive with basic groups of protein carriers, the principles described by Goldstein et al.[5] for the preparations of fluorescent antibody can be applied to the preparation of hapten–protein conjugates with a narrow distribution of substituent groups.

Since the variability of the sites of substitution on the carrier protein may influence the apparent relative association constants of a series of haptens it may be desirable for some studies to use high molecular weight

[5] G. Goldstein, I. S. Slizys, and M. W. Chase, *J. Exptl. Med.* **114**, 89 (1961).

poly-L-lysine as a carrier. The only groups available for substitution in this synthetic polymer are amino groups. A conjugate of poly-L-lysine and angiotensin, described by Haber et al.[6] is an example of such a conjugated antigen.

A stock solution of test antigen is prepared so that 0.1 to 0.2 ml contains the amount of antigen required to give maximal precipitation of the antibody in 0.5 ml of the stock immunoglobulin solution. This amount of antigen is determined by quantitative precipitation as described in Chapter 13, Sections A.3 or D. If the haptenic groups have a characteristic absorption, this can be used to determine the contribution of the antigen to the precipitate and hence the absolute amount of antibody precipitated.

ii. Stock Solutions of Haptens

The haptens are accurately weighed out and dissolved in the appropriate buffer to give stock solutions of 10^{-2}, 10^{-3}, and 10^{-4} M. Adjustment of the pH may be necessary, especially if the hapten is in the form of a free acid or base. Heating or titration with acid or base may be required to dissolve the hapten to the required concentration. The range of inhibitor concentrations to be used in the quantitative study may be approximated by setting up a preliminary, qualitative set of tests as described in Chapter 13, Section B.4.a.iv. Ordinarily, molar concentrations of hapten required to affect precipitation are 10^1 to 10^3 times greater than the molar concentration of antibody used.

b. QUANTITATIVE INHIBITION TEST PROCEDURE

The volume and order of adding the immunoglobulin, hapten inhibitor, and conjugated test antigen, and the treatment of the reaction mixture and resulting precipitates are described in Chapter 13, Section B.4.b. The section on inhibition of protein systems also describes necessary control tests applicable to hapten inhibition measurements and relevant limitations and precautions to be taken with the inhibition assay.

4. CALCULATION OF RELATIVE ASSOCIATION CONSTANTS AND DIFFERENCES IN FREE ENERGY CHANGE OF COMBINATION

a. RELATIONSHIPS NECESSARY FOR THE TREATMENT OF THE EXPERIMENTAL DATA

The necessary mathematical relationships were derived by Pauling et al.[2] Antibody molecules of a particular specificity were assumed to

---

[6] E. Haber, L. B. Page, and G. A. Jacoby, *Biochemistry* **4**, 693 (1965).

be heterogeneous with respect to their free energy change of combination with hapten. Thus, the combining constants of particular antibodies in a given population would deviate from the average combining constant, K_0. The distribution of values of the natural logarithm of the particular constants (K_1, K_2, etc.) about the natural logarithm of the mean combining constant (K_0) was taken to be Gaussian, and the probability, $f(\sigma)$, that the deviation from the mean is ln (K/K_0) is given by:

$$f(\sigma) = \frac{1}{\sqrt{\pi}\,\sigma} e^{-\{\ln\,(K/K_0)\}^2/\sigma^2} \tag{1}$$

where K is any particular combining constant for the formation of antibody–hapten complex.

Now the fraction (dn/N) of the total population of antibody (N) made up of molecules having values for K that lie between $K_{1+\epsilon}$ and $K_{1-\epsilon}$, where K_1 departs from the average constant, K_0, is:

$$\frac{dn}{N} = \frac{1}{\sqrt{\pi}\,\sigma} e^{-\{\ln\,(K/K_0)\}^2/\sigma^2} \cdot d\{\ln\,(K/K^\circ)\} \tag{2}$$

Pauling et al. further showed that the relationship between precipitation and inhibitor concentration for a *homogeneous* population of antibodies could be reduced to the following after making some simplifying assumptions:

$$P = 1 - K[I] \tag{3}$$

where $[I]$ is the concentration of hapten and precipitation, P, is the amount of precipitate formed in presence of inhibitor divided by the amount of precipitate formed in the absence of inhibitor.

If antibodies are heterogeneous, then the infinitesimally small part of the total precipitate, dP, given by that fraction of antibodies having K values in a differential region removed from K_0 is:

$$dP = (1 - K[I]) \frac{dN}{N} \tag{4}$$

Substituting the expression for dn/N given in Eq. (2) and summing up all contributions to the total precipitate given by antibodies having all possible K values, the following is obtained:

$$P = \int_0^{'} dP = \frac{1}{\sqrt{\pi}\,\sigma} \int_{-\infty}^{*} (1 - K[I])e^{-\{\ln\,(K/K_0)\}^2/\sigma^2} \cdot d\{\ln\,(K/K_0)\} \tag{5}$$

The lower limit is set by that class of molecules which do not bind hapten at all; hence ln $(K/K_0) = -\infty$. The upper limit (*) is set by that class of molecules having values for K just large enough to prevent precipitation, and is $\ln (1/K_0[I])$. If the substitution $u^2 = \{\ln (K/K_0)\}^2/\sigma^2$ is made, then the form of Eq. (5) is simplified to:

$$P = \frac{1}{\sqrt{\pi}} \int_{-\infty}^{u^*} (1 - K_0 e^{u\sigma}[I]) e^{-u^2} \, du \tag{6}$$

where $u^* = (1/\sigma)\{\ln (1/K_0[I])\}$.

Now values for the integral of the error function, $H(x)$, have been computed and tabulated for many values of x.[7] The form of $H(x)$ is:

$$H(x) = \frac{2}{\sqrt{\pi}} \int_0^x e^{-\alpha^2} \, d\alpha \tag{7}$$

Values for precipitation, P, at any given hapten concentration can therefore be computed using the tables of values for $H(x)$ after Eq. (6) is rewritten, utilizing the definition of $H(x)$ given in Eq. (7), to become:

$$P = \tfrac{1}{2}\{1 + H(u^*)\} - \tfrac{1}{2}K_0[I]e^{\sigma^2/4}\{1 + H(u^* - \sigma/2)\} \tag{8}$$

If σ, sometimes called the heterogeneity constant or heterogeneity index, equals zero, then Eq. (8) reduces to the simple form of Eq. (3), since $H(\infty) = 1$.

When P is plotted against $\log [I]$, the effect of different values of K_0 for different hapten inhibitors is merely to shift the plots along the $\log [I]$ axis since K_0 and $[I]$ always would appear as the logarithm of their product, as seen from Eq. (8) above. Variation of the value of the heterogeneity constant, σ, would cause variation in the slope of the plot of P against $\log [I]$. Hence, if two such plots are parallel, then equal degrees of heterogeneity with respect to two different haptens is indicated for a given antibody population.

b. Graphical and Mathematical Treatment of the Data

The amount of precipitate formed in the presence of different concentrations of hapten is usually expressed as "percent inhibition" [1.0 − (amount of precipitate in presence of hapten/amount of precipitate in absence of hapten)] × 100 or as "fraction of maximum precipitation" (amount of precipitate in presence of hapten/amount of precipitate in absence of hapten), which is the P of Eqs. (3), (5), and (8). If P or percent inhibition is plotted vs. inhibitor concentration, then one can obtain a rough comparison of the effectiveness of members of a series of inhibitors.

[7] A. N. Lowan, "Tables of Probability Functions." The Federal Works Agency, Works Projects Administration, New York, 1941.

Some interpretations of such plots for inhibition of protein systems are given in Chapter 13, Section B.4.

The discussion following Eq. (8) above pointed out that if P (or percent inhibition) were plotted vs. logarithm of inhibitor concentration, then the effect of different values of K_0 was to shift the plots obtained for different haptens along the log $[I]$ axis. Thus, relative association constants, $K_0(\text{rel})$, may be calculated for a series of haptens affecting the *same* antibody–conjugate system from plots of P, or percent inhibition vs. the logarithm of the inhibitor concentration. The linear distance along the log $[I]$ axis (abscissa) is then a relative measure of log K_0 at the temperature used for the inhibition assay (3° to 5°). One hapten, often the homologous hapten, is defined as a standard with $K_0 = 1$ and log K_0 $= 0$. The linear distance between curves is measured between each curve and the standard curve at the ordinate $P = 0.5$, or at 50% inhibition, to minimize the effects of variation of antibody heterogeneity constant, σ, with respect to the different inhibitors. Figure 1 and the following section indicate that the plots are least sensitive to variations in σ over the range 0 to 3.0 at values near $P = 0.5$. Usually, the *same* antibody population shows little variation in σ for the different members of a series of haptens.

A value for $\Delta(\Delta F^\circ)$, which represents the difference in change in standard free energy for the combination of two different haptens with antibody, can be calculated from:

$$\Delta(\Delta F^\circ) = -2.3RT \log (K_{0(1)}/K_{0(2)}) \tag{9}$$

where $K_{0(1)}$ and $K_{0(2)}$ are the average combining constants for two different haptens, $R = 1.99$ cal/mole $\cdot \,^\circ K$, and T is the absolute temperature of the assay ($^\circ$K). Of course, the $K_0(\text{rel})$ value for any hapten can be used in place of $K_{0(1)}/K_{0(2)}$ to compare that hapten with the standard. Two haptens, not including the standard, can be compared using their $K_0(\text{rel})$ values in Eq. (9).

c. The Heterogeneity Index (Constant)

The value of σ for any given population of antibodies reacting with a particular hapten may be approximated by fitting a theoretical curve, given by Eq. (8), to the experimental data for a P or percent inhibition vs. log $[I]$ plot. A family of curves can be constructed, as shown in Fig. 1, which show the effect of variation of σ on the shape of the curve. The theoretical curves can be constructed from Eq. (8) by setting $K_0 = 1$ and using tables to obtain values for $H(x)$.[7] To obtain the theoretical curve for a population of antibodies having a particular value of σ, $[I]$ is varied and the corresponding values for $H(u^*)$, $H(u^* - \sigma/2)$, and

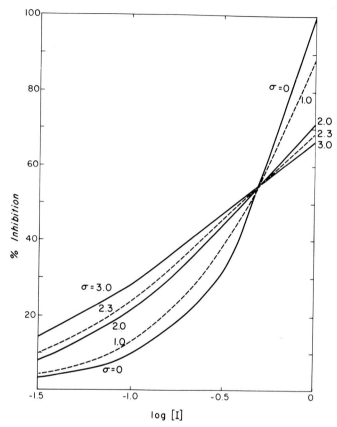

Fig. 1. Theoretical curves showing the effect of different values of σ on plots of percentage inhibition vs. log $[I]$.

$e^{\sigma^2/4}$ are computed and used to determine P or percent inhibition. P is then plotted vs. log $[I]$ using the same scales for the abscissa and ordinates that are employed to plot the experimental data. The value of σ which allows construction of the theoretical curve giving closest fit to the experimental data is taken as the heterogeneity index of the actual antibody population. The absolute values of the experimental points along the log $[I]$ axis are unimportant for the curve-fitting process. One easy procedure to determine the best-fitting theoretical curve is to plot the experimental points on transparent graph paper and then to attempt to superimpose them onto each of a series of theoretical curves (each obtained for a different value of σ as in Fig. 1) in turn by lining up ordinates (P, or percent inhibition) and by shifting the curves along the abscissa.

F. Thermodynamic and Kinetic Investigation of the Antigen–Antibody Reaction by Fluorescence Labeling Techniques* †

1. INTRODUCTION

Fluorescence labeling techniques provide powerful new approaches for exploring the thermodynamic and kinetic parameters of antigen–antibody interactions. The technique[1, 2] described in this chapter possesses two distinctive features: (1) One component, either the hapten, antigen, or antibody, must be obtained in a purified and fluorescent labeled form. The fluorescent label may be entirely unrelated and foreign to the antigen–antibody reaction in question. (2) Measurements of fluorescence polarization or intensity on solutions of the labeled component together with its unlabeled immunologically complementary partner are then related to the extent of the reaction. Of prime importance is the fact that the unlabeled component need not be in a purified form.

The analysis results in the determination of both thermodynamic and kinetic parameters, viz., (1) binding site concentration, (2) association constant, (3) heterogeneity constant, (4) order of reaction, and (5) rate constants.

The technique lends itself to a study of these quantities under a wide variety of conditions of pH, ionic strength, solvent composition, and temperature.

The essential feature of the method consists of first labeling either the antigen or antibody molecule with a fluorescent label, and then in following the fluorescence polarization and molar fluorescence when measured quantities of the labeled partner are mixed with the unlabeled one.

The dependence of polarization and the molar fluorescence upon the extent of reaction between the antigen and antibody forms the basis for the quantification of the antigen–antibody reaction. Reaction between the antigen and antibody results in an increase in size of the kinetic unit and in a retardation of the rotary Brownian motion, which in turn is manifested by an increase in the polarization of fluorescence. The first additions of labeled component result in high values of polarization. As the additions are continued, the polarization drops off and approaches,

* Sections 15.F.1–7 were contributed by Walter B. Dandliker.

† Supported by The John A. Hartford Foundation, Inc., the National Science Foundation (GB-4288), and the National Institute of Arthritis and Metabolic Diseases (AM 07508).

1 W. B. Dandliker and G. Feigen, *Biochem. Biophys. Res. Commun.* **5**, 299 (1961).
2 W. B. Dandliker, H. C. Schapiro, J. W. Meduski, R. Alonso, G. A. Feigen, and J. R. Hamrick, Jr., *Immunochemistry* **1**, 165 (1964).

as a limit, that of the labeled partner alone. Changes in polarization may usually be expected as long as the antigen–antibody combination results in appreciable changes in the rotary Brownian motion of the labeled molecule.

Concomitant with these changes, the alteration in environment of the fluorescent label (which occurs as a result of the antigen–antibody reaction) may simultaneously produce changes in the molar fluorescence. If such changes occur, they may be used as well as the polarization to quantify the reaction.

2. THEORY

a. Absorption, Fluorescence, and Phosphorescence

Absorption of radiation in the visible or ultraviolet region results in excitation of the absorbing molecule to one of the vibrational levels of an excited state. Thereafter, vibrational relaxation to the lowest vibrational level of the first excited singlet state takes place in about 10^{-12} second. The subsequent fate of the electronic excitation energy depends both upon the structure of the molecule and the nature of its environment. The molecule may return by a radiationless path to the ground state (ordinary absorption); fluorescence emission may occur during the lifetime of the excited state (10^{-8} second) by a transition to one of the vibrational levels adjacent to the ground state, or phosphorescence may result if the molecule has a low-lying triplet state accessible from the excited singlet state. (The long-lived triplet state usually becomes deactivated by collisions in liquid media, but the protective environment of solid media at low temperatures often allows emission to appear.)

b. Polarization of Fluorescence

In classic terms, the emission from a single molecule may be regarded as radiation from a single oscillating dipole; this radiation has an oscillating electric field parallel to the oscillation of the dipole and is said to be polarized in the same direction.

If a randomly oriented assembly of |molecules| is| excited |by fully polarized light, their fluorescence is only "partially" polarized even if the molecules are prevented from Brownian rotation in solution, as may be seen by the following considerations. (Partially polarized light may be thought of as being a mixture of polarized light and unpolarized light.) For simplicity, assume that the directions of the absorption and emission oscillators in a single molecule are the same and that they are rigidly fixed with respect to the geometric axes of the molecule. Furthermore, assume the molecules to be rigidly fixed in position during the interval between absorption and emission (typically 10^{-8} second). The probability of absorption of light is proportional to the square of the magnitude of the component of the electric vector of the exciting light in the direction of the oscillator.[3] From Fig. 1, this probability is proportional to $\cos^2 \theta$, where θ is the angle between the incident electric field E, which is parallel to the z axis, and the direction of the absorption oscillator. Because the probability of absorption falls off as θ increases, molecules oriented so that θ is small are preferentially excited, while those with large θ have little chance of absorbing. Since the absorption and emission oscillators

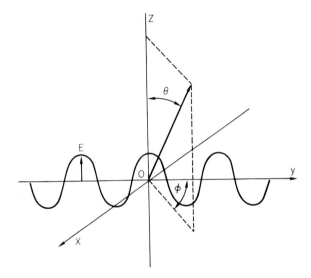

FIG. 1. Excitation of randomly oriented oscillators by polarized light. The absorption (and emission) oscillators make an angle θ with the direction of the incident electric field. The maximum value of the polarization observed at any angle ϕ in the xy plane is $\frac{1}{2}$.

are parallel, the emitted light will be partially polarized with a degree of polarization, P. This quantity is defined in terms of the intensities, I, polarized parallel or perpendicular to the incident electric field:

$$P = (I_{\parallel} - I_{\perp})/(I_{\parallel} + I_{\perp})$$

Integration over the angles θ and ϕ shows that the maximum value of P observed in the xy plane with linearly polarized incident light is $\frac{1}{2}$. If,

[3] P. P. Feofilov, "The Physical Basis of Polarized Emission." Consultants Bureau, New York, 1961.

instead of being rigidly fixed, the molecules are subject to Brownian motion, then the molecular rotation taking place between absorption and emission may be expected to result in values of P lying between $\frac{1}{2}$ and zero. The extent of this rotation is a function of molecular dimensions and structure, solvent and temperature. Low molecular weight compounds, such as inorganic ions, will give rise to virtually completely depolarized fluorescence. Some polarization will be retained as molecular size increases, and between two molecules of equal size the fluorescence of the more asymmetric rigid structure will be more polarized. If there is considerable internal flexibility within a molecule, very little polarization may be retained, since the fluorescent label may assume a wide range of positions within the 10^{-8} second lifetime of the excited state, even if the entire structure does not rotate significantly as a unit.

The polarization of fluorescent light from solutions has provided information concerning molecular size, shape, and conformation,[4-15] molecular anisotropy,[16] electronic energy transfer,[17] and molecular interaction including dye and coenzyme binding,[18-20] and the antigen–antibody reaction.[1, 2, 21-26]

[4] G. Weber, *Biochem. J.* **51**, 145 (1952).
[5] R. F. Steiner and A. J. McAlister, *J. Polymer Sci.* **24**, 105 (1957).
[6] R. F. Steiner and H. Edelhoch, *J, Am. Chem. Soc.* **84**, 2139 (1962).
[7] R. F. Steiner and H. Edelhoch, *Chem. Rev.* **62**, 457 (1962).
[8] D. M. Young and J. T. Potts, Jr., *J. Biol. Chem.* **238**, 1995 (1963).
[9] G. Fasman, K. Norland, and A. Pesce, *Biopolymers, Symp.* **1**, 325 (1964).
[10] D. B. S. Millar, III, R. Cukier, and M. Nirenberg, *Biochemistry* **4**, 976 (1965).
[11] D. B. S. Millar and R. F. Steiner, *Biochim. Biophys. Acta* **102**, 571 (1965).
[12] T. J. Gill and G. S. Omenn, *J. Am. Chem. Soc.* **87**, 4188 (1965).
[13] D. B. S. Millar and R. F. Steiner, *Biochemistry* **5**, 2289 (1966).
[14] M. Frey and G. Weill, *Biopolymers* **5**, 185 (1967).
[15] J. Knopp and G. Weber, *J. Biol. Chem.* **242**, 1353 (1967).
[16] A. Albrecht, *J. Mol. Spectry.* **6**, 84 (1961).
[17] G. Weber and F. W. J. Teale, *in* "The Proteins" (H. Neurath, ed.), Vol. 3, p. 445. Academic Press, New York, 1965.
[18] D. J. R. Laurence, *Biochem. J.* **51**, 168 (1952).
[19] G. Weber and E. Daniel, *Biochemistry* **5**, 1900 (1966).
[20] J. E. Churchich, *Biochim. Biophys. Acta* **147**, 32 (1967).
[21] E. Haber and J. C. Bennett, *Proc. Nat. Acad. Sci. U.S.* **48**, 1935 (1962).
[22] W. B. Dandliker, S. P. Halbert, M. C. Florin, R. Alonso, and H. C. Schapiro, *J. Exptl. Med.* **122**, 1029 (1965).
[23] R. P. Tengerdy, *Immunochemistry* **3**, 463 (1966).
[24] R. P. Tengerdy, *J. Immunol.* **99**, 126 (1967).
[25] W. B. Dandliker, R. Alonso, and C. Y. Meyers, *Immunochemistry* **4**, 295 (1967).
[26] W. B. Dandliker and S. A. Levison, *Immunochemistry* **5**, 171 (1968); see also *Federation Proc.* **26**, 579 (1967); *Pacific Slope Biochem. Conf.* 16 (1968).

c. QUANTUM YIELD AND MOLAR FLUORESCENCE

The classic measure of fluorescence intensity is in terms of quantum yield, i.e., number of photons emitted/number of photons absorbed.

An intensity measure more easily determined is the molar fluorescence, i.e., the fluorescence intensity in arbitrary units (referred to a constant incident intensity) divided by the molar concentration of dye.

A variety of factors may affect the molar fluorescence and give rise either to quenching or enhancement of fluorescence. A full discussion of these factors is found in Section 15.C.

The quenching by collision with heavy ions such as iodide is well known. Heavy atom substituents in a molecule may either favor inter-system crossing or enhance deactivation by favoring internal conversion. Quenching by oxygen is a very efficient process for many excited molecules. The intense fluorescence of the fluorescein dyes has been attributed to planarity and restricted molecular flexibility when compared with the structurally related but nonfluorescent triphenylmethane dyes. The influence of the solvent environment forms the basis for the current use of fluorescence enhancement as a hydrophobic probe.

On theoretical grounds, it may be anticipated that quenching or enhancement of fluorescence will usually require some intimate role of the fluorescent label in the antigen–antibody reaction, e.g., as a hapten[1, 2, 23, 24, 27, 28] or perhaps being located adjacent to an active site or determinant group. If the label is carried along on the antigen, hapten, or antibody molecule in a purely passive role, changes in fluorescence intensity may be absent.[22, 25]

Situations giving rise to large intensity changes will unavoidably greatly modify the observed polarization change. However, the equations given below take into account in a simple way the complex interrelationships existing between the polarization, decay time, and intensity.

3. EVALUATION OF THERMODYNAMIC PARAMETERS*

a. GENERAL ASSUMPTIONS

Our quantitative treatment of the antigen–antibody reaction is based upon the assumption of a reversible chemical reaction between a fluores-

---

[27] M. Winkler, *J. Mol. Biol.* **4**, 118 (1962).

[28] D. S. Berns and S. J. Singer, *Immunochemistry* **1**, 209 (1964).

* *Symbols:* Relative intensities of the vertically polarized and horizontally polarized components in the fluorescent light are denoted by V and H, respectively, and correspond to the z and y vibration directions of Fig. 1, with the observer located on the x axis. The symbol Δ is used to denote the "excess fluorescence"; ΔV and ΔH are

cent labeled antigen, hapten, or antibody, $\mathfrak{F}$, and the receptor sites of the complementary unlabeled partner, $\mathfrak{R}$, according to Eq. (1).

$$\mathfrak{F} + \mathfrak{R} \underset{k_{-1}}{\overset{k_1}{\rightleftarrows}} \mathfrak{F}\mathfrak{R} \tag{1}$$

The rate constants for the forward and reverse reactions are indicated by k_1 and k_{-1}, respectively. The association constant is expressed as

$$K_{\text{assoc.}} = \frac{(\mathfrak{F}\mathfrak{R})}{(\mathfrak{F})(\mathfrak{R})} \tag{2}$$

assuming that one "molecule" of $\mathfrak{F}\mathfrak{R}$ is formed for each molecule of $\mathfrak{F}$ which is bound by a receptor site of $\mathfrak{R}$.

Thus a molecule of $\mathfrak{F}$ can be assumed to be in one of two chemical states, i.e., either "free" or "bound" (to $\mathfrak{R}$). Since the method of detection

---

obtained from the solution reading by subtracting the respective values of V and H for the blank.

Subscripts

    e, equilibrium value of parameter

    f, b, free and bound forms, respectively, of fluorescent-labeled material

    0, at time approaching zero

a, heterogeneity constant defined by Eq. (7)

F, molar concentration of fluorescent-labeled material (in either free or bound state)

$UF_{b,\max}$, maximum value of F_b (taken to be equal to the total receptor site concentration)

dF_f/dt, rate of change of the molar concentration of free, fluorescent-labeled material

dF_b/dt, rate of change of the molar concentration of bound fluorescent-labeled material

K_0, average association constant defined by Eq. 7

k_1, bimolecular rate constant defined by Eq. 1

k_{-1}, unimolecular rate constant defined by Eq. 1

M, total concentration of labeled component equal to $F_b + F_f$

n_1, order of reaction with respect to the unlabeled component, $\mathfrak{R}$

n_2, order of reaction with respect to the labeled component, $\mathfrak{F}$

p, polarization of fluorescence equal to $(\Delta V - \Delta H)/(\Delta V + \Delta H)$

p', limiting value of p as $M \to 0$

dp/dt, rate of change of polarization

Q, molar fluorescence equal to $(\Delta V + \Delta H)/M$

R, molar concentration of receptor (unlabeled component). If antibody, this quantity might be determined, e.g., from precipitin analysis

t, time in seconds

U, relative concentration of receptor (unlabeled component) normalized to unity for the lowest receptor concentration in a set of experiments

of the reaction depends upon fluorescence, the reaction between antigen and antibody is measured by the rate of binding and the degree of binding of $\mathfrak{F}$.

b. ANALYTICAL EQUATIONS

The total concentration of fluorescent labeled material, M, will be divided between that which is uncombined, F_f, and that which is bound to its complementary immunological reactant, F_b.

$$M = F_f + F_b \tag{3}$$

The concentrations of free and bound labeled material, may be determined from the degree of fluorescence polarization and quenching. Both these quantities are computed from the "polarized components of the excess fluorescence" in the vertical and horizontal directions. For any given concentration of labeled material, part of which may be free and part bound, the polarization, p, is given by the following expression:

$$p = \frac{\Delta V - \Delta H}{\Delta V + \Delta H} \tag{4}$$

where ΔV and ΔH are the excess fluorescences polarized in the vertical and horizontal directions compared with the values obtained for an appropriate blank. Similarly, the molar fluorescence, which may be either quenched or enhanced when compared to a preparation of the labeled material alone, may be obtained from the total excess fluorescence:

$$Q = \frac{\Delta V + \Delta H}{M} \tag{5}$$

Both p and Q must be determined for the totally free and totally bound material, and the values, p_f and Q_f, and p_b and Q_b, used as constants in the final calculations:

$$\frac{F_b}{F_f} = \frac{Q_f}{Q_b}\left(\frac{p - p_f}{p_b - p}\right) = \frac{Q_f - Q}{Q - Q_b} \tag{6}$$

The evaluation of the ratio of bound to free labeled material by measuring changes in molar fluorescence alone has already been discussed in Section 15.C. Equation (6) permits computation of this ratio, however, even when $Q_f = Q = Q_b$.

Even in a purified antibody preparation, considerable heterogeneity may still be present, implying a range of affinities for the antigen. A

satisfactory approximation for the distribution of binding free energies is
based upon the equation of Sips.[29]

$$\log F_f = \frac{1}{a} \log \left(\frac{F_b}{UF_{b,max} - F_b} \right) - \log K_0 \qquad (7)$$

While there is little information to indicate that the actual distribution
of binding affinities is that described by Sips' equation, a great deal of
evidence indicates that this distribution is often "compatible" with
experimental results.

c. Calculations

i. Preliminary Estimates of Q_b, p_b, and $F_{b,max}$

For each experimental curve obtained for p as a function of M, values
of p are extrapolated to $M = 0$ to find the limiting value of the polarization, viz. p'. A similar extrapolation for the curves of Q vs. M yields
values of Q'. The values of Q' are then plotted[2] according to Eq. (8).

$$Q' = Q_b + \frac{Q_f - Q'}{KF_{b,max}} \qquad (8)$$

Since only relative values of $KF_{b,max}$ are needed to use this equation,
one may simply insert for $KF_{b,max}$ the relative concentrations, U, of
the unlabeled component, for the different curves. An extrapolation of
the points to $1/U = 0$, gives an approximate value of Q_b. A similar plot
of the values of p' according to Eq. (9), furnishes an estimate of p_b.

$$p' = p_b - \frac{Q_f(p' - p_f)}{Q_b KF_{b,max}} \qquad (9)$$

The normal control (containing all components except Ⓡ) plotted as p
or Q vs. M is usually found to yield straight lines parallel to the M axis.
These lines give p_f and Q_f directly. These measured values of Q_f and p_f,
the estimates of Q_b and p_b, together with the measured p's or Q's are
used to calculate F_b/F_f and F_b from Eqs. (3) and (6). A Scatchard plot
(F_b/F_f vs. F_b) furnishes an estimate of $F_{b,max}$. Normally, the Scatchard
plots are quite curved and the extrapolations are uncertain, but quite
sufficient.

ii. Final Calculations for Equilibrium Polarization Data

The experimental data consisting of the measured values of Q_f and
p_f and of p and M at several different values of U, and the estimates of

[29] A. Nisonoff and D. Pressman, *J. Immunol.* **80**, 417 (1958).

Q_b, p_b, and $F_{b,max}$, are all processed by computer, using the program given in the appendix (Section 15.F.7). This program searches over specified values of the variables Q_b, p_b, and $F_{b,max}$, and gives the best least squares fit between the experimental and calculated p vs. M curve. It is by this means that any inaccuracies in estimating the tentative values of Q_b, p_b, and $F_{b,max}$ are unimportant, since the final criterion is the fit between observed and calculated values of p.

4. EVALUATION OF KINETIC PARAMETERS

The strong affinity of antibodies for the antigens used to elicit their production is accompanied by an extremely large rate constant for the combination of antibody and antigen. Only techniques and permit measurement of rapid reaction rates, or which are sensitive enough to detect the reactants in extremely dilute solution, in which they will combine more slowly, are adequate for evaluation of kinetic parameters in the antigen–antibody reaction. The former approach, measuring rapid rates, has been discussed in Section 15.D for the hapten–antibody reaction. Fluorescence techniques are sufficiently sensitive, however, to permit kinetic measurements on protein antigens or hapten-labeled carriers in a concentration range which slows the effective rate of combination sufficiently to obtain data from simple manual mixing. Results from this technique have demonstrated that the antigen–antibody reaction (in contrast to the hapten reaction) is not diffusion controlled and may involve solvent and ion relaxation processes as well as conformational changes.[26]

a. INITIAL RATE EQUATIONS*

Order of reaction with respect to $\mathfrak{F}$:

$$\log \left(\frac{dp}{dt}\right)_0 = (n_2 - 1)(\log F_{f0}) + \text{const.} \tag{10}$$

Order of reaction with respect to $\mathfrak{R}$:

$$\log \left(\frac{dp}{dt}\right)_0 = n_1(\log R_{f0}) + \text{const.}' \tag{11}$$

b. INTEGRATED RATE EQUATION

For an excess of receptor, $\mathfrak{R}$, so large that its concentration remains substantially constant at R_{f0} throughout the reaction, and for $Q_f = Q_b$:

$$\log (p_e - p) = \log (p_e - p_f) - \left(\frac{k_1 R_{f0}^{n_1} + k_{-1}}{2.3}\right) t \tag{12}$$

* The kinetic equations were derived and applied by Dr. S. A. Levison.[26]

Hence, a plot of log $(p_e - p)$ vs. t should be linear with a slope of $(-1/2.3)$ $(k_1 R_{f0}^{n_1} + k_{-1})$. A plot of this latter quantity vs. R_{f0} will be linear if the order with respect to receptor concentration is 1 and the rate constants k_1 and k_{-1} can be obtained from the slope and intercept. The rate constant, k_1, can also be evaluated from initial rates[26] regardless of the relationship between Q_f and Q_b.

c. Calculation of Kinetic Results

The order of the reaction with respect to $\mathfrak{F}$ and $\mathfrak{R}$ may be found by plotting data according to Eqs. (10) and (11). It may be noted that relative concentrations of $\mathfrak{F}$ and $\mathfrak{R}$ are sufficient for this purpose.

Measurements in large excess concentrations of $\mathfrak{R}$ enable the determination of k_1 and k_{-1} from Eq. (12), if $Q_f = Q_b$. First the slope of a plot of log $(p_e - p)$ vs. t is determined for different values of R_{f0}. By standard least-squares techniques, both k_1 and k_{-1} can be evaluated. A simpler procedure if $n_1 = 1$ is to plot the slopes of the log $(p_e - p)$ vs. t curves against the corresponding values of R_{f0} whereupon k_1 and k_{-1} are obtained as slope and intercept.

5. PROCEDURES

a. Instrumentation

i. Basic Requirements

The simplest type of fluorescence polarometer consists of a conventional fluorometer or spectrofluorometer with an added polarizer oriented vertically in the incident beam, and a second polarizer which may be rotated to either the vertical or horizontal position in the fluorescent beam. In this way, V and H readings for the solution and for the blank may be used to calculate p from Eq. (4). A more elegant type of arrangement permits a direct and separate readout of both $(\Delta V + \Delta H)$ and p.

ii. Standards

A solution of 10^{-4} to 10^{-3} M uranyl acetate in water is a reliable standard with $p \approx 0$. Uranium glass standards* have a polarization of about 0.1 and can be used with an absorbing filter to monitor the intensity. Both uranyl acetate in water and uranium glass have negative temperature coefficients of fluorescence intensity ($\sim -1\%/°C$). Slightly turbid glass blocks have negligible temperature coefficients of scattering and make excellent standards. They suffer from the disadvantage that the rejection filter in the fluorescent beam must be removed to utilize them.

* Carl Zeiss, New York.

iii. Performance Tests

(a) *Short-Term Precision.* A series of intensity readings, taken in rapid succession over a total period of a few minutes using a fluorescence standard, should have a coefficient of variance (% C.V.) of 0.2 or less. (% C. V. = 100 × standard deviation/mean).

(b) *Long-Term Stability.* This property is less critical than the short-term precision, since a standard can be used to compensate for long-term drift.

(c) *Linearity.* Linearity of response can be tested by using a series of fluorescein solutions, buffered at pH 9 or above (all in the dianion form). Only relative fluorescein concentrations need be known, and the ratio of $(\Delta V + \Delta H)$ divided by concentration should be constant from about $10^{-10}M$ by $10^{-7}M$ fluorescein.

(d) *Response of the Phototube to V and H.* The response of phototubes usually depends upon the state of polarization of the impinging light. A depolarizer over the phototube eliminates errors arising from this source. The Lyot, three-element quartz depolarizer* is effective (if the wavelength band is not too narrow) and is also transparent. Opal glass varies in its ability to depolarize, and its use entails a considerable loss in intensity. Finely ground crystals of ammonium dihydrogen phosphate mounted in a transparent medium between glass plates can also be used.[29a]

Alternatively, often the polarization effect can be eliminated by suitable orientation of the phototube about the optical axis of the detecting system.[29a] Absence of the polarization effect can be checked by allowing the phototube to view the light from an unpolarized source, through the polarizer, first in the V and then in the H position. An illuminated solution of fluorescein in the cell compartment, with a piece of opal glass between the solution and the polarizer, furnishes unpolarized light.

(e) *Rejection Ratio.* In order to permit measurements at relatively low fluorescence intensities, scattered or reflected light of the incident wavelength must be removed from the fluorescent beam. A convenient means for determining the efficiency of rejection is to measure the relative response to fluorescence and to scattering. As an example, the readings $(\Delta V + \Delta H)$ on an instrument employing interference filters peaked at 487 mμ and 520 mμ were 503 for 10^{-9} M fluorescein at pH 9.2 and 214 for 15% Ludox† (in water), which had an optical density of 0.090 cm^{-1} at 487 mμ. Ludox is particularly suitable since it is nearly a Rayleigh scatterer at low concentrations.

---

* Crystal Optics Co., Chicago, Illinois.
[29a] D. E. Williamson, personal communication, Cordis Corporation, Miami, Florida (1966).
† E. I. DuPont de Nemours and Co., Wilmington, Delaware.

Spurious results, leading to entirely erroneous conclusions, can be obtained if the rejection ratio is not sufficiently high. Polarization results on fluorescein-labeled BSA and antiBSA showing a maximum in p at the antigen–antibody equivalence ratio were interpreted[21] as being analogous to the precipitin curve. The correct interpretation most probably is that scattered light was not rejected because of the limitations of the instrument used, and the authors were unaware of this pitfall.

(*f*) *Temperature Control.* Since both the fluorescence intensity and polarization vary with the temperature, thermostatting of the cell assembly to within a few tenths of a degree is necessary for precise work.

iv. Availability of Instrumentation

Several types of fluorescence polarometers have been described.[30–35] A number of commercially available instruments appear to be satisfactory*; one† provides direct and separate readouts of $(\Delta V + \Delta H)$ and of p.

b. ANTIGEN OR ANTIBODY PREPARATIONS

Labeled preparations. Depending upon the nature of the problem, either the antigen or the antibody must be purified as highly as possible and then labeled with a fluorescent dye.[7, 36]

If both the antigen and antibody are highly purified, it may be possible to utilize the ultraviolet fluorescence of the tryptophan residues in the protein so that no labeling would be necessary.

Unlabeled component. This may consist of serum, a globulin fraction, purified antibody, or some crude antigen preparation. Whether the antibody is the labeled or unlabeled component, a normal control should always be included for comparison. This control contains all components except the unlabeled receptor ℜ. Generally, the unlabeled component does not have to be purified, but any purification is an advantage since the background fluorescence intensity will then be lower.

[30] G. Weber, *J. Opt. Soc. Am.* **46**, 962 (1956).

[31] P. Johnson and E. Richards, *Arch. Biochem. Biophys.* **97**, 250 (1962).

[32] W. B. Dandliker, H. C. Schapiro, R. Alonso, and D. E. Williamson, *San Diego Symp. Biomed. Eng.* **3**, 127 (1963).

[33] R. F. Chen and L. Bowman, *Science* **147**, 729 (1965).

[34] G. Weber and B. Bablouzian, *J. Biol. Chem.* **241**, 2558 (1966).

[35] J. U. White, D. E. Williamson, W. B. Dandliker, and S. A. Levison, in preparation.

* Perkin-Elmer Corp., Norwalk, Connecticut; Phoenix Precision Instrument Co., Philadelphia, Pennsylvania; G. K. Turner Associates, Palo Alto, California.

† Cordis Corporation, Miami, Florida.

[36] R. C. Nairn, "Fluorescent Protein Tracing." Livingstone, Edinburgh and London, 1962.

c. Titration and the Recording of Results

To the unlabeled component, $\mathcal{R}$, contained in a cuvette, a series of additions of the labeled component, $\mathcal{F}$, is made, starting at a fluorescent intensity of about 3 times background. "Background" includes the intrinsic fluorescence of the unlabeled receptor $\mathcal{R}$ alone.

A micrometer-driven precision-bore syringe is suitable for equilibrium measurements; for kinetic measurements of slow reactions, additions can be made manually with a syringe. In either case, the solutions can be mixed with a footed Teflon rod.

In order to determine an equilibrium constant, measurements must be carried out in a "sensitive" range. This range is in the general region at which the ratio of "bound/free" is 1 for both ligand and receptor. For uniform sites of association constant, K, this condition implies that $M = F_{b,max} = 2/K$. For the evaluation of p_b, Q_b, and $F_{b,max}$, M must also extend to the region at which $p \rightarrow p_f$ and $Q \rightarrow Q_f$.

Three or more concentrations of $\mathcal{R}$ in the sensitive range are chosen for complete titration curves. A normal control must be included. If time effects are noted, a sufficient interval must be allowed between additions for equilibrium to be reached. The resulting primary equilibrium data consist of a series of values of p or Q vs. M, at different values of U.

For kinetic measurements the proper concentration region is largely dictated by the speed of mixing and the speed of response of the detector and recorder. For the determination of reaction order or rate constants, concentrations should be varied over at least a factor of 100. The primary data consist of values of p or Q as a function of t at different values of M and either R or of $UF_{b,max}$.

6. RESULTS AND DISCUSSION OF METHOD

Representative equilibrium results[2] are shown in Fig. 2, for a typical antigen–antibody reaction, and in Fig. 3, for a hapten–antibody reaction.[22] A summary of the calculations for the data of Fig. 3 is shown in Table I.

Figure 4 illustrates the evaluation of the kinetic constants[26] according to Eq. (12).

a. Accuracy, Precision, and Sensitivity

i. *Accuracy and Reproducibility of Measurement*

As a test of the accuracy of polarization measurements, Eq. (6) was applied to mixtures of fluorescein-labeled ovalbumin (FO) and of fluorescein itself (F). Mixtures of FO and F constitute a good test system in that they can be thought of as mixtures of the bound and free form of fluorescein. The results are shown in Table II, in which $(F_b/F_f)_{known}$ was calculated from the known concentrations of FO and F, while $(F_b/F_f)_{calc}$ was computed from the measured values of the polarization

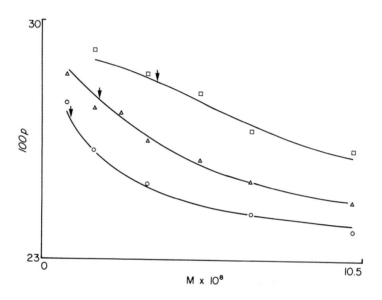

Fig. 2. Fluorescence polarization titration of rabbit antiovalbumin with fluorescein-labeled ovalbumin (FO). Ordinate: polarization of fluorescence. Abscissa: molarity of FO. Antibody concentrations (μg/ml) from precipitation with ovalbumin: O, 3.3; $\triangle$, 6.6; $\square$, 13.2. Vertical arrows indicate points at which the antigen–antibody ratio equals that found in precipitates at maximum precipitation. Solid curves calculated by computer from : $Q_f = 4.36$; $Q_b = 3.90$; $p_f = 0.234$; $p_b = 0.293$; $K_0 = 1.83 \times 10^{-8}\ M^{-1}$; $a = 0.65$; $F_{b,max} = 1.5 \times 10^{-8}\ M$ for the lowest antibody concentration. From W. B. Dandliker, H. C. Schapiro, J. W. Meduski, R. Alonso, G. A. Feigen, and J. R. Hamrick, Jr., *Immunochemistry* **1,** 165 (1964).

p, and from the measured values of Q_f, p_f, Q_b, and p_b. The coefficient of variation for the entire set is 7%; the ratios F_b/F_f range from 0.1 to 13.

Duplicate sets of data obtained 10 days apart with the same materials (human antipenicilloyl globulin and a fluorescent penicilloyl hapten) gave the following results, respectively: $Q_f = 3.55, 3.65$; $p_f = 0.0283, 0.0296$; $Q_b = 3.73, 3.73$; $p_b = 0.197, 0.228$; $10^{-7}K_0 = 2.33, 2.95$; $a = 0.90, 0.95$; $10^8 F_{b,max} = 1.2, 1.1$; $S = 0.13, 0.28$.

ii. Extent of Agreement between Theory and Experiment

An additional measure of accuracy which includes the agreement between theory and experiment can be applied to the data of Table I. The value of

$$S = \frac{100}{N} \left[\sum_{i=1}^{N} \left(\frac{p_i - p_{\text{calc}}}{p_i} \right)^2 \right]^{\frac{1}{2}}$$

is 0.3 for the entire set of data. This measure includes additional sources of error above and beyond the accuracy of measurement, since it involves

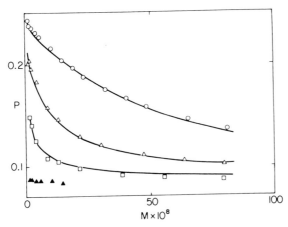

FIG. 3. Fluorescence polarization titration of rabbit anti-penicilloyl rabbit serum albumin with a fluorescent penicilloyl hapten (PDABF). PDABF is made by the condensation of fluorescein isothiocyanate, 1,4-diaminobutane, and penicillin. Ordinate: polarization of fluorescence. Abscissa: molarity of PDABF. Total globulin concentrations (mg/ml): □, 0.13; △, 0.40; ○, 1.2. , ▲, 0.40, normal globulin control. Solid curves computer calculated from $K_0 = 8.7 \times 10^6 \ M^{-1}$; $a = 0.711$; $F_{b,\text{max}} = 4.32 \times 10^{-8} \ M$ (for lowest curve); $Q_f = 6.84$; $Q_b = 5.00$; $p_f = 0.0844$; $p_b = 0.250$. From W. B. Dandliker, S. P. Halbert, M. C. Florin, R. Alonso, and H. C. Schapiro, *J. Exptl. Med.* **122**, 1029 (1965).

the interpretation of results within the framework of an assumed mass law.

iii. Sensitivity Range

A variety of experimental factors, such as magnitude of the background, instrument stability and linearity, and the reproducibility of solutions, all impose limits on the signal-to-noise ratio. In addition, an

TABLE I
Calculations for Data of Figure 3

U^a	$10^8 M^b$	$10^4 p_{exp}{}^c$	Approximate values of $F_b/F_f{}^d$	$10^4 p_{calc}{}^e$
1	0.895	1477	0.571	1478
1	1.788	1391	0.461	1362
1	3.572	1238	0.297	1246
1	8.008	1071	0.153	1118
1	12.42	1033	0.125	1056
1	21.15	974	0.117	994
3	0.448	1996	1.817	2120
3	0.895	2013	1.890	2028
3	1.788	1938	1.592	1914
3	3.572	1807	1.194	1772
3	8.008	1561	0.695	1564
3	12.42	1449	0.534	1436
3	21.15	1279	0.337	1281
3	29.77	1190	0.252	1192
3	46.66	1092	0.170	1092
3	63.14	1042	0.132	1038
9	0.448	2419	6.360	2398
9	0.895	2368	5.180	2366
9	1.788	2344	4.745	2324
9	3.572	2296	4.033	2265
9	5.351	2255	3.550	2219
9	9.774	2144	2.606	2123
9	14.17	2028	1.957	2037
9	18.54	1951	1.639	1958
9	22.88	1859	1.337	1884
9	31.47	1734	1.019	1752
9	39.96	1644	0.837	1642
9	48.33	1567	0.705	1551
9	64.75	1446	0.530	1417
9	80.76	1351	0.414	1325

[a] U = relative concentration of the unlabeled component (antibody).

[b] M = total molar concentration of labeled material (a fluorescent penicilloyl hapten, PDABF).

[c] p_{exp} = experimental values of p.

[d] Calculated from Eq. (6) with $Q_f = 6.84$, $p_f = 0.0844$, $Q_b = 6.25$, $p_b = 0.269$.

[e] p_{calc} = final values of p calculated by computer from the best values of parameters: $Q_b = 5.00$, $p_b = 0.250$, $F_{b,max} = 4.32 \times 10^{-8} M$, $K_0 = 8.7 \times 10^6\ M^{-1}$ and $a = 0.711$ (Q_f and p_f as above). p_{calc} can be used to check operation of the computer program.

inherent limit on sensitivity is imposed by the magnitude of the association constant.

In comparison with other immunological methods, the fluorescence polarization technique lies in the midrange of sensitivities, i.e., somewhat more sensitive than the precipitin test. For "penicillin" antibodies it is

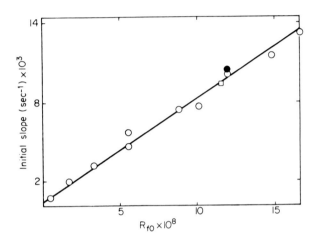

FIG. 4. Kinetics of the reaction between rabbit antiovalbumin and fluorescein-labeled ovalbumin at $1.5 \pm 0.5°$ [W. B. Dandliker and S. A. Levison, *Immunochemistry* **5**, 171 (1968)]. Ordinate: Initial slopes of pseudo first-order plots graphed according to Eq. (12). Abscissa: antiovalbumin concentrations as determined by precipitin analysis. Reaction solutions contained $0.15 M$ NaCl, $0.009 M$ Tris acid, and $0.001 M$ Tris base, pH 7.0. Fluorescein-labeled ovalbumin concentrations were: ○, 6.4×10^{-10}; ●, 6.4×10^{-9}; and □, $3.2 \times 10^{-8} M$. From the slope and intercept of this curve $k_1 = 2.0 \times 10^5$ l mole^{-1} sec^{-1} and $k_{-1} = 0.71 \times 10^{-3}$ sec^{-1}.

more sensitive[22] than immunodiffusion and compares favorably with hemagglutination.

iv. Other Factors Affecting Accuracy

(a) *Relative Molecular Sizes of Antigen and Antibody.* In order to obtain an appreciable change in polarization when the antigen–antibody reaction occurs, the molecular size of the labeled component must not be large compared to that of the unlabeled one. The size of the molecule carrying the label should be as small as possible in order to maximize the difference between p_f and p_b.

(b) *Choice of the Fluorescent Label.* (1) *Decay time of the excited state.* This parameter must be suited to the relaxation time for rotary Brownian

452 HAPTEN REACTIONS 15.F.6.a]

motion of the molecule to be labeled. Ideally, the decay time should be long compared to the relaxation time of rotation of the labeled molecule alone, but short when compared to that of the antigen–antibody complex. Under these conditions ($p_b - p_f$) is maximized as before. An additional factor to be considered is the limiting maximum value of the polarization in the absence of any Brownian motion. This value may be expected to decrease as the decay time is lengthened.

TABLE II
VALIDITY OF EQUATION (6)[a]

$10^8 M_{FO}$	$10^8 M_F$	$(F_b/F_f)_{known}$	$10^4 p$	$(F_b/F_f)_{calc}$	calc/known
0.531	5.055	0.105	297	0.108	1.029
0.545	2.593	0.210	411	0.220	1.048
0.552	1.314	0.420	537	0.361	0.860
2.113	5.031	0.420	606	0.448	1.067
0.555	0.661	0.840	842	0.813	0.968
2.168	2.581	0.840	847	0.823	0.980
0.557	0.332	1.678	1173	1.633	0.973
2.196	1.307	1.680	1180	1.635	0.973
2.211	0.658	3.360	1524	3.330	0.991
0.558	0.166	3.361	1462	2.906	0.865
2.218	0.330	6.721	1810	7.095	1.056
2.221	0.165	13.46	1971	13.60	1.010

[a] Polarizations and intensities were measured for mixtures of fluorescein (F) and fluorescein-labeled ovalbumin (FO).
Known values of $(F_b/F_f) = (M_{FO}/M_F)$ are compared with the values calculated from Eq. (6).
Accessory optical constants measured include: $Q_f = 12.13$; $p_f = 0.0172$; $Q_b = 7.43$; $p_b = 0.219$.

(2) *Emission wavelength.* If possible, the fluorescent label should emit in a wavelength region where the background contributed by the unlabeled component is low. Having a choice of emission wavelengths makes it possible to control the level of the background and constitutes a key advantage to the methods described here.

(3) *Immunochemical effect of the label.* The introduction of a fluorescent label into a molecule may alter its immunological properties. The experience of many workers using the Coons fluorescent antibody technique indicates that this effect is not very important, especially with light labeling. However, if a change in reactivity is suspected, its effect may be nullified by an extrapolation to zero extent of labeling. A more elegant

approach is to measure the inhibition of the reaction between labeled component α and unlabeled component β by unlabeled component α.[37]

b. CONSIDERATION OF OTHER FACTORS

i. *Underlying Assumptions*

The fluorescence polarization method is based upon the assumption that the labeled partner can exist in either of only two chemical states, that is, either free or combined (with antigen or antibody, as the case may be). This amounts to saying that all types of binding between the antigen and antibody are lumped together and averaged so that no attempt is made to gain more intimate information about the size, nature, or distribution of complexes which may be present. This is analogous to representing the structure of water by the formula H_2O, although it is common knowledge that a wide variety of polymers actually exist in liquid water. The assumption of only two chemical states leads to the characterization of the labeled partner by the optical constants Q_f, p_f, Q_b, and p_b. This compensates automatically for any changes in free rotation, anisotropy, lifetime and fluorescence yield occurring upon antigen–antibody combination.

Systematic errors could possibly be introduced into the measurements if binding sites existed which produce no change in polarization or intensity.

ii. *Primary Combination Measured*

The change in polarization, produced by the antigen–antibody reaction, occurs rapidly; practically all the effect should be realized by the primary combination alone, with little additional rise in polarization as the complexes grow larger (cf. "Rejection ratio," under Section 15.F.5.a). This factor contributes to making the method rapid, since it is not dependent upon the occurrence of subsequent changes. Other immunological methods, which also focus prime attention on the initial combination, include the Farr ammonium sulfate technique, equilibrium dialysis, and the fluorescence quenching method of Velick *et al.*[38]

ACKNOWLEDGMENTS

The author gratefully acknowledges invaluable and pleasant collaboration with Dr. G. A. Feigen of Stanford University, Dr. S. P. Halbert of the University of Miami, Drs. V. A. de Saussure, F. Kierszenbaum, and H. C. Schapiro, and Mr. R. Alonso.

[37] F. Kierszenbaum, J. Dandliker, and W. B. Dandliker, *Immunochemistry* **6**, 125 (1969); see also *Federation Proc.* **27**, 260 (1968).
[38] S. Velick, C. Parker, and H. Eisen, *Proc. Nat. Acad. Sci. U.S.* **46**, 1470 (1960).

7. APPENDIX: USER'S EXPLANATION OF PROGRAM WD*

a. Method

Given values of p vs. M for different U, measured values of Q_f and p_f, and estimates of Q_b, p_b, and $F_{b,max}$, the program finds a and K_0 by straight-line fit and calculates the quantity

$$\text{SUM} = \frac{100}{N} \left[\sum_{i=1}^{N} \left(\frac{p_i - p_{calc}}{p_i} \right)^2 \right]^{1/2}$$

By variation of the input parameters Q_b, p_b, and $F_{b,max}$, one can experiment with optimizing the choice of those parameters to minimize SUM. The basic equations used are

$$M_i = F_{fi} + F_{bi} \tag{1}$$

$$\frac{F_{bi}}{F_{fi}} = \frac{Q_f}{Q_b} \left[\frac{p_i - p_f}{p_b - p_i} \right] \tag{2}$$

$$\frac{U_i \cdot F_{b,max}}{F_{bi}} = \frac{1}{(K_0 F_{fi})^a} + 1 \tag{3}$$

subject to

$$p_i > p_f$$
$$p_b > p_i$$
$$F_{b,max} > F_{bi} > 0$$
$$a, K_0, F_{fi} > 0$$

b. Program Listings

Listings of the FORTRAN instructions (written for the CDC 3600 at UCSD in FORTRAN '63) for PROGRAM WD, SUBROUTINE FIT, and FUNCTION COUNT are included at the end of the Appendix. Cards may be punched directly from these listings. It is advisable to have a programmer check the instructions for compatibility with the FORTRAN compiler to be used. Necessary modification, if any, will be minor.

* Prepared by Computer Applications, Inc., 3045 Rosecrans, San Diego, California.

The names of the variables as used by the program are as follows:

Variable	Program name
M	AM
p	P
p_b	PB
p_f	PF
Q_b	BK
Q_f	FK
$F_{b,max}$	FBMAX
U	AB

c. Data Deck Organization

The organization of the data deck to be adjoined to the program deck is as follows:

Card 1—Identification information (alpha-numeric characters in columns 2–72)

For cards 2–6, data field 1 is columns 1–6, data field 2 is columns 7–12, . . . , data field 6 is columns 31–36. Each data field may contain a five digit number with decimal point. At least one value is required on each card.

Card 2—from 1–6 values of Q_f in data fields 1–6

Card 3—from 1–6 values of Q_b in data fields 1–6

Card 4—from 1–6 values of p_f in data fields 1–6

Card 5—from 1–6 values of p_b in data fields 1–6

Card 6—from 1–6 values of $F_{b,max}$ in data fields 1–6

Cards 7—$(7 + N)$, p in columns 1–8

    M in columns 9–16

    U in columns 17–24

Use one card for each of the N data triples (p, M, U).

Last Card—blank

It should be noted that $M \times 10^8$ and $F_{b,max} \times 10^8$ are entered on the data cards, and that $K_0 \times 10^{-8}$ is listed on the output.

d. Output Listing

The output listing consists of columns of data with appropriate heading information to identify the listed quantities. Most of these headings are self-explanatory and correspond to those listed in Sections a and b above. In addition, the following measure of precision is given:

SD = standard deviation of the straight line fit used to determine a and K_0 from the equation

$$Y_i = \frac{1}{a}\left(X_i\right) - \log\left(K_0\right)$$

where

$$Y_i = \log F_{ti}$$

$$X_i = \log \left(\frac{F_{bi}}{U_i F_{b,\max} - F_{bi}} \right)$$

FORTRAN Instructions

```
        PROGRAM WD
        DIMENSION AB(50), P(50), AM(50), X(50), Y(50), COE(9),
       1FF(50), FB(50), FBMAX(12), HEAD(12), BK(12), PB(12),
       2FK1(12), PF1(12), ITER8IND(50)
        TYPE INTEGER COUNT
90      CONTINUE
        ICNT = 0
        READ 15,(HEAD(I),I = 1,12)
        IF(EOF,50) 92,95
92      STOP
95      READ 10,(FK1(I),I = 1,12)
        KF = COUNT(FK1)
        READ 10,(BK(I),I = 1,12)
        KB = COUNT(BK)
        READ 10,(PF1(I),I = 1,12)
        IPF = COUNT(PF1)
        READ 10,(PB(I),I = 1,12)
        IPB = COUNT(PB)
        READ 10,(FBMAX(I),I = 1,12)
        IFBMAX = COUNT(FBMAX)
100     CONTINUE
        READ 18,X1,X2,X3
        IF(X1+X2+X3) 110,120,110
110     ICNT = ICNT + 1
        P(ICNT) = X1
        AM(ICNT) = X2
        AB(ICNT) = X3
        GO TO 100
C
120     CONTINUE
        JTAG = 0
129     DO 190 IFK = 1,KF
        FK = FK1(IFK)
        DO 190 IP = 1,IPF
```

```
        PF = PF1(IP)
        DO 190 N = 1,KB
        DO 180 M = 1,IPB
        DO 170 K = 1,IFBMAX
        NFIT = 0
        DO 130 I = 1,ICNT
        FF(I) = BK(N)*AM(I)/(BK(N)+FK*((P(I) − PF)/(PB(M) −
           P(I))))
        FB(I) = AM(I) − FF(I)
        Y(I) = LOGF(FF(I))
        XX = FB(I)/(AB(I)*FBMAX(K) − FB(I))
        IF(XX) 130,130,131
131     X(I) = LOGF(XX)
        NFIT = NFIT + 1
130     CONTINUE
C
        COE(1) = 0.
        COE(2) = 0.
        CALL FIT (X,Y,NFIT,1,SD,IM,COE)
        IF(IM) 140,150,140
140     PRINT 11,IM
        GO TO 170
150     CONTINUE
        IF(COE(2)) 22,22,25
22      PRINT 20
        GO TO 170
25      AK = EXPF(−COE(1))
        A = 1./COE(2)
C
        SUM = 0.
        DO 160 I = 1,ICNT
        DO 155 J = 1,10
        FBB = FB(I)
        FB(I) = FB(I) − (LOGF(ABSF(AM(I) − FB(I))) − COE(2)*
           LOGF(ABSF(FB(I)/
        1(AB(I)*FBMAX(K) − FB(I)))) − COE(1))/(1./(FB(I) − AM
           (I)) − COE(2)*AB(I)*
        2FBMAX(K)/(FB(I)*(AB(I)*FBMAX(K) − FB(I))))
        IF(ABSF((FB(I) − FBB)/FB(I)).LT..001) 156,155
155     CONTINUE
        ITER8IND(I) = 1H*
        GO TO 157
```

```
156  ITER8IND(I) = 1H
157  FF(I) = AM(I) − FB(I)
     X(I) = (FB(I)*BK(N)*PB(M) + FF(I)*FK*PF)/(FB(I)*BK
     (N)+FF(I)*FK)
     SUM = ((P(I)−X(I))/P(I))**2 + SUM
160  CONTINUE
     SUM = SQRTF(SUM)/FLOATF(ICNT)*100.
     IF (JTAG) 92,162,166
162  PRINT 16,(HEAD(I),I=1,12)
     PRINT 12
     PRINT 13,(P(I),AM(I),AB(I),X(I),ITER8IND(I),I=1,ICNT)
     SUMLAST = SUM
163  PRINT 17
164  PRINT 14,PB(M),BK(N),FBMAX(K),A,AK,PF,FK,SD,SUM
     JTAG = 1
     GO TO 170
166  IF (SUM − SUMLAST) 168,164,164
168  SUMLAST = SUM
     PRINT 19
     DO 169 I=1,ICNT
169  Y(I) = (P(I) − X(I))/P(I)
     PRINT 21, (P(I),X(I),Y(I), I=1,ICNT)
     GO TO 163
C
170  CONTINUE
180  CONTINUE
190  CONTINUE
     GO TO 90
C
10   FORMAT (12F6)
11   FORMAT (1H1,2X,5HIM = I2)
12   FORMAT(1H0,3X,10HOBSERVED P,13X,1HM,15X, 1 HU,
     13X,12HCALCULATED P/)
13   FORMAT(F17.7,E17.7,2F17.7,A1)
14   FORMAT (9F12.7)
15   FORMAT (12A6)
16   FORMAT (1H1 /// 23X,12A6 /// )
17   FORMAT (/1H0,6X,2HPB,10X,2HQB,7X,5HFBMAX,11X,
     1HA,10X,2HKO,10X,2HPF
     1,10X,2HQF,10X,2HSD,9X,3HSUM)
18   FORMAT (3F8)
```

```
 19  FORMAT (1H0,2X,10HOBSERVED P,3X,12HCALCULATED
     P,3X,35HRELATIVE ERR
     1OR (=(OBS.−CALC.)/OBS.))
 20  FORMAT (31H1NEGATIVE A---PROBABLY BAD DATA )
 21  FORMAT (F12.7,F14.7,F15.7)
     END
```

116 CARDS

```
     SUBROUTINE FIT(X,Y,N1,I1,SD,IM,COE)        FIT  001
C                                               FIT  002
C    X=X ARRAY LOCATION                         FIT  003
C    Y=Y ARRAY LOCATION                         FIT  004
C    N1=NUMBER OF POINTS IN X AND Y ARRAYS (50 OR
       LESS)                                    FIT  005
C    I1=ORDER OF FIT DESIRED (8 OR LESS)        FIT  006
C    SD=STANDARD DEVIATION (RETURNED FROM
       SUBROUTINE)                              FIT  007
C    IM=0 WORKED,=1 DATA ERROR,=2 XSIMEQ ERROR  FIT  008
C    COE=COEFFICIENTS OF EQUATION (I1+1 VALUES) FIT  009
C                                               FIT  010
     DIMENSION XI(50,17),XIS(17),YIS(9),A(8,8),B(8,1),COE(9),
       X(50),Y(50
     1),XIP(50),IPIVOT(8),INDEX(8,2),PIVOT(8)   FIT  011
     EQUIVALENCE(XI,A),(XIS,B)                   FIT  013
C                                               FIT  014
     N=N1                                       FIT  015
     IO=I1                                      FIT  016
     IOR=IO+1                                   FIT  017
C                                               FIT  018
C    TESTS TO SEE IF DATA IS SUFFICIENT         FIT  019
C                                               FIT  020
     IF(N−10)1,1,2                              FIT  021
   1 IM=1                                       FIT  022
     RETURN                                     FIT  023
   2 CONTINUE                                   FIT  024
C                                               FIT  025
C    SCALES ALL VALUES OF X AND Y               FIT  026
C                                               FIT  027
     XMAX=ABSF(X(1))                            FIT  028
     YMAX=ABSF(Y(1))                            FIT  029
     DO 3 I=2,N                                 FIT  030
     XMAX=MAX1F(XMAX,ABSF(X(I)))                FIT  031
```

```
      YMAX = MAX1F(YMAX,ABSF(Y(I)))        FIT  032
  3   CONTINUE                             FIT  033
      DO 4 I=1,N                           FIT  034
      X(I) = X(I)/XMAX                     FIT  035
      Y(I) = Y(I)/YMAX                     FIT  036
  4   CONTINUE                             FIT  037
C                                          FIT  038
C     COMPUTES(X**N)TERMS                  FIT  039
C                                          FIT  040
      XIS(1) = N                           FIT  041
      IORD = IO*2+1                        FIT  042
      XIS(2) = 0.0                         FIT  043
      DO 5 J=1,N                           FIT  044
      XI(J,2) = X(J)                       FIT  045
      XIS(2) = XIS(2) + XI(J,2)            FIT  046
  5   CONTINUE                             FIT  047
      ASD = XIS(1)                         FIT  048
      DO 6 I=3,IORD                        FIT  049
      XIS(I) = 0.0                         FIT  050
      DO 6 J=1,N                           FIT  051
      XI(J,I) = XI(J,I-1)*X(J)             FIT  052
      XIS(I) = XIS(I) + XI(J,I)            FIT  053
  6   CONTINUE                             FIT  054
C                                          FIT  055
C     COMPUTES SUM OF (Y*X**N) TERMS       FIT  056
C                                          FIT  057
      YIS(1) = 0.0                         FIT  058
      DO 7 J=1,N                           FIT  059
      YIS(1) = YIS(1) + Y(J)               FIT  060
  7   CONTINUE                             FIT  061
      DO 8 I=2,IOR                         FIT  062
      YIS(I) = 0.0                         FIT  063
      DO 8 J=1,N                           FIT  064
      XI(J,I) = XI(J,I)*Y(J)               FIT  065
      YIS(I) = YIS(I) + XI(J,I)            FIT  066
  8   CONTINUE                             FIT  067
C                                          FIT  068
C                                          FIT  070
      DO 9 I=1,IOR                         FIT  071
      DO 9 J=1,IOR                         FIT  072
      J1 = I+J-1                           FIT  073
      A(I,J) = XIS(J1)                     FIT  074
```

```
     9  CONTINUE                                         FIT  075
        DO 10 I=1,IOR                                    FIT  076
        B(I,1) = YIS(I)                                  FIT  077
    10  CONTINUE                                         FIT  078
C                                                        FIT  079
C                                                        FIT  087
        D = A(1,1)*A(2,2) - A(2,1)*A(1,2)
        IF (D) 12,11,12
    11  IM = 2                                           FIT  089
        RETURN                                           FIT  090
    12  CONTINUE                                         FIT  091
        COE(1) = (B(1,1)*A(2,2) - B(2,1)*A(1,2))/D
        COE(2) = (A(1,1)*B(2,1) - A(2,1)*B(1,1))/D
C                                                        FIT  095
C       RESCALE X,Y AND COE                              FIT  096
C                                                        FIT  097
        DO 14 I=1,N                                      FIT  098
        X(I) = X(I)*XMAX                                 FIT  099
        Y(I) = Y(I)*YMAX                                 FIT  100
    14  CONTINUE                                         FIT  101
        DO 17 I=1,IOR                                    FIT  102
        IF(I-1)15,15,16                                  FIT  103
    15  COE(I) = COE(I)*YMAX                             FIT  104
        GO TO 17                                         FIT  105
    16  COE(I) = COE(I)*(YMAX/(XMAX**(I-1)))             FIT  106
    17  CONTINUE                                         FIT  107
C                                                        FIT  108
C       COMPUTES STANDARD DEVIATION                      FIT  109
C                                                        FIT  110
        SUM = 0.0                                        FIT  111
        DO 21 J=1,N                                      FIT  112
        P = X(J)                                         FIT  113
    18  XIP(J) = COE(1)                                  FIT  114
        P1 = 1.                                          FIT  115
        DO 20 I=2,IOR                                    FIT  116
    19  P1 = P1*P                                        FIT  117
        XIP(J) = XIP(J) + (P1*COE(I))                    FIT  118
    20  CONTINUE                                         FIT  119
        ERR = Y(J) - XIP(J)                              FIT  120
        SUM = SUM + ERR*ERR                              FIT  121
    21  CONTINUE                                         FIT  122
        SD = SQRTF(SUM/ASD)                              FIT  123
```

```
      IM = 0                                              FIT   124
      RETURN                                              FIT   125
      END                                                 FIT   126
      FUNCTION COUNT(X)
      DIMENSION X(10)
      TYPE INTEGER COUNT
      I = 0
    5 IA = X(I+1).AND.77777777B
      IB = X(I+1).AND.7777777700000000B
      IF(IA.EQ.77777777B) 6,10
    6 IF(IB.EQ.7777777700000000B) 15,10
   10 I = I+1
      GO TO 5
   15 COUNT = 1
      END
```

APPENDIX I

Identification of Multiple Antibody Components by Radioimmunoelectrophoresis and Radioimmunodiffusion*

A. Introduction

Recent studies have revealed the multiplicity of antibody components in biological fluids such as serum. The radioimmunoelectrophoresis (RIE) and radioimmunodiffusion (RID) techniques[1,2] provide simple means for directly identifying these antibody components in unfractionated biological fluids. The methods depend on the fact that antibody globulins retain their ability to combine with antigens even after precipitation by antiserum against these globulins. Thus, when a sample is subjected to regular immunoelectrophoresis or immunodiffusion utilizing antiglobulin sera and is then (or simultaneously) treated with the corresponding radiolabeled antigen, the specific precipitate arcs due to antibody-active components are labeled with radioactive antigen. These radioactive arcs are visualized by autoradiography and distinguished from other nonradioactive arcs representing nonantibody components. Factors which prevent antigen–antibody complexes from precipitating, such as univalency of antigen or antibody and high solubility of the complexes, do not interfere with the method.

For identifying arcs of antibody-active components produced by antiglobulin serum, two methods can be used (Fig. 1). When the sample does not form precipitate arcs directly with the radiolabeled antigen,† antigen is diffused simultaneously with antiglobulin antiserum (Fig. 1, one-step method).[1,2] Otherwise, radiolabeled antigen is reacted with the pre-

* Appendix I was contributed by Yasuo Yagi.

† This can be tested readily by using a mixture of radioantigen and normal serum instead of a mixture of radioantigen and antiglobulin antiserum for diffusion against the sample. If precipitation occurs directly between radioantigen and corresponding antibody in the sample, the image of the arc will be registered on the autoradiograph, although no arc will appear on the stained slide because of low amounts of radioantigens used. The arc due to direct precipitation of radioantigen shifts further from the trough when the concentration of radioantigen (or radioantigen plus nonlabeled antigen) is increased.

[1] Y. Yagi, P. Maier, and D. Pressman, *J. Immunol.* **89**, 736 (1962).

[2] J. H. Morse and J. F. Heremans, *J. Lab. Clin. Med.* **59**, 891 (1962).

cipitate arcs developed with antiglobulin antiserum after soluble proteins containing precipitating antibody are thoroughly washed out from the gel (Fig. 1, two-step method).[3]

For detecting multiple antibody components in complex mixtures, RIE is preferable to RID because of its superior resolving power. RID is particularly useful in detecting minute amounts of antibody when monospecific antiglobulin sera are available. Monospecific antiglobulin antisera are also useful in RIE for final identification of antibody components.

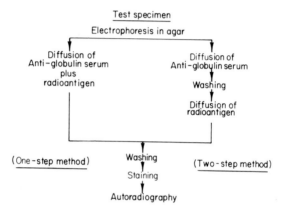

Fig. 1. Two methods of radioimmunoelectrophoretic analysis.

The following description is given for practical aspects of RIE and RID based on the techniques currently used in our laboratory.

B. Reagents

Radioiodinated Antigens and Carriers. Protein and peptide antigens are normally labeled directly by introducing radioiodine atoms into their tyrosine or histidine residues.

In the case of antihapten antibodies, hapten–protein conjugates are used rather than haptens themselves.[4] The protein part of the conjugate is labeled with radioiodine, to avoid possible disturbance of structure around the hapten group which might occur if the iodine atom were intro-

[3] Y. Yagi, P. Maier, D. Pressman, C. E. Arbesman, and R. E. Reisman, *J. Immunol.* **91**, 83 (1963).

[4] K. Onoue, Y. Yagi, and D. Pressman, *J. Immunol.* **92**, 173 (1964).

duced directly into a simple hapten molecule. The protein portion of *test conjugates* must not be related to the protein moiety of conjugates which have been used as immunizing antigens. Proteins of smaller molecular size are preferable, such as insulin or ribonuclease, since the protein carrier should not interfere in combination of the haptenic group with the antihapten antibody, which is precipitated by antiglobulin sera. (The preparation of radioiodinated insulin is described below.) The number of hapten groups on a protein molecule should be limited to 1 to 2 groups to avoid the possibility of direct precipitation with antihapten antibodies. This light coupling permits use of the one-step method, which is much simpler than the two-step method.

Antigens are generally labeled by iodination to the extent of 1–10 μCi/μg for ^{131}I or 10–50 μCi/μg for ^{125}I.* The ratio of iodine to protein should be limited, i.e., only a few atoms of iodine per mole of protein should be used so that antigenic determinants are not damaged by introducing iodine atoms. In order to avoid the use of unnecessarily large amounts of radioisotopes, iodination is carried out usually with 30–200 μg protein. The radioiodine solution should be carrier-free and of biochemical grade, and be prepared without any preservative. ^{131}I or ^{125}I with an activity of 25 mCi/ml is received at the time of delivery. These solutions can be used for 2 to 3 weeks for ^{131}I and up to 2 months for ^{125}I without any effect on the efficiency of iodination. At this concentration of protein, the method of Greenwood *et al.* utilizing chloramine-T[5] appears to give most efficient iodination. Details of radioiodination procedures are given in Vol. I, p. 391. It is important to carry out iodination in the smallest practical volume (less than 1 ml). Normally 60–90% of added iodine becomes coupled to protein antigens.†

After iodination, radioiodinated antigens should be stored frozen in small portions in the presence of unrelated protein carrier (e.g., 1% BSA or 10% normal serum of the same animal species as used for producing

---

* Other iodine-containing reagents, such as *p*-iodophenylsulfonyl(pipsyl) chloride and 3-nitro-4-hydroxy-5-iodophenylacetyl (NIP) azide, may also be used to label N-terminal α-amino groups or ϵ-amino groups of protein, but such reagents must be prepared specifically for this purpose since the method requires reagents of a much higher specific radioactivity than those available from commercial sources.

[5] F. C. Greenwood, W. M. Hunter, and J. S. Glover, *Biochem. J.* **89**, 114 (1963).

† Purified ragweed antigen (Pool C) [Y. Yagi, P. Maier, D. Pressman, C. E. Arbesman, and R. E. Reisman, *J. Immunol* **91**, 83 (1963)] and coccidioidin [Y. Sawaki, M. Huppert, J. W. Bailey, and Y. Yagi, *J. Bact.* **91**, 422 (1966)] show much lower efficiency of iodination (<30%) than other protein antigens, as insulin, ribonuclease, serum albumin, various immunoglobulins, and their derivatives. The reason for the low efficiency is not clear, but may be due to contaminating materials such as saccharides or lipids which rapidly react with iodine.

antiglobulin sera) to minimize radiation damage. Once thawed, radio-antigen solution should be kept in a refrigerator and used within one week.

Preparation of Radioiodinated Insulin. Methods for external labeling of proteins with ^{131}I and ^{125}I are given in Section 4.A.2 of Volume I. With insulin, however, we introduce some changes in procedure.*

a. REAGENTS

1. Bovine insulin solution: 5×10^{-5} M in borate buffer pH 8.0, described below (300 μg of Zn-free insulin/ml).

2. KI aqueous solution: 10^{-4} M

3. ^{131}I or ^{125}I solution: Carrier-free iodide solution, less than 1 mCi/ml for ^{131}I or 5 mCi/ml for ^{125}I.

4. Chloramine-T solution:† 2.5×10^{-3} M in borate buffer (0.70 mg/ml). Prepare fresh before use.

5. NaHSO$_3$ solution: 5×10^{-3} M in distilled water (0.51 mg/ml). Prepare fresh before use.

6. Sephadex G-25. Prepare a column (approx. 10 mm i.d.) with 2 gm G-25 (fine) in borate buffer pH 8.0. Pass 2 ml of 1% solution of bovine serum albumin to saturate protein-binding sites of Sephadex and wash the column with borate buffer.

7. 1 and 2% bovine serum albumin (BSA) solution in borate buffer.

b. PROCEDURES

1. To 0.2 ml of insulin solution (60 μg, 10^{-8} mole) in a small test tube, add radioiodide solution of desired radioactivity and 0.1 ml of KI (10^{-8} mole).

2. Add 0.1 ml of chloramine T (2.5×10^{-7} mole) while stirring. Check the presence of excess chloramine T in the mixture by testing a small portion with a starch–KI indicator paper (pale purple color).

3. After 5 minutes, add 0.1 ml of NaHSO$_3$ (5×10^{-7} mole) and test with a starch–KI paper (no color change).

4. Apply the mixture on Sephadex G-25 column with a capillary pipette, rinse the tube and pipette twice with 0.2 ml of borate buffer, and elute the column with the same buffer. Collect 1 ml fractions in test tubes (13 × 100 mm) and determine the radioactivity of each fraction. (The radioactivity can be estimated approximately by placing a fraction

---

* For other proteins, amounts of KI and radioiodine are adjusted according to the amount of protein used and the molecular weight of the protein. Amounts of chlor-amine-T and NaHSO$_3$ are fixed at the stated concentration since further reduction of their amounts often results in lower efficiency of iodination.

† Chloramine-T deteriorates in the presence of moisture. Do not use the contents of a bottle with clumps.

at a predetermined fixed position in relation to a survey meter at an appropriate distance.) Elution volume for protein is usually around 4 to 7 ml of effluent and that for unreacted iodide is around 8 to 13 ml.

5. Pool two or three fractions around the summit of the protein peak. [The efficiency of iodination is estimated by comparing the radioactivity under the protein peak and the iodide peak. The concentration of insulin in the pool is estimated roughly from the radioactivity of the pool and the total radioactivity under the protein peak (assuming no loss during the procedure).]

6. Mix the pooled radioinsulin solution with $\frac{1}{3}$ volume of 2% BSA and assay the radioactivity after an appropriate dilution (e.g., 10,000 times) with 1% BSA.

c. STORAGE

Divide radioinsulin solution into 0.5 ml portions and store in a freezer with appropriate shielding. Once thawed, that portion should be discarded after a week in a refrigerator.

Antiglobulin Antisera. Antiimmunoglobulin antisera produced in goat, sheep, rabbit, horse, and guinea pig are used successfully in RIE and RID. Horse antisera tend to give more nonspecific arcs on autoradiographs than antisera of other animal species. The reason is not clear; it may be due in part to the extreme sharpness of the arcs produced, resulting in formation of ridges in dried agar which can cause mechanical artefacts (Section 14.E.4.c) of false image on the film due to uneven pressure of contact.

Specimens. Formation of sharp precipitate arcs is essential for maximum sensitivity. Generally, serum or plasma specimens are subjected directly to immunoelectrophoresis. For immunodiffusion, the specimens should be adjusted in concentration to produce sharp arcs with the antiglobulin sera. For example, under the condition described below, sharp arcs are produced with good antiglobulin sera (1–3 mg antibody/ml) at a concentration of around 200 μg/ml for IgG and IgA and 1 mg/ml for IgM. However, for IgD and IgE, dilution of anti-δ or anti-ε sera rather than dilution of the sample may be necessary to avoid a condition of extreme antibody excess. Samples with fairly high or unduly low salt concentrations (e.g., M NaCl, or H_2O as diluent) may be used in both methods so long as antibody components will remain soluble in the buffer used, even though the electrophoretic mobility of the components may appear slower or faster than under normal conditions.

Supporting Media. Agar (1.5%, Difco Noble) or agarose (1.2%, Fisher Scientific Co.) is normally used. Solutions are made by heating agar or agarose suspended in Buffer B (see below) in a boiling water bath. Several batches of about 100 ml each are prepared at one time, stored in a refrigerator, and used as required after remelting in a boiling water bath. Excessive heating should be avoided.

Choice between agar and agarose depends on the system. Although agarose seems in general to give a somewhat lower background of radioactivity than agar, agar is definitely better than agarose when radioiodinated insulin is used.

Buffers. Barbital (Veronal) buffers are used for immunoelectrophoresis. Buffers of different concentrations are used for electrode chambers (A) and for supporting medium (B). Stock concentrated buffer is prepared by dissolving 30.9 gm of barbital sodium, 5.52 gm of barbital and 12.3 gm of sodium acetate in about 800 ml of distilled water at 50 to 60°C and bringing the total volume to 1000 ml with water at room temperature. Buffer A is made by diluting the stock buffer with 2 volumes of water and Buffer B with 11 volumes of water. pH should be approximately 8.6 for both A and B; the ionic strength of A is 0.1* and of B is 0.025.

Borate buffer is prepared by adding NaOH to a solution of 12.4 gm H_3BO_3 and 8.1 gm NaCl to raise the pH to 8.0, then bringing the total volume to 1000 ml with water.

C. Diffusion Procedures

Immunodiffusion. Microimmunodiffusion with microscope slides is normally used. Usually, the agar (1.5%) or agarose (1.2%) layer is 1 mm in thickness and the center well (for antiglobulin serum and radioantigen) and peripheral wells (for test samples) are 3 mm in diameter. The distance between the edges of the central and peripheral wells is 5 mm. It is advisable not to use more than 3 peripheral wells (triangle position) for test samples, for reasons discussed below. Two sets of wells are accommodated on a single slide (1 × 3 inch).

Immunoelectrophoresis. A micro modification of Scheidegger's technique is normally used. Although any IEA apparatus may be used, the apparatus we found most convenient is the older Immunophor Model LKB-6800A of LKB-Produkter AB, Stockholm, Sweden, presently marketed by Gelman. It accommodates several slide frames (5.5 × 27.0 cm) of high impact polystyrene, each with 2 rows of 3 slides (1 × 3 inch, 1 mm thick, Gelman No. 51459). Ten ml of agar are used for each row. Up to 3 frames or a total of 18 slides can be used for a single run. No peeling of agar from the surface of the glass slides is encountered during the washing procedure. If samples are to be tested with different radioantigens,

* Buffer A is buffer **11A**, Vol. II, Appendix II.

separate frames should be used for each antigen and each frame should be washed separately. (Other types of apparatus for gel electrophoresis are described in Section 14.D.2.)

Electrophoresis is performed in agar or agarose layer (1 mm in thickness) on microscope slides in the usual manner. Usually, two samples are added to wells of 1.5 or 3 mm in diameter (1.8 or 7 μl, respectively). These wells are placed in the middle of the slide, for agar, and 1 cm towards the cathode, for agarose, at a distance of 6 mm from the center line. Electric potential is applied for 60 min at room temperature (225 volts on meter and approximately 5 volts/cm in agar).

Reaction of Samples with Antiglobulin Sera and Radioantigen. Procedures used for RIE are described below. RID is performed similarly but the samples are not subjected to electrophoresis.

(a) *One-Step Method* (to be used when samples do not form precipitate arcs directly with radioantigen). After electrophoresis, a trough of 1 or 2 mm wide and 6.5 cm long is cut in the center and a mixture (65 or 130 μl) of antiglobulin antiserum and radioiodinated antigen (normally 0.5 to 1 μg of antigen*/ml serum) is diffused from the trough. After diffusion in a moist chamber (usually overnight at room temperature), the slides are soaked in borate-buffered saline and washed thoroughly by several changes of borate buffer for at least 24 hr. Proper precautions must be used during washing to avoid contamination of the laboratory bench and personnel by radioisotopes. Washing trays should be clearly marked and placed on absorbent paper within a large overflow tray. The buffer used for washing should be removed by means of an aspirator rather than by decantation. After washing, the slides are soaked in distilled water for 1 hr and taken out on absorbent paper. A strip of thoroughly wetted filter paper (Whatman No. 1 roll, 1 inch wide) is placed on the agar. Drying is accomplished by leaving at 20° or 37° overnight or by placing under a fan for 4 to 5 hr. Filter paper can be removed readily when the slides are dry.

(b) *Two-Step Method* (to be used when samples form precipitate arcs directly with radioantigen). The sole difference from the one-step method is that antiglobulin antiserum and radioantigen are reacted with the sample in separate steps.

After electrophoresis, an antiglobulin antiserum is diffused from the trough to develop precipitate arcs. The slides are then washed at least

* For detection of minor antibody components in samples containing very high concentration of other antibody components such as specifically purified antibody preparations, radioantigen concentration should be increased (e.g., 10 μg antigen/ml antiglobulin serum). If the amount of radioantigen is not sufficient, the radioantigen may be exhausted by the major antibody component it first encounters and may not be able to react with the minor antibody components.

for 24 hr by several changes of borate-buffered saline to remove soluble proteins in agar. After washing, the buffer remaining in the trough is removed by a piece of absorbent paper and the slides are allowed to stand in the air for 15–30 min to remove excess moisture. A mixture of radio-iodinated antigen and normal serum (of the same species as used for production of antiglobulin serum) is then added to the trough* and the slides are placed in a moist chamber. After diffusion overnight, the slides are washed and dried as in the one-step method.

Staining. The dried slides are then removed from the carrier frame, cleaned with a razor blade to remove excess agar on the back and sides of the slides, and then stained for 15 min with 0.6% Naphthol blue black which is dissolved in methanol:acetic acid:water (45:10:45). Excess dye is removed by rinsing repeatedly with methanol:acetic acid:water (45:10:45) and the slides are dried overnight or under a fan.

Autoradiography. (a) *Means of Contact with Films.* The slides are subjected to autoradiography either singly or in groups. Brown light (15 watt bulb with Kodak Safelight Filter, Wratten Series 6B, used no closer than 4 feet from the working surface) may be used for these X-ray films. For individual slides, a piece of X-ray film (e.g., Kodak No-Screen Medical X-Ray Film NS54T)† previously cut to the size of the slide (1 × 3 inch) is placed between the stained slide and a blank slide, wrapped together with Parafilm, and placed in an X-ray exposure holder. For exposure as groups of slides, a series of slides are mounted on a sheet of Lucite plate (8 × 10 × ⅛ inch) by double-coated Scotch tape and put into contact with an 8 × 10-inch sheet of X-ray film by sandwiching under a blank Lucite plate. After the Lucite plates are fixed with adhesive tape, the sandwich is placed in a large envelope lined with a black paper and placed in an X-ray exposure holder. The latter procedure insures a better comparison of the several slides since exposure and further processing of X-ray film is more uniform than when many pieces of film are handled separately. In addition, the Lucite plate with mounted slides

---

* Alternatively, the slides may be immersed in a solution of radioantigen containing 10% normal serum for a few hours and then washed [K. Onoue, Y. Yagi, and D. Pressman, *J. Immunol.* **92**, 173 (1964)]. For routine work, the diffusion method is preferable to the immersion method since a much smaller amount of radioantigen solution is required and the removal of radioantigen after the second step is easier. However, the immersion method has the advantage of excluding completely the possibility of the formation of precipitate arcs between radioantigen and the antibodies which may still remain in the agar due to incomplete washing after the first step.

† Kodak No-Screen Industrial Type-KK X-ray film, previously used by us, has been discontinued. Both KK and No-Screen Medical X-Ray films are coated with emulsion on both sides and contact can be made with either side. On special order, Kodak will supply No-Screen and Type A emulsions on pre-cut glass plates, see Section 14.E.4.b.*ii.*

can be kept for future reference. When permanent mounting of slides is not desired (and economy is at stake),* one may use Lucite plates divided with Lucite strips $\frac{1}{32}$-inch thick to accommodate many 1 × 3-inch slides.

Light pressure is applied on the sandwich by placing the holder simply under a pile of books or by placing it in a cassette made of two wooden boards having inner linings of polyurethane foam sheets. Pressure is regulated by screw nuts at the four corners.

(b) *Exposure.* Time of contact required for proper exposure is dependent on a number of factors, such as antibody content of the test specimens, the specific radioactivity, the type of radioiodine (^{131}I or ^{125}I), and the purity of radioiodinated antigens. Sharpness of precipitate arcs is also an important factor. The film is about 5 times more sensitive to ^{131}I than to [125]I. For the sake of convenience, the amount of exposure (Ex) is defined as a product of time of contact (hours) and the average specific radioactivity of the test antigen (μCi/μg antigen) during the contact period. Proper exposure for the major antibody component may be obtained in several hours when a test sample contains over a few hundred μg of antibody per ml and a test antigen having a sufficiently high specific radioactivity is used (over 1 μCi/μg for ^{131}I or over 5 μCi/μg for ^{125}I). For the detection of antibody components present in low concentrations (e.g., reaginic sera), much higher exposure is required (e.g., Ex = 600 for ^{131}I and 3000 for ^{125}I). Normally, we expose the slide for 1–2 days and ascertain the time required for proper exposure from the autoradiograph obtained.

(c) *Processing of Films.* A two-step developer, Diafine (Bauman Photochem Corp., Chicago, Illinois), is used for developing exposed films. This developer, consisting of two developing solutions, A and B, is relatively insensitive to the temperature and time of development, gives very reproducible results, and has an unusually long working life. Alternatively, a regular X-ray developer may be used. After fixation with an X-ray fixer, films are washed and dried.

Observation and Interpretation of Results. Identification of radioactive arcs is made by superimposing on the stained slide the film bearing the autoradiograph. The exact positions can be determined readily by the image of troughs registered by the radioantigen remaining in the surrounding area (Fig. 2). With human sera, precipitate arcs due to IgG, IgA, and IgM are readily identified on stained slides even with use of multispecific antiglobulin antisera in RIE. Arcs due to IgD and IgE, however, are not normally visible on stained slides; yet they may be registered on the auto-

---

* Once fixed with double-coated Scotch tape, slides cannot be removed readily from the Lucite plate. Lucite plates of the above dimension cost 40 to 50 cents per sheet.

radiograph if antibodies belonging to IgD or IgE are present and a proper dilution of anti-δ or anti-ε serum is used. Addition of nonantibody carrier IgD or IgE to the test specimen prior to the run and use of class-specific antisera would facilitate the detection and identification of these antibody components. Amounts of carrier and antiglobulin sera should be chosen to produce sharp visible arcs on stained slides. Much higher sensitivity (by a factor of as much as 10) may be achieved by using carrier under appropriate conditions.

When arcs are seen on autoradiographs only and not on the corresponding slides, these arcs may be due to direct precipitation of radioantigen by precipitating antibodies in the test sample even when the two-step method is used. This possibility should be rigorously excluded by procedures described in the footnote of page 463 and the footnote of page 470.

When multispecific antiglobulin sera are used, radioactive arcs due to minor antibody components are often masked by strongly radioactive arcs of major antibody components (e.g., IgG) on autoradiographs. Monospecific antisera, or at least antisera from which antibodies against the globulin possessing a major portion of antibody activity are eliminated (e.g., by absorption with normal IgG), should be used for detection of minor antibody components (Fig. 2).

Radioantigen may be located in only a portion of the precipitate arcs.[6] This is seen frequently with antihapten antibodies and is generally considered to be due to the limited heterogeneity of antibody globulin. Use of other antiglobulin sera, which have more discriminating antibodies with respect to the class, subclass, and type of immunoglobulin components, may reveal that the antibody actually belongs to only one of these components.*

After satisfactory results are obtained by autoradiography, stained slides may be sprayed with a clear plastic spray (available in stationery stores for coating drawings and blue prints, etc.) to avoid disintegration of dried agar upon standing. Slides mounted on Lucite plates are permanently filed with the corresponding autoradiograph. Both slides and autographs can be photographed on a light box or used as negatives to maintain permanent records. Alternatively, most of the precipitate arcs on stained slides can be copied directly by a Xerox copier.

---

[6] C. A. Mattioli, Y. Yagi, and D. Pressman, J. Immunol. **101**, 939 (1968).

* For example, when anti-κ- or anti-λ-chain serum is used for immunoelectrophoresis, they will form a long precipitate arc spanning the area from γ_2- to the α-globulin region. If the specimen contains only antibody of the IgA, IgM, IgD, or IgE class, radioantigen is bound on only the faster migrating portion of this long arc. The immunoglobulin class of the antibody can be identified with certainty only when class-specific antisera are used.

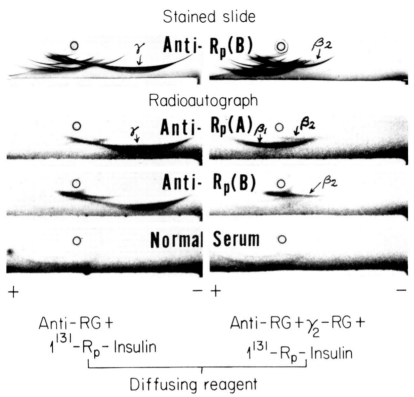

FIG. 2. Radioimmunoelectrophoresis of rabbit anti-*p*-azobenzenearsonate (Rp) serum [after K. Onoue, Y. Yagi, and D. Pressman, *J. Immunol.* **92**, 173 (1964)]. Immunoelectrophoretic pattern for an anti-Rp serum (B) is shown in the upper portion (other sera showed similar patterns). In the lower portion are shown autoradiographs for two anti-Rp sera (A and B) and normal rabbit serum. Plates on the left were obtained with a mixture of horse anti-rabbit globulin serum (anti-RG) and ^{131}I-Rp-insulin as diffusing reagent. Plates on the right were obtained similarly except that normal rabbit IgG had been added to the above mixture to remove anti-IgG antibody. The exposure factor (Ex) was 41. Note that minor antibody components, β_2 (IgM) and β_1, are more clearly seen after removal of anti-IgG antibody from anti-RG serum. A very significant increase of the image density was observed for the β_1-antibody arc after removal of anti-IgG antibody [compare autoradiographs for anti-Rp (A)]. This is probably due to the fact that the absorbed anti-RG serum produced a better-defined β_1-arc than the original anti-RG serum did. The original anti-RG serum appears to contain an excessive concentration of β_1-reactive antibody since the β_1-arc was more clearly seen along with the γ-arc, when the anti-RG serum was used after 4-fold dilution. Absorption of anti-RG serum with IgG would remove antibody cross-reactive to both IgG and β_1-immunoglobulin component, thus reducing the concentration of β_1-reactive antibody. Faint arcs seen on autoradiographs of normal serum and anti-Rp sera in β_1 to α-globulin region are due to nonspecific fixation of radioiodinated antigen because similar arcs were observed with ^{131}I-insulin, ^{131}I-dinitrophenyl-insulin, or ^{131}I-Rp-ribonuclease. (Reproduced by permission of The Williams & Wilkins Co., Baltimore, Maryland.)

Controls. In order to determine that fixation of radioantigen is due to specific interaction of antigen and antibody, three types of controls are necessary. First, autoradiographs obtained with test samples should be compared with those obtained with normal serum or antiserum of unrelated specificity. Second, the specificity of the antigen–antibody system should be tested by substituting the radioantigen with similarly labeled non-crossreacting proteins. In case of antihapten antibodies, proteins used for preparing the hapten–protein conjugate, conjugates of unrelated carrier protein with the same hapten group, and conjugates of the same carrier proteins with non-crossreacting groups, would serve as control antigens. Third, radioantigen is mixed with an unrelated antigen (nonradioactive) and reacted with antiserum against the latter antigen.

A few precipitate arcs, especially those in the β_1- and α-globulin regions, fix radioantigens nonspecifically to a minor extent (Fig. 2). These arcs are readily identified on stained slides and are distinguishable from arcs due to IgG, IgA, and IgM. Although nonspecific fixation of radioantigens by normal immunoglobulin arcs is negligible in most cases, control serum should be included in each run. Comparison between the test sample and the control serum is essential especially when one deals with samples of low antibody content such as reaginic sera.

Fixation of radioantigens by normal immunoglobulin arcs as an artefact occurs more often in RID than in RIE. This situation can be found especially when a sample of high antibody content is placed adjacent to control serum.[7] It represents fixation of antibody globulin in the adjacent well to the arc of normal globulin during the process of immunodiffusion and subsequent washing. This type of artefact can be recognized sometimes by the density change of the normal globulin arc on the autoradiograph, such as being darker on the side nearer the antibody globulin arc. In RID, not more than three samples should be placed around a center well from which antiglobulin serum and radioantigen are diffused. Several control procedures are described in Section 14.E.4.c.*iii.*

D. Quantitative Aspects

Estimation of antibody components belonging to different immunoglobulin classes is nearly impossible because the method is based upon the immunodiffusion and immunoelectrophoresis techniques which are basically qualitative in nature. However, relative antibody contents of a particular immunoglobulin component (e.g., IgG) among different samples can be estimated roughly by the density of images on the autoradiographs,

[7] P. Minden, H. M. Grey, and R. S. Farr, *J. Immunol.* **99**, 304 (1967).

providing the experiments are carried out under the same conditions with one particular batch of antiglobulin serum and the concentration of the particular immunoglobulin component is similar in the samples. More accurate estimations can be made if samples are diluted serially with a particular batch of normal serum or with a solution of normal immunoglobulin and the end point dilutions of the respective autoradiographs are compared.

Even under such conditions, however, the lowest concentration of antibody which gives a detectable image on the autoradiograph is dependent upon the affinity of antibody. In RIE of rabbit anti-dinitrophenyl antibodies, the limit of detection varied from 0.2 μg/ml for high affinity antibodies ($K \doteqdot 10^8\ M^{-1}$ for ϵ-DNP-lysine) to 2.0 μg/ml for low affinity antibodies ($K \doteqdot 10^5$–$10^6\ M^{-1}$).* Similar difference (0.03–0.16 μg antibody/ml) was found among guinea pig antiinsulin antibodies of high ($K \doteqdot 10^9\ M^{-1}$) and low affinity ($K \doteqdot 10^7\ M^{-1}$).[1]

E. Other Applications

Both methods can be used not only for antibody and its derivatives (chemically and physically modified antibodies, subunits,[8] fragments,[2,9] component chains,[10] etc.), but also for components which specifically bind radioactive compounds and which are precipitated specifically by antiserum against the component or by other reagents. These applications are listed in Section 14.E.4.d.

* Unpublished results.
[8] K. Onoue, Y. Yagi, P. Stelos, and D. Pressman, Science 146, 404 (1964).
[9] P. Stelos, Y. Yagi, and D. Pressman, J. Immunol. 93, 106 (1964).
[10] O. Roholt, K. Onoue, and D. Pressman, Proc. Natl. Acad. Sci. U.S. 51, 173 (1964).

Author Index

Numbers in parentheses are reference numbers and indicate that an author's work is referred to although his name is not cited in the text.

A

Abrams, B., 288
Ackers, G. K., 193, 194
Adair, M. E., 54
Adams, J., 25
Adler, F. L., 30
Agostoni, A., 173, 224
Ainbender, E., 351
Aisenberg, A. C., 16
Aitken, I. D., 7, 33
Aladjem, F., 15, 112, 116, 117 (5, 9, 10), 190
Alberty, R. A., 184, 186(5), 424
Albrecht, A., 438
Allison, A. C., 160, 189, 190, 192, 193, 194, 197, 359
Alonso, R., 435, 438 (2, 22), 439 (2, 22, 25), 446, 447 (2, 22), 451 (22)
Amano, T., 108
Ambrose, E. J., 339
Amdur, I., 381
Amin, A. H., 287, 288(6)
Anacker, R. L., 15, 16(44)
Andrews, P., 196
Antoine, B., 235, 358
Aoki, T., 264
Araki, C., 365
Arbesman, C. E., 351, 464, 465
Arnon, R., 7, 25
Ashley, B. B., 421
Asofsky, R., 344, 353(5, 28, 29, 31) 354 (5, 28), 355(29), 356(31), 357
Augustin, R., 121, 123(6), 175, 214
Avery, O. T., 51
Avrameas, S., 296, 303, 306, 307, 308, 310, 314(35), 315(22), 316(29, 38), 317 (29), 365

B

Bablouzian, B., 446
Baier, J. G., 94, 100
Bailey, J. W., 465

Baldwin, R. L., 184, 186
Banovitz, J., 34
Barbu, E., 25
Bar-Eli, A., 60
Barnes, A. E., 67
Barnett, E. V., 352
Barron, A. L., 370, 371(4)
Bartholomew, R., 311
Bata, J. E., 27, 28
Bauer, S. C., 5
Bechhold, H., 103
Becker, E. L., 17, 32, 112, 122, 124(8), 175, 228, 230, 231(2, 5), 232(2), 234
Becker, M., 412
Becker, W., 237
Beckman, L., 311
Bednarik, T., 343
Beiser, S. M., 24
Benacerraf, B., 7, 15(21), 106, 157, 158
Bendich, C. H., 22, 25(67)
Benedict, A. A., 32
Benjamini, E., 66
Bennett, J. C., 438, 446(21)
Berg, D., 4, 6(5), 15(5)
Bergdoll, M. S., 161
Berger, R., 351
Berges, J., 310, 313(33), 320(28a)
Bernovská, J., 365
Berns, D. S., 439
Berson, S. A., 412
Bezer, A. E., 22, 25(67)
Bier, M., 57
Binaghi, R. A., 7, 15(21)
Bittman, R., 427
Bjorklund, B., 25, 295
Blumberg, B. S., 352
Boltz, D. F., 422
Bornstein, P., 128
Bowden, F. C., 19
Bowen, E. J., 397
Bowman, L., 446
Boyd, W. C., 9, 23, 59, 87, 229

Eberlein, W. S., 424
Eddy, J., 47
Edelhock, H., 438, 446(7)
Edelman, G. M., 107, 157
Edsall, J. T., 75
Ehrenpreis, S., 56
Eigen, M., 412, 413(6), 415(6), 419, 421 (12), 425(12), 427
Eisen, H. N., 39, 43, 45, 46(114), 377, 378, 384, 393, 395, 397, 400, 402, 403 (12, 13, 14), 412, 453
Elek, S. D., 147, 148
Engelberg, J., 190
Erlanger, B. F., 24
Exum, E. D., 351
Eyring, H., 380, 381(13)

F

Fahey, J. L., 214, 218(6), 222
Farah, F. S., 19, 45, 46
Farr, R. S., 66, 67(1, 6, 8) 68(1, 6, 14, 15) 70(1), 72(1), 351, 474
Fasman, G., 438
Faure, F., 20
Feigen, G. A., 435, 438(1, 2), 439(1, 2), 447(2)
Feigl, F., 300, 304
Feinberg, J. G., 174, 201, 203, 214
Feinberg, R., 7, 19
Felgenhauer, K., 236
Fenton, E. L., 9, 51(31)
Feofilov, P. P., 437
Ferris, T. G., 359
Finger, I. H., 143, 144, 229, 230(1, 4), 233
Florin, M. C., 438, 439(22), 447(22), 451 (22)
Forster, O., 17
Freeman, T., 287, 288(6, 8–13), 290(4)
Freter, R., 67
Freund, J., 11, 16(35), 30(35)
Frey, M., 438
Fric, I., 74
Fricke, H., 88, 89, 90
Friedman, A., 370
Friedman, D. F., 51
Froese, A., 382, 419, 420(10, 15), 421(12), 424, 425(12), 426(10)
Frost, A. A., 380
Fuchs, S., 15, 29, 60

Fujio, H., 108
Fulthorpe, A. J., 145, 147, 148, 180, 181

G

Gallop, R. C., 367, 369
Ganoza, M. C., 344, 353(8, 9), 354(8, 9, 32), 356(9)
Garner, A. C., 120
Geissman, T. A., 422
Gell, P. G. H., 200
Genereaux, B. D., 235
Gengozian, N., 33, 34(98, 100, 103)
Gerulat, B. F., 5, 7(9, 9a), 21(9a)
Ghetie, V., 365
Gibb, T. R. P., Jr., 96
Giblett, E. R., 352
Gilden, R. V., 30
Gill, T. J., 11(37), 12, 13(37), 15, 16(37, 38), 22(38), 28(37), 29(37), 58, 438
Gitlin, D., 9, 30, 31, 43, 51
Givol, D., 27, 60
Glasstone, S., 380, 381(13)
Glenn, A., 174
Glenn, W. G., 120
Glick, D., 47
Glover, J. S., 465
Götz, H., 237, 239, 240
Goldberg, R., 32, 34(96)
Goldin, M., 174
Goldsack, D. E., 424
Goldstein, G., 429
Goldwater, S. G., 378, 424
Good, R. A., 47
Goodman, H. C., 351
Goodman, J. W., 25, 61
Goodman, M., 32, 33, 34(96), 149, 159, 360
Gonder, M. T., 310
Gordon, A. H., 234
Gosting, L. J., 184, 186(5)
Gotz, H., 304
Gould, H. J., 11, 12, 13, 16, 28(37), 29, 58
Goullet, P., 268
Grabar, P., 13, 27, 107, 157, 235, 237, 240, 265, 287, 295, 296, 297(2), 298(2), 300(2), 301, 302(13), 304, 310, 314 (36), 365
Grant, R. A., 27
Greenberg, L. J., 47

480   AUTHOR INDEX

Greenwood, F. C., 465
Grey, H. M., 67, 72(3), 73(7), 351, 412, 474
Gronwall, A., 300
Gropper, L., 405
Grossberg, A. L., 426, 427
Grumbach, M. M., 353
Guilbert, B., 310, 313(33)
Gynes, L., 27, 28(81)

H

Haber, E., 430, 438, 446(21)
Hafleigh, A. S., 28, 45
Halbert, S. P., 361, 438, 439(22), 447(22), 451(22)
Hamilton, J., 54
Hamilton, J. R., 352, 353(24)
Hammes, G., 381
Hampton, J. W. F., 186
Hamrick, J. R., Jr., 435, 438(2), 439(2), 447(2)
Hanlon, S., 405
Hanson, L. A., 236
Hassid, W. Z., 16
Haughland, R. P., 396
Haurowitz, F., 23
Hawkins, J. D., 30
Hayden, A. R., 231
Hayward, B. J., 214
Haywood, B. J., 237, 239
Heck, Y. S. L., 201
Heidelberger, M., 1, 2, 3, 4(2, 3, 3a, 6), 5, 6(2, 4, 11, 12), 9(27, 33), 11, 13, 14, 15(2), 16(2, 3, 35, 45), 18, 19, 20, 21, 22, 24(2), 25(76, 77), 27(4, 6), 30(35), 42, 45, 46, 51, 52(27), 53(12), 54(12, 127, 128, 129), 58(3), 82
Heller, C., 143, 144, 230, 233
Heremans, J. F., 107, 157, 214, 215(8), 216(8), 218(8), 220(8), 222, 224, 237, 344, 350(4)
Heremans, M. T., 107, 157
Hermann, G., 311
Hersh, R. T., 32
Heulle, H., 222
Hevizy, M. M., 351
Hickman, C. G., 352
Hirs, C. H. W., 61
Hirschfeld, J., 154, 353

Hirsch-Marie, H., 310, 319(39)
Hjertén, S., 358, 365
Hochwald, G. M., 344, 353(5, 6, 29), 354(5), 355(6, 29, 33)
Hodes, H. L., 351
Hoeffgen, B., 353
Hogan, M. D., 161
Hokama, Y., 279
Holm, S. E., 154
Hooker, S. B., 9, 59
Hotchkiss, R. D. A., 300
Hu, C. C., 359
Hughes, A., 344
Hughes, T. R., 385
Hultin, T., 355, 356
Humphrey, J. H., 160, 189, 190, 192, 193, 359
Hunter, W. M., 465
Huppert, M., 465
Hurlimann, J., 352
Hurwitz, E., 29
Hÿmans, W., 356

I

Ishizaka, K., 156, 158(15)
Ishizaka, T., 156, 158(15)

J

Jackson, R., 152
Jacobson, E. B., 344, 353(6, 29) 355(6)
Jacoby, G. A., 430
Jahrmarker, H., 25
Jameson, J. G., 278
Janeway, C. A., 51
Jaross, R. W., 116, 190
Jennings, R. K., 147, 148
Jerne, N. K., 16
Johanson, B. J., 352
Johansson, B. G., 236
Johnson, P., 446
Jones, V. E., 7

K

Kabat, E. A., 4, 6(5, 11, 15), 15(5), 22, 24, 25(67, 74), 26, 42(15), 43, 44, 46, 49 (15), 50, 51(15, 122), 54, 61, 229, 230
Kaiser, S. J., 18, 19(54)
Kaminski, M., 59, 149, 159, 237
Kaplan, S. L., 353

482

Subject Index

Page numbers in italic type refer to figures, tables, or reaction schemes.

A

ABC, see Antigen binding capacity
Absorbancy values, 378, 399, 421, see also Vol. II
  azoproteins, 45
  purified anti-DNP antibody, 46, 396
Absorption spectrum, rabbit antiserum, 97
Acetamide, effect on precipitin reaction, 29
Acetone, effect on precipitin reaction, 29
Acetonitrile, effect on precipitin reaction, 29
Acetylcholinesterase, color reaction, 309, 313
Acetylglucosaminidase, identification of precipitate in gels, 309
Acid phosphatases, color reactions, 309, 313
Acrylamide, see Polyacrylamide
Adjuvants
  charcoal, blood, 59
  Freund's W/O type, 75, 201
Affinity
  anti-hapten antibody, 395, 398, 399, 401, 402, 403, 405, 422, 425, 426, 441, 475
  antiprotein antibody, 23, 39, 72, 73
  high and low affinity anti-DNP, 401, 402, 403, 475
  labeling of Ab site, 428
Affinity constant, see Association constant, Binding constant
Agar (Agar-agar), 118, 119, 139, 147, 148, 163, 176, 189, 192, 193, 203, 217, 228, 231, 284, 341, 467, 469, see also Agarose; Diffusion in Gels; Immunoelectrophoretic analysis
  characteristics, 296, 358, 364ff.;
    changes from repeated melting, 228
  charge effects, 193, 251

dried films for subbing, 118, 139, 161, 163
dry weight, 363
handling, 192, 216, 228, 246, 296, 361, 467
immunoelectrophoresis, 251, 361, 362
infrared lamp for temperature control, 140, 163
preservatives: merthiolate, 118, 139, 148, 161, 201, 210; sodium azide, 118, 148, 217
purification, 246, 361ff.
superiority for IEA with radioinsulin, 468
Agar gel diffusion (AGD), see Diffusion in gels
Agaropectin (compound of agar), 364, 358
  properties, 364
Agarose, 147, 182, 183, 189, 193, 196, 358, 365, 467, 469
  advantages for precipitation in gels, 182, 189, 296, 356
  characteristics, 364, 365
  charge effect on electroosmosis, 251
  gel diffusion, 361
  immunoelectrophoresis, 251, 361, 362
  preparation, 365
AGD, Agar gel diffusion, see Diffusion in gels
Alanine dehydrogenase, color reaction, 308, 309
Albumin, egg, see Ovalbumin
Albumin, methylated, 21, see Vol. II
Albumin, serum, 122, 125, 197, 223, 256, 290, 291
  aggregation on storage, 223
  antigenic fragments (by proteolysis), 59
  bovine: antigen binding capacity, 33, 66, 67ff.; chemically modified, 56, 57; diazobenzidine derivative, 5; external labeling (^{131}I), 68, 348, 349, 351; fluorescein labeled, 146; [131]I- BSA in gel precipitates, 351;

488 SUBJECT INDEX

Antibodies, general, *continued*
concentration
absolute units, 229ff.
equivalence proportions, 2, 4ff., 11,
19, 27, *48*, 62: determination by
diffusion in gels, 181, 191, 200, 201,
205, 207–210, *211*, 212, 233
relative units, 225ff.
conformational changes during reaction: haptens, 426; proteins, 443
coprecipitating, *see* nonprecipitating
cross reactions, 53, *87*; 222
inhibition studies: antigen fragments, 59, 61, *63*, 66, haptens,
427ff., 431, 432
quantitative precipitation, 53, 180ff.,
236
detection: autoradiography, 350,
463ff.; deflection of band positions, 209, 262; gel diffusion tests,
see Diffusion in gels; precipitin
tests, *see* Precipitin tests: qualitative, 35ff., 40
diffusion coefficient (gels), 116, 122
dissociation from Ag, 67, 383, 425
enzymatic degradation, 25
equivalence zone, 2, 4ff., 11, 19, 27
fluorescence (tryptophan) quenched by
hapten, 380, 395
heterogeneity, 4, 7, 9, 23, 24, 35, 48, *51*,
64, 66, 377, 379, 401, 425, 427, 428,
431, 441, 472
heterogeneity index (constant), 390,
392, 398, 401, 432, 433, *434*, 435
homogeneity in Ag excess, 52
inhibition tests, 58ff., 427ff.
labeled, 224, *see* Vol. I
molecular size, methods: diffusion in
dense agar, gelatin, 192, *193*; Sephadex columns, 193ff.; Sephadex
TLC, 197
multiplicity of Ab's in antisera, tests,
463ff.
nonprecipitating, 7, 19, 35, *52*, 66ff.,
125, *see also* Vol. I
Ag/Ab complexes: diffusion coefficients, 190
effect on precipitation in gels, 125,
229
in simple diffusion, 125

precipitins, *see* Precipitin tests
purification, *see also* Vol. II
necessity for fluorescence quenching,
396, 397, 420
tests for impurities, 469
radiolabeled, 224, *see* Vol. I
rate constant, 435, 443
ratios (Ab:Ag): antibody excess, 2;
antigen excess, 2, 19; equivalence,
see Antigen-antibody reactions
resolution of complex mixtures, 50, 91,
94, 127, 164, 168, 185
sensitivity of detection
affinity dependence, 475
antigen binding capacity method, 67
autoradiography: guinea pig antiinsulin, 351; rabbit Ab, 351; rabbit
anti-DNP, 475
diffusion in gels: double diffusion,
158, 159, 230, simple diffusion,
37
precipitin reaction (fluid): Folin-
Ciocalteu, 45; Kjeldahl, 40; ninhydrin, 47, *see also* Vol. II
ring test, 36
species, *see* individual species
size (effective), 192ff.
structure, 59, 63, 472
synthesis *in vitro*, 355
tryptophan fluorescence, 380, 395:
quenching by antigens, haptens,
395
univalent, 463, *see* nonprecipitating
weight: absolute values, 1ff., microgram level, 73; estimates (by antigen binding capacity), 73ff.
Antibodies, hapten-specific, 400, *see also*
Hapten-antibody reactions, Hap-
tens, Fluorescence quenching, Fluorescence
active site, 428
affinity, 395, 398, 399, *401*, 402, 403,
405
anti-*p*-azobenzenearsonate, 473
anti-dinitrophenyl (purified), 377, 400,
403, 475: absorption and emission
spectra, *396*, 397; high affinity,
401, *403*, *475*; low affinity, *401*,
403, *475*; Q_{max} value, 403

α-1-Antitrypsin, two-dimensional IEA,
291
Apoferritin, 50
Association constant (Ag/Ab), 398, 425,
427, 428, 431, 435, 440, 447, 451, *475*
relative, 428, 429, 430, 433
Autoradiography of Ag/Ab bands, 195,
343ff., 466ff., see Radioimmunoelectrophoresis, see also Vol. II
applications
antibody formation *in vitro*, 355
coprecipitation (nonimmunological):
in Ag-cold Ab arc, 355, 473; hemo-
globin-haptoglobin, 356; lipoproteins, 355; α-2-macroglobulin, 355,
473, 474; protein-protein (nonimmunological), 353, 356, *473*, 474
detection of Ab in trace amounts,
350: sensitivity, 351, 472, 475
labeled antigens, 348, 349
multiple Ab's in serum, 463, 464
nonimmunological binding of proteins: growth hormone, 352, 353;
metal-binding (Fe), 352, 353;
insulin (^{131}I), 350, 352; thyroxine,
353; vitamin B_{12}, 352
nonprecipitating Ag/Ab, 350
tissue sites of protein synthesis,
353ff.
choice of isotope, 196, 344, 345
^{14}C, 196, 345
^{60}Co, 351
^{125}I, 196, 345, 466
^{131}I, 196, 345, 466
^{32}P, 345, 351
controls required, 347, *349*, 350, 351,
354, 356, 463, 470, 472, 474
coprecipitation effects, 351, 355
equivalence proportions (Ag/Ab) used,
347
film (photographic), 195, 345, 470, 471
emulsion characteristics, 345
exposure proportional to radioactivity briefly, 356
exposure time, 195, 346, 352, 471
handling, 350
lantern plates, 345
marking film, 349
pressure artifacts, 349

relative sensitivity to ^{131}I and ^{125}I,
471
sheet film, 345
stripping film, see Vol. II
X-ray sheet films, 195, 345, 470
gels stained: after autoradiography,
347; before autoradiography, 470
Ouchterlony plates (RID), 468, see also
Diffusion in gels
photography (autoradiographs), 350,
472
precipitates in Sephadex TLC plates,
195
densitometry of photographic X-ray
film, 196
radioimmunodiffusion (RID), 463ff.,
474
antibody detected in minute
amounts, 464
diffusion: artifacts, 474; procedures,
468, 474
preservation of slides, 472
principles, 463
radioimmunoelectrophoresis (RIE),
344, 463ff., *464*, see also Radioimmunoelectrophoresis
sensitivity, 343, *356*, 357, 472, *475*
detection of impurities, 343, 344, of
trace amounts of Ab's, *356*, 472,
475
Avidity, see Affinity
Azide, see sodium azide
Azobenzene arsonate as hapten, 397, 473
Azocarmine, stain for protein precipitates, 297ff.
Azodyes (dye-hapten), 419, 420, 423, 424
Azoproteins, detection in precipitates by
absorbancy, 45

B

Bacterial antigens, 172, see also Vol. I
somatic O antigens, soluble Ab complexes precipitated, 67
Bacterial species
E. coli, 320
pneumococci, 54, *55*
streptococci, 67, 174
S. typhi, 125